ANIMAL REPRODUCTION IN
VETERINARY MEDICINE

Animal Reproduction in Veterinary Medicine

Principles and Practices

Noah Thompson
Violet Burke
Sophie Cooper

Kruger Brentt
Publishers
2026

Kruger Brentt Publishers UK. LTD.
Company Number 9728962

Regd. Office: 68 St Margarets Road, Edgware, Middlesex HA8 9UU

ISBN: 978-1-78715-599-2

For information on all our publications visit our website at http://krugerbrentt.com/

PREFACE

Reproduction is the cornerstone of animal production, genetic improvement, and species survival. In veterinary medicine, a thorough understanding of reproductive biology and its practical applications is essential not only for enhancing livestock productivity but also for ensuring animal welfare and supporting sustainable breeding programs.

This book, Animal Reproduction in Veterinary Medicine: Principles and Practices, is designed to provide a balanced integration of theoretical foundations with clinical applications. It explores the anatomy, physiology, endocrinology, and reproductive cycles of major domestic animals while also addressing modern advances in reproductive technologies such as artificial insemination, embryo transfer, and in vitro fertilization.

Special attention has been given to species-specific reproductive management, diagnostic approaches to infertility, and strategies for treating reproductive disorders. The book also emphasizes the role of veterinarians in improving fertility, optimizing breeding systems, and contributing to animal genetic resources.

We have attempted to present complex scientific concepts in a clear and structured manner, supported by practical insights, case studies, and recent research developments. This text aims to serve as a reliable resource for veterinary students, practicing veterinarians, animal scientists, and researchers engaged in the field of animal reproduction.

It is our hope that this work will not only aid in academic learning but also guide veterinary practitioners in addressing real-world reproductive challenges, thereby contributing to advancements in veterinary medicine and livestock development.

Noah Thompson

Violet Burke

Sophie Cooper

CONTENTS

1
Chapter

PHYSIOLOGICAL AND CLINICAL ASPECTS OF EQUINE ESTROUS CYCLE AND PREGNANCY ENDOCRINOLOGY

1. INTRODUCTION: AN OVERVIEW

Gestation in the mare commences with the fertilization of the ovum, followed by the implantation of the blastocyst in the uterus, and then the development of the placenta and fetus until parturition. Gestation is a dynamic and coordinated process that entails systemic and local alterations in the mare, facilitating the provision of nutrition and oxygen to the fetus for its growth and development within the uterus. [1]. In part, these changes occur through the secretion of hormones in the placenta, which in turn interact with each other and exert extensive effects on maternal tissues during gestation [2]. These endocrine changes in maternal physiology adaptations to gestational status result from modifications in the maternal environment of steroids such as progesterone (P4), estrogens, androgens, and other hormones such as relaxin and prostaglandins (PG). However, an inadequate adaptation of maternal physiology can lead to gestational complications, such as restriction or overgrowth of the fetus and premature delivery [3].

This chapter provides a fundamental review of endocrinology in horse species, emphasizing its relevance for hormone treatment in cyclic and pregnant mares, along with clinical therapeutic applications. This chapter intends to outline the endocrine alterations that transpire in the mare during gestation and to examine the pivotal function of hormones in facilitating pathological processes.

2. NEUROENDOCRINE CONTROL OF THE ESTRUS CYCLE IN CYCLING MARES

The estrous cycle is defined as the interval of time between two consecutive ovulations. The approximate length varies between 18 and 22 days, considering on average a period of 21 days [4, 5]. The current nomenclature stipulates that the estrous cycle consists of two differentiated stages: estrus or follicular phase and diestrus or luteal phase. These phases are characterized by internal modifications of the sexual organs and glandular system as well as behavioral alterations based on the levels of oestradiol (E2) and P4 [6, 7].

2.1 Follicular phase

Estrus, heat or follicular phase is characterized by the presence of follicles at different stages of development, and the simultaneous increase in the secretion of E2. It has a duration of about 5–7 days, with a variability of 3–9 days related to the season. Thus, estrus is extended in autumn (7–10 days) and is shortened considerably, in late spring and early summer (4–5 days). During this period the mare is sexually receptive to the stallion genital tract and is ready to receive and transport of sperm and finally culminates with ovulation [5, 6, 8].

2.1.1 Follicular dynamics

Ovarian follicular development is a complex dynamic process, characterized by marked proliferation and differentiation of follicular cells, providing an optimal environment for oocyte maturation and preparation for fertilization after ovulation [9]. Among the recruited follicles in each follicular wave, dominance takes place and one follicle of the cohort acquires the ability to continue growing while others undergo atresia. The regulation of each wave and follicular selection involves interactions between specific circulating gonadotropins and intrafollicular factors, ensuring that each follicle is properly stimulated to grow or regress at any stage of development [8]. From an experimental point of view, the occurrence of a wave is defined as follicular growth or simultaneous emergence of a variable number of follicles below 6–13 mm in diameter [10, 11]. In the mare, these follicular waves are classified depending on their ability to develop the dominant follicle (primary-waves) or, in contrast, generate only small follicles (smaller waves). Thus, the main waves or greater originate several follicles subordinate and a dominant follicle, while smaller waves, the follicles are not larger than 30 mm in diameter and then regress [12, 13].

During each cycle produces 1 or 2 major follicular waves, differentiated according to time of onset at primary and secondary. The primary major wave occurs near the middle of the diestrus, in which the dominant follicle ovulates at the end or near the end of estrus. The largest wave precedes the previous secondary and emerges during late estrus or early diestrus. There are two anovulatory follicular waves followed by an ovulatory surge during the estrous cycle [14, 15].

Steroidogenesis in the ovaries involves both theca and granulosa cells. The antral follicles acquire receptors for follicle-stimulating (FSH) and luteinizing (LH) hormones in the membranes of the granular cells and theca, respectively. Cholesterol passes through theca cell plasma membrane attached to a lipoprotein, is stored in cytoplasmic vacuoles, and is transported to the outer membrane of the mitochondria. The LH is released in a pulsating form from the anterior pituitary gland and binds to its receptor in the theca cell membrane, mobilizing cholesterol. Inside theca cells, the StAR protein helps transfer cholesterol to the internal mitochondrial membrane, where the cytochrome P450 (CYP) enzyme system divides cholesterol into pregnenalone (P5), and subsequently, P5 becomes to androstenedione (A4). The A4 produced in theca cells is transported through the basal membrane to the granulose cells. There FSH supports the steroidogenic pathway and converts A4 into E2 [16].

Increased concentrations of estrogen stimulate the secretion of LH, which in turn induces greater estrogen synthesis. This progressive increase in estrogen also promotes the onset of LH receptors in granulosa cells, which facilitates the transition from the antral stage to the preovulatory stage, when the oocyte reaches the final stage of maturation. At 6 days after the emergence of major follicular wave deviation occurs. This event relates to the growth rate difference of the preovulatory follicle size (22.5 mm) compared to the subordinate follicles (19 mm) [12, 13, 17]. Deviation is related to inhibin secretion [12] and insulin-like growth factor-1 (IGF-1) [13, 17]. Specifically, inhibin reduces FSH secretion, making it impossible to continue the development of the subordinate follicle. However, the dominant follicle continues to grow at a constant rate of 2.3 mm per day until reaching a size of 40 mm in response to the increased sensitivity to FSH. As has been mentioned, at this stage of development, granulosa cells also develop receptors for LH required for final oocyte maturation and ovulation after the LH surge [18].

As has been demonstrated in different horse breeds such as Quarter Horse, Arabian, Thoroughbred, and Spanish Purebred, the maximum diameter of the ovulatory follicle usually varies between 40 and 45 mm [19], although the range may be higher (30–70 mm) [7, 20]. Moreover, size differences were established concerning the breeding season or the presence of multiple ovulations. Thus, the follicles reach a size 5–8 mm higher in spring than in summer or autumn and are 4–9 mm lower in multiple ovulations compared to the simple [20, 21].

The highest concentrations of estrogen secreted by the granulosa cells of the preovulatory follicle also induce the appearance of typical behavioral manifestations of estrus. Estrogens are also responsible for reproductive changes that ensure the reception, transport of sperm and oocyte fertilization [4, 6]. After the preovulatory LH surge, ovulation occurs spontaneously 24–48 h before the end of the follicular phase. The ovulatory process brings rapid evacuation of the oocyte and follicular fluid after follicular rupture at ovulation fossa. Once completed, E2 concentrations return to basal levels and at the same time completing the oestrus behavior in mares [11, 22–24].

2.2 Luteal phase

The diestrus or luteal phase begins at the time of ovulation with the formation of CL, which is responsible for the synthesis of P4. Unlike the follicular phase, the insensitivity of the corpus luteum (CL) photoperiod makes the length of this period more constant. Most research estimates an average duration of 14–15 days but can be more durable in mid-summer (16 days) than in spring or autumn (13 days) [5, 6].

2.2.1 Formation of corpus luteum

The disorganization of the follicular wall after ovulation allows blood vessels and fibroblasts invade the follicular cavity. Luteinization involves structural and functional changes in granulosa and theca cells. These are the same cells that initially produced E2 and become into luteal cells that produce P4. P4 remains high from day 5 post-ovulation until the end of the diestrus and exerts specific functions related to the preparation of the endometrium to accept and maintain pregnancy, endometrial gland development and inhibition of myometrial contractility [24].

Have been described two types of CL regarding the presence or absence of central blood clot. In a high percentage of cases (50–70%) in place of ovulation, a core clot develops surrounded by luteal tissue. This type of condition is defined as a corpus hemorrhagic. The cavity begins to fill with blood, fibrin, and transudate for the first 24 h, reaching the maximum size at 3 days. Around day 5 post-ovulation CLs that develop a central cavity usually, have a significantly higher size (32.8 mm) to those without it (26.0 mm). The ratio of the maximum diameter of the CL is 65–80% compared to pre-ovulatory follicle size and has an outer wall thickness of 4–7 mm corresponding to the portion of luteinized tissue. As happens with the size, texture also changes depending on the type of CL. The CL that develops the central cavity is denser than those that lack it, in which the structure is more spongy [25]. Usually, the ratio of non-luteal luteal tissue of the corpus hemorrhagic is minimal during the early diestrus and maximum in halfway of diestrus. These events are associated with the gradual decrease of fluid as a result of the production and organization of connective tissue associated with the clotting mechanism [26, 27]. Notably, the formation of one type or another of CL is a random event. The morphology luteal repeatability is not always observed in subsequent ovulation [26–28].

Furthermore, continuous P4 levels during diestrus reduce the frequency and intensity of gonadotrophin-releasing factor (GnRH) pulses by a feedback mechanism. However, because the pulses of FSH are higher than those of LH, a new follicular wave is developed during this period. In the absence of pregnancy, the end luteal phase culminates with the lysis of CL induced by the PGF2α of endometrial origin and decreased concentrations of P4 [5, 6]. Luteal regression involves several structural and functional events characterized by decreased vascularization, an increase of connective tissue, hyalinization, atrophy and fibrosis [29].

2.3 Neuroendocrine control of the estrus cycle

Physiological events that occur during the estrous cycle are regulated by the coordinated interaction of various hormones and releasing factors like GnRH, FSH, LH, E2, P4, and PGF2α, among others [22]. In this section we will describe a synthesis of the most notable changes and the physiological participation that all these factors have during the estral cycle in the mare.

2.3.1 Gonadotrophin releasing factor

The increased photoperiod during spring and summer causes decreased secretion of melatonin. This signal has a positive effect on the pulses of hypothalamic GnRH, which in turn controls the release of gonadotropins [27]. GnRH pulses produced every 45 min originate predominantly LH secretion whereas those occur every 6 h stimulate the secretion of FSH. The high-frequency pulses of GnRH (2 pulses per hour) during estrus favors an increase in LH and FSH decline, while reducing the frequency to 2 pulses per day, leads an increase of FSH and LH inhibition [30]. These endocrine events, allowing the emergence of follicular waves, E2 synthesis, and ovulation during estrus and appearance of the CL with P4 release during diestrus [24].

2.3.2 Follicle stimulating hormone

Follicle-stimulating hormone describes two types of secretion patterns during the estrous cycle in the mare: uni or bimodal. The bimodal pattern occurs frequently during the spring transition period and the ovulatory season. The first peak of FHS appears between the 8th and 14th day of the cycle, the moment in which the largest follicle reached a diameter of 13 mm [18]. This initial increase precedes the beginning of the deviation and is associated with increased synthesis of inhibin by the largest follicle [8, 13, 15, 18, 31] and persists until the preovulatory follicle reaches 22 mm of diameter. The second peak of FSH begins on day 15 of the cycle and it is necessary to complete the development of the preovulatory follicle [19, 31]. Unlike the bimodal pattern, the first peak of FSH would be absent in the unimodal pattern [18]. In the latter pattern, FSH levels remain low during estrus, rise in times around ovulation, maintaining increased during diestrus [31].

FSH is also involved in the development of the LH receptors in the preovulatory follicle [32, 33]. At the start of follicular growth, low levels of estradiol exert negative feedback on the hypothalamic-hypophysis axis (HHA) controlling the tonic or basal release of gonadotropin. This mechanism controls the follicular growth and E2 synthesis continuously preventing ovarian overstimulation. After the period of follicular growth, once the dominant follicle has been selected, the E2 and inhibin levels are significantly increased. This elevation of E2 is responsible for the characteristic changes of the genital tract and signs of heat during estrus. Furthermore, this response exerts positive feedback on the HHA, favoring the emergence of preovulatory LH surge, necessary to produce the ovulation. Additionally, the stimulatory effects of E2 on LH combined to the inhibitory action of inhibin on FSH create the ideal microenvironment for the final maturation of the oocyte, inhibiting the development of immature follicles [4].

2.3.3 Luteinizing hormone

LH levels gradually increase from day 5 to the day of ovulation, when it reaches the maximum concentration [7, 34]. The pre-ovulatory LH surge occurs as a result of the positive feedback mechanism exerted in the adenohypophysis by E2 concentrations secreted by the granulosa cells of the preovulatory follicle. However, the peak of E2 is reached 2 days before the LH surge. During diestrus, LH is released in a pulsatile manner, with a frequency of 1.4 pulses per 24 h and for a period of 20–40 min at the central level, or 2–4 h per pulse at the peripheral level [34]. Therefore, P4 secretion is maintained by basal levels of LH. The decline of LH at the end of diestrus is a result of the combined effect of decreased estrogen positive feedback, and the resurgence of negative feedback induced by P4 on the HHA. This gonadotropin not only participates in the development and maturation of the primary follicles but also in the development and maintenance of CL during the luteal phase [8, 13, 22].

2.3.4 Estradiol-17β

The ability of estrogen synthesis is dependent on the effect of FSH on granulosa cells. In the absence of P4, estrogens begin to be actively secreted by the preovulatory follicle 5–7 days before ovulation. This event coincides with the time of departure and reaches the peak 2 days before ovulation [5, 22], and will be responsible for the preovulatory release of LH. After ovulation, E2 levels begin to decrease, reaching basal levels at day 5 post-ovulation [13, 19].

Although estrogen levels are directly related to the degree of ovarian activity, sexual receptivity and reproductive tract changes [4, 6, 13, 31, 35] there is no evidence of a direct relationship between the intensity of endometrial edema and E2 concentration. This situation is much clearer on P4. Swelling occurs when P4 levels are <1 ng/ml, so this hormone could be responsible in principle on the intensity of edema, among other behavioral and morphological changes of the cervix and uterus [35]. However, at the time of ovulation inverse correlations are established between E2 and FSH levels associated with the negative feedback effect of inhibin, as previously referred [31].

2.3.5 Progesterone

The steroidogenic activity of P4 depends on the action of LH on theca cells. As noted above, levels of P4 are <1 ng/ml during estrus [19, 36]. After ovulation, it increases progressively and significantly to the 5th or 6th day, with values similar to those of pregnant mares during the first 14 days of gestation. At this time the CL is fully functional and P4 levels remain high until day 9 [35, 37], consistent with the maximum diameter reached by the CL [7, 20, 35, 37]. However, peripheral concentrations of P4 are highly variable between mares. This variability is associated with secretory capacity CL and hormonal catabolic rate. Perhaps this fact may explain the differences in P4 levels between different breeds during the first 5 days of the luteal period, despite the similarity in length of estrous cycles. Among other factors related to variations in levels of P4 highlights the number of ovulations. In fact, double ovulations induce higher concentrations of P4 compared to simple ones [35].

P4 inhibits the secretion and pulsatile release of GnRH and LH but does not modify the pattern of FSH [7, 13, 15]. This event, unlike what happens in other species, enabling a new wave of follicular growth and in some cases the presence of ovulation during diestrus related to high levels of this hormone [18, 22, 38]. After lysis of the CL at the end of diestrus, P4 is drastically reduced to levels <1 ng/ml, a fact which promotes the mare returns to estrus [19, 36].

2.3.6 Prostaglandin F2α

In the absence of pregnancy, the average life span of the CL is controlled by the release of endometrial PGF2α source, establishing a bimodal pattern of discharge around day 13–16 of diestrus. While the first 4-h peak precedes the decline of P4, the second occurs during and after luteolysis. Luteolysis involves decreased blood supply, leukocyte infiltration, cell disruption and loss of lutein steroidogenic capacity by apoptotic or non-apoptotic mechanisms intended to disintegrate the CL and therefore secretion P4 [39, 40].

3. RECENT ADVANCES IN HORMONAL CONTROL OF ESTROUS CYCLE

In mares, the natural breeding season extends from spring to early autumn. Until now, various methods have been used to advance the onset of the breeding season or to synchronize the estrus during the reproductive season. Ovulation induction protocols have also been developed for use in artificial insemination or embryo transfer programs [41, 42].

3.1 Gonadotropin releasing hormone

Seasonal reproductive inactivity in mares is due to reduced synthesis and storage in the hypothalamus of GnRH and decreased amounts of FSH and LH in the anterior pituitary gland [27]. Taking this physiological basis into account, it would be expected that the administration of gonadotropins to anestrous mares will restart reproductive capacity.

The administration of a single dose of GnRH to mares causes an increase in the circulating concentrations of FSH and LH [43]. However, constant infusions result in a continuous release of both hormones [44]. An experience conducted in the late 1980s reported that 50% of mares treated during the seasonal anestrous had fertile estrous after infusion of GnRH for 28 days (100 ng/kg; SC). However, thissame experiment showed that mares with transitional anestrous were more likely to respond to GnRH than mares with deep anestrous [45].

In another study, daily but not continuous administration of GnRH to induce ovulation in anestrous mares only induced the development of preovulatory follicles [46]. Also, another report [47] showed that the administration of 0.5 mg GnRH three times daily for 7 or 7.5 days induced normal follicular maturation and normal luteinization in anestrous mares. From these studies, it has been demonstrated that the administration of GnRH in diverse protocols is not profitable and requires a lot of manpower. It also results in variable response to treatment among mares, especially deep anestrous mares.

3.2 GnRH agonists

GnRH is known to be responsible for the secretion of FSH and LH, but studies performed to evaluate the efficacy of GnRH-agonists are conflicting. GnRH agonists were used as injections or slow-releasing implants to induce estrus and ovulation in anestrous and transitional mares. The GnRH agonists available for mares include deslorelin, buserelin, and historelin [48].

According to Allen et al. [49] two injections of GnRH agonists each day or continuous administration of GnRH agonists were able to induce follicular development and ovulation in acyclic mares. In the same way, Bergfelt and Ginther [26], demonstrate the same result where mares where about 60% of treated mares with GnRH-agonist ovulated within a 21-day long treatment.

In a study conducted in transition mares for 28 days, Harrison et al. [50] administered buserelin twice daily (40 µg, IM, q 12 h) for 28 days, or as SC implants releasing 100 µg/day. 45% of the mares ovulated between the 10th and 25th day after the start of treatment, in response to the two daily injections.

However, 60% of the mares ovulated between 4 and 30 days after implant treatment. The same results were observed when the GnRH agonist was combined with E2 [51].

Deslorelin has also been used to induce cycle and ovulation in mares. Slow liberation subcutaneous deslorelin implants are effective in increasing LH and accelerating ovulation in mares [52, 53].

It is important to indicate that the response is in correlation with the follicular size at the beginning of the treatment and the depth of anestrus. This means that due to the insensitivity of GnRH, mares that are already in the transition period are more likely to respond to the treatment compared to those who are in deep anestrus [54]. Another negative aspect of GnRH treatment in anestrous mares is the risk of early pregnancy losses due to inadequate luteal function [26].

3.3 Progesterone and progestins

The administration of P4 suppresses the release of LH from the anterior pituitary gland. Once P4 supplementation ceases, the so-called "rebound effect" induces follicular maturation and ovulation. Its use in equine reproduction is a common practice and the available protocols include progestogens administered orally or parenterally. However, its use in mares with seasonal anestrous is questionable.

Different studies indicate that mares in deep anestrous or early transition do not anticipate the first ovulation of the year with P4 treatments [30, 55]. However, it has been shown that, if treatment is carried out at the end of the transition period and the mares have at least one follicle of more than 20 mm in diameter in the ovaries, they show regular post-treatment cycles [56].

Intravaginal devices containing P4 (CIDR, PRID, and intravaginal sponges) have been used in mares. Indeed, Hanlon and Firth [57] examined the effect of intravaginal devices placed during 10 days in transitional Thoroughbred mares. The results of the experiment showed that the use of P4 has a positive effect in bringing forward the first estral cycle of the breeding season. Compared to control mares, in the first 21 days of the season, 95.2% treated mares were served and conceived sooner after the start of the breeding season.

Regumate is the most commonly used orally administered progestogen. Its active ingredient is allyl trenbolone, also called Altrenogest. Allen et al. [55] evaluated the effect of oral P4 treatment in mares with seasonal anestrous. Within 8 days, 88% of the treated mares showed estrous behavior and within 18 days of treatment interruption, 84% had ovulated. Based on these figures, the treatment gave a positive result in the acceleration of cyclicity in mares, but its response depends on the depth of the anestrus.

3.4 Recombinant equine FSH (reFSH) and LH (reLH)

The use of recombinant equine FSH (reFSH) has been reported to induce follicular growth in cyclic mares [58, 59]. A study reviewed in 2013 however determined the efficacy of it in deep anestrous mares to be very successful with ovulation rate of 76.7% in response to FSH treatment followed by human chorionic gonadotropin (hCG) administration [60].

Mares in deep anestrous treated with reFSH alone or reFSH and reLH in combination under natural photoperiod showed a significant increase in follicular development within 6 days on average and all of them ovulated within 10 days. In comparison, the control group needed a significantly longer time for follicular growth and only 30% of the control mares had ovulated at the end of the 14 days used for the experiment [61].

3.5 Dopamine antagonists and prolactin

Studies in sheep found that dopamine antagonists are effective in increasing LH secretion during estrus by inhibiting the release of dopamine in the brain [62]. In mares, the increased release of dopamine during winter anestrous has been confirmed in studies measuring a higher concentration of dopamine in the cerebrospinal fluid during deep anestrous. It has also been shown that inhibition of dopamine D2 receptors may accelerate the onset of the ovulatory season in mares. Sulpiride, domperidone, and perphenazine have been studied [63].

Mari et al. [64] compared the efficacy of sulpiride and domperidone, two longacting dopamine antagonists, to induce ovarian activity in mares with deep anestrous. The results showed that sulpiride administration was effective in accelerating the transition period and first ovulation in mares with deep anestrous.

On the other hand, as daylight increases, the concentration of prolactin (PRL) also increases. Dopamine is an inhibitor of PRL release, and it has been suggested that the administration of this hormone may help stimulate cycling in mares in anestrus [65]. Various studies have confirmed that the administration of recombinant prolactin from different animal species (equine, porcine and ovine) has a stimulating effect on mares in anestrus. Thompson et al. [66] examined the effect of subcutaneous administration of recombinant porcine prolactin (rpPRL) pony mares for 45 days. About 17 days after the start of treatment, a high percentage of treated mares showed signs of heat and ovulation accelerated by more than 1 month. However, another study examined the effect of a single dose of recombinant ovine prolactin (ovPRL). As a result, significant stimulation of follicular development was observed, but only one mare ovulated [67].

3.6 Induction of ovulation in mares

A reliable ovulation-inducing drug is one that can trigger ovulation within a certain "fixed" period of time. This pharmacological action can provide enormous advantages in anticipating the right time for artificial insemination. Several pharmacological agents such as GnRH and GnRH agonist, hCG, recombinant equine LH, and equine pituitary extracts, prostaglandins and kisspeptin have been used to determine their efficacy in ovulation induction [68].

3.6.1 GnRH

The frequency of GnRH pulses is the main regulator of LH secretion by the adenohypophysis [69]. Because of this stimulation, they can be used as an ovulatory agent and therefore can be used to induce ovulation in mares. On the other hand, due to its natural origin, it does not cause an immune response after being administered in several sessions. There is also little risk of contamination as GnRH is a synthetic product. In the 1990s, several experiments were conducted to evaluate the efficacy of GnRH in ovulation induction in cyclic mares [70, 71]. In one of them, the effect of a single administration of 2 mg of synthetic GnRH was tested but did not affect ovulation induction. However, daily injections of the same compound from day 2 of heat to ovulation resulted in a shortening of the duration of heat and the time for ovulation [72]. Likewise, Duchamp et al. [73] conducted a study to try to identify a more suitable ovulatory agent. To do that, they compared the effect of an intramuscular injection of 2.500 i.u. hCG and 2 mg GnRH (not synthetic). The use of hCG, injected when the follicle reached 35 mm in diameter, induced ovulation in 24 or 48 h. However, GnRH was not effective in shortening ovulation time compared to the control group.

On the other hand, the pulsatile infusion of endogenous GnRH was effective in advancing ovulation time in cyclic mares [70]. Treatments with low doses of endogenous GnRH (2.5 µg) continuous infusion for 14 days demonstrated increased LH and ovulation in all treated mares compared to controls [74].

3.6.2 GnRH-agonist

Deslorelin (ovuplant and other products)

Deslorelin is a potent GnRH agonist and is marketed as a controlled-release subcutaneous implant under the trade name Ovuplant™. In the past, several authors have investigated the efficacy of Deslorelin in inducing ovulation in mares [29, 75, 76].

It has been shown that between 84 and 93% of mares ovulate after 2 or 3 days of treatment, respectively [77]. However, adverse effects have been reported for this drug. Mares treated with Ovuplant™ showed a prolonged interovulatory interval and estrual cycles of 3–7 days longer than controls [78]. In this sense, it was suggested that the GnRH agonist may cause a decrease in the regulation of the pituitary gonadotropic cells [79]. Besides, additional studies reported suppression of follicular growth and decreased FSH levels in mares treated with Ovuplant™ [80]. A study conducted by McCue et al. [81] showed that the extraction of Ovuplant™ after 48 h prevented a prolonged interovulatory interval. These authors also observed an alteration in ovulation rates. However, Ovupant™ is currently not commercially available.

A short-term release product of deslorelin was developed in a biocompatible liquid vehicle called BioRelease™ [82]. This product releases deslorelin for approximately 6–36 h. An increase in the number of ovulations within 48 h has been demonstrated

(75% vs. 7% for controls). There was also no effect of fertility and the number of coverages per conception decreased in treated mares (1.6 vs. 2.9).

Subsequently, a greater number of injectable deslorelin products have been developed. Many of them are suspensions in saline or sterile water and do not contain any slow-release mechanism. McCue et al. [83] compared several deslorelin formulations and reported that all of the formulations tested in their study resulted in a shortening of the follicular phase, acceleration of ovulation and a similar response to human chorionic gonadotropin (hCG). It is important to note that these studies were conducted in the middle of the breeding season.

3.6.2.2 Buserelin

Different works have also tested Buserelin for its effect of inducing ovulation in mares [84]. Treatment with 40 µg de buserelin (4 doses/12 h) caused ovulation without altering fertility in mares [84, 85]. Also, the effect of treatments with 20 µg or 13.3 µg of buserelin (4 doses/12 h; or 3 doses/6 h respectively) was comparable with treatment with 2.500 IU of hCG (iv).

However, some problems with Buserelin to induce ovulation were also reported [86]. Mares treated with 40 µg iv. of Buserelin (2 times daily), 2.500 IU of hCG (single dose iv) and 2 ml of water distilled as placebo (iv) were compared. The highest ovulation rate was found in hCG treatments where 88% of the mares ovulated between 36 and 48 h. However, Buserelin treatment caused only 22.7% ovulation within 48 h.

Buserelin has also been given during early diestrus to pregnant mares as a means of improving pregnancy rates [87, 88]. These studies used doses of 20–40 mg of Buserelin between days 8 and 12. The results showed that pregnancy rates after ovulation increased by approximately 10%. The exact mechanism of how GnRH increases pregnancy rates is unclear since P4 does not appear to be increased.

3.6.2.3 Human chorionic gonadotropin

hCG is a glycoprotein hormone and has a biological function like LH. It is composed of two subunits (α-subunit and β-subunit). The biological activity of hCG is determined by β-subunit, which is composed of 145 amino acids [89]. Several experiments have been conducted to test the efficacy of hCG in ovulation induction [73, 90, 91]. The results of these studies showed that administration of 1.500–3.300 IU of hCG to mares with a follicle in the ovary 35 mm in diameter, or after estrus day 2, induced ovulation within 48 h. The administration of hCG to mares with a follicle in the ovary 35 mm in diameter, or after estrus day 2, induced ovulation within 48 h. The administration of hCG to mares with a follicle in the ovary 35 mm in diameter, or after estrus day 2, induced ovulation within 48 h. However, the adverse effect of consecutive administration of hCG has been reported. The results demonstrate a null effect from the second administration of hCG.

On the other hand, significant levels of antibodies to hCG were also observed after repeated injections [91, 92]. However, there is much conflicting evidence as to whether antibody formation affects the efficacy of hCG [93].

3.6.2.4 Equine recombinant LH

The recombinant equine LH (reLH) was successfully developed and tested for both in vitro and in vivo efficacy [94, 95]. To test the efficacy of reLH in ovulation induction, a study was performed in mares with 35 mm follicles that were treated with 0.3, 0.6, 0.75, 0.9 mg reLH, 2.500 IU hCG and the number of ovulations within 48 h of injection was monitored. With a total of 84 mares of various breeds 28.6, 50, 90, and 80% ovulated within 48 h in response to 0.3, 0.6, 0.75, and 0.9 mg reLH, respectively. Changes in hormonal profiles (LH, FSH, P4, E2) in response to 5, 0.65, or 10 mg reLH were similar to those of mares of the control group, except for the early increase in LH after reLH injection. The result of this study indicates that reLH is a drug that induces ovulation in mares with a follicle size of 35 mm in 48 h. It is important to point out that as a synthetic product it offers good potential by having, for example, a low production cost.

3.6.2.5 Equine pituitary extracts

The raw extract of equine gonadotropin (CEG) from the pituitary, contains FSH and LH. These extracts have been tested to determine if they can be used as agents to control the estrual cycles of mares. Also, due to their LH content, the effect of CEG for ovulation induction has been tested. Duchamp et al. [73] showed that 80% of ponies and 57% of mares ovulated 2 days after the administration of 50 mg and 25 mg of CEG, respectively. However, there is one major obstacle to these results; the FSH and LH relationship in cEG is not always consistent. Another important factor to keep in mind is that CEG may be contaminated with other pituitary hormones. Also, the potential transmission of certain associated diseases between animals or between animals and humans [96–98].

3.6.2.6 Prostaglandins

Savage and Liptrap [99], reported on the use of PGF2α was able to induce ovulation in mares. By administering 250 μg PGF2α synthetic (Fenprostalene) 60 h after the onset of estrus, the interval between treatment and ovulation and the duration of estrus were significantly reduced.

Despite these good results, no other PGF2α could be found that could give similar results [100]. It is therefore believed that the prolonged action of Fenprostalene was responsible for these results. Another PGF2α (Luprostiol), has also been shown to induce a release of LH from the anterior pituitary gland [101].

3.6.2.7 *Kisspeptin*

Kisspeptin is a neuropeptide that induces the secretion of gonadotropins through the stimulation of GnRH secretion and has also been described as having a role in triggering the onset of puberty [102, 103]. A study in pony mares demonstrated the anticipated ovulation when treated with 10 mg of kisspeptin. Another report identified that the administration of 500 μg and 1.0 mg of kisspeptin induces indistinguishable LH and FSH responses to 25 μg GnRH. However, a single injection of 1.0 mg of kisspeptin (iv) was insufficient to induce ovulation in the mare in heat [104].

4. HORMONAL REGULATION OF PREGNANCY IN NORMAL MARES

4.1 Progesterone

"Maternal recognition of gestation-MGR" it is essential to establish a complete and uninterrupted interaction between the uterus and the conceptus to prevent the regression of primary CL as a result of the blocking of luteolysis. The mobility of the conceptus within the uterine lumen between days 11 and 15 (or "first luteal response of pregnancy"); [27] seem to compensate for the reduced contact surface due to the relatively small size of the equine trophoblast, demonstrating that restriction of movement only partially leads to early embryo loss [105]. The PGs synthesized and secreted by the concept itself stimulate myometrial contractions that promote their migration through the uterus, avoiding premature regression of CL. Additionally, the longitudinal direction of the uterine folds, as well as the spherical shape of the embryo due to the persistence of the glycoprotein capsule, contribute to facilitating this movement [106, 107]. During the mobility phase and its subsequent fixation uterine high amounts of estrogen, mainly oestrone sulfate (E1S) by the equine conceptus are synthesized, related to the development of the embryonic and endometrial vasculature and local effects on myometrial activity, uterine mobility and endometrial gland secretion [108, 109].

Embryo implantation begins around day 36 post-ovulation and involves the development of the chorionic band from the trophoblast, whose cells invade the maternal endometrium giving rise to endometrial cups [110]. Ginther [28] reported that the embryonic cup cells produce a hormone called equine chorionic gonadotropin (eCG), formerly known as pregnant mare's serum gonadotropin. This hormone is first detectable systemically between days 35 and 40 of pregnancy. The cups are mature and robustly secreting eCG at approximately days 50–60, but they will subsequently undergo sloughing by days 100–150 in most mares This resurgence phase of P4 secretion by the primary CL is termed the "secondary luteal phase or output 2," whereas the production by supplementary CL is termed the "third luteal phase" or "output 3". These accessory CLs formed, respectively, causing an increase in P4 secretion around the 75th day of gestation [27, 28, 111]. Thus, during this period, two secretion peaks of P4 are described, which gradually decreasing to undetectable levels at the 200 days of gestation [112, 113].

Ovarian P4 is necessary for the early maintenance of gestation in the mare until 150 days of pregnancy. After the regression of CLs, the placenta is then the organ in charge of maintaining gestation [114]. Several studies describe maximum levels of P4 during the second and third months of gestation, followed by a significant decrease to minimum values (<1 ng/ml) from mid-gestation to term [115]. Additionally, the presence of eCG causes a change in luteal steroidogenesis. In this case, CL changes from synthesizing only P4 to secreting also estrogens and androgens, increasing plasma levels rapidly and tripling the basal values [116].

However, it is not until approximately day 35 that systemic estrogen rises. The source of this estrogen is the ovary, more specifically, the CL and possibly follicles. The stimulation of the ovaries by eCG is responsible for the timing of this increase in estrogen. It appears that estrogen is not actually necessary for pregnancy maintenance, because ovariectomized mares administered only exogenous progestins will maintain pregnancy without the administration of estrogens [28]. The origin of both steroids is found in the primary CL, since their increase takes place before the formation of the secondary CLs and is absent in mares without functional CL. Although the mechanism by which gonadotropin exerts this activity is unknown, an increase in the expression of the enzyme 17α-hydroxylase in charge of the conversion of P5 into dehydroepiandrosterone (DHEA) and P4 into A4 has been described. Both events coincide with the secretion of eCG, they seem to be limited to the first period since they are not detected towards the middle of gestation [116]. The increase in P4 responds primarily to the growth of primary CL and the development of secondary and accessory CLs [4, 117].

During the period of endometrial cups activity, secretion peaks are described for testosterone (T) and A4 [118, 119], whose activity may be decisive in uterine processes related to cell transformation associated with decidualization [120]. In addition, estrogen production depends on the increased synthesis and availability of androgens that are subsequently metabolized by the enzyme aromatase, present in luteal tissue even before eCG secretion. Thus, total estrogen levels are like right-handed during the first 35 days of gestation and increase around day 40 due to follicular development before the formation of CL [121]. Additionally, primary gestational CL produces E1S in response to eCG stimulation [113, 115, 118].

The regression of the endometrial cups to 100–120 days of gestation causes the cessation of eCG secretion and luteal development, observing a progressive decrease in plasma levels of P4 to reach basal values around 200 days of gestation [115]. Currently, all the luteal structures present in the ovary have completely involuted [27]. From this moment onwards, various metabolites derived from P4 (progestins) increase in the systemic circulation, that exceed 500 ng/ml during the last weeks of gestation, which subsequently fall in the 24–48 h prior to birth [122].

4.2 Progestagens

Progestins can be subclassified as pregnenes and 5α-pregnenes. The pregnenes includes P5, P4 and 5-pregnene-3β,20β-diol (P5ββ), while 5α-pregnenes includes 5α-pregnane-3,20-dione (5αDHP), 3β-hydroxy-5α-pregnan-3-one (3β5P), 20α-hydroxy-5α-pregnan-3-one (20α5P), 5α-pregnane-3β,20β-diol (ββ-diol) and 5α-pregnane-3β,20α-diol (βα-diol). Of them, the most important ones in maternal plasma during this period are the 5αDHP and its derivatives, 20α5P, and βα-diol.

The origin of all of them is found in P5, synthesized mainly in the fetal adrenal gland, with a production rate exceeding 10 μmol/min. In the placenta, P5 is converted to P4 and this is transformed into 5αDHP in the endometrium [123]. The pattern of secretion of 5αDHP at beginning of gestation runs parallel to that of P4, while around 90 days the onset of P4 decline gives way to fetoplacental synthesis of the different progestogens whose concentrations continue to increase during the second half of gestation. Thus, 20α5P, which is initially at 5 ng/ml, reaches 69 ng/ml at 200 days of gestation and 300 ng/ml at term. In addition, the concentrations of βα-diol increase to 484 ng/ml [112], while 3β5P, P5ββ and ββ-diol reach values of 100, 10 and 100 ng/ml, respectively, towards the end of gestation [124].

The 5αDHP is found primarily at the uterine level during midgestation, but as labor approaches, its distribution changes and is predominantly in fetal circulation. This metabolite is an immediate precursor of allopregnanolone, a potent gamma-aminobutyric acid (GABA) receptor agonist with activity on myometrial relaxation in other species [125–127]. Serum allopregnanolone increases similarly to its precursor, reaching maximum values at the middle of gestation and a term [112]. However, both P4 and 5αDHP prevent weakly myometrial contractions induced by oxytocin in vitro, suggesting the intervention of the other hormones in the maintenance of uterine quiescence [128]. On the other hand, an umbilical increase of P4 after 300 days of gestation related to a greater expression in the trophoblast of the enzyme necessary for the conversion of P5 into P4 has been described [129].

Simultaneously with the production of progestagens, the feto-placental unit (FPU) synthesizes phenolic estrogens, E1S and E2 17β and 17α, through the aromatization of dihydroandrosterone (DHA), DHEA and its precursors (3β-hydroxyl

C-19). The estrogens β unsaturated, equilin and echinelin, specific to the equine species, derive from farnesyl pyrophosphate, through a noncholesterol-dependent pathway. In general, the pattern of estrogen secretion during gestation is characterized by the first peak of secretion around day 40 in relation to follicular development before the formation of secondary and accessory CLs and a subsequent increase from day 80, reaching maximum levels around 210 days of gestation [130–132]. Thus, the initial plasma concentrations of E1S, corresponding to ovarian synthesis and are affected by ovariectomy. On the contrary, the subsequent peak of liberation comes only from fetoplacental synthesis, descending drastically after fetal death [108, 113, 115, 133].

This increase in estrogens temporarily coincides with the hypertrophy of fetal gonads, which together with local expression of the enzyme 17α-hydroxylase, lead to elevated umbilical levels of P5, T and DHEA [134]. At the same time, maternal plasma concentrations of T and DHEA increase after 100 days of gestation, reaching maximum values at 6 months [116, 135] to promote greater perfusion in the fetal compartment and the uterine tonicity [27, 136]. Legacki et al. [112] describe DHEA values that increase since the first 2 months of gestation to at 6–8 months, decreasing afterward.

The mitochondrial cytochrome P450 side-chain cleavage enzyme (P450scc), necessary for the conversion of cholesterol into P5 is present in the glomerulosa and reticularis zone of the fetal adrenals from 150 days of gestation. However, its expression increases noticeably at the end of gestation, is also found in the fasciculata zone, in the placenta, and the utero-placental tissues. At the same time, fetal plasma levels of P5 and its uteroplacental diffusion are doubled and tripled between 200 and 300 days of gestation and that subsequently descend in the days prior to birth [132, 137]. One of the main metabolites of P4, the 5α-DHP, returns to umbilical circulation after synthesis in the endometrium, excreting only 30% of its production to the maternal circulation. Thus, it has been suggested that it could play a relevant role within fetoplacental tissues [137].

4.3 Estrogens

Estrogen production can likewise be determined in serum obtained from the mare and used as an indicator of feto-placental health [136]. Although total estrogen levels decrease in term gestation, E2 increases dramatically hours before parturition with accentuated myoelectric activity at the uterine level, suggesting the involvement of E2 in myometrial activation [132, 138]. In fact, estrogens promote PGs synthesis and increase endometrial sensitivity to oxytocin, stimulating myometrial contractile activity during delivery [137].

4.4 Cortisol

A few days before parturition, fetal adrenals change from mainly synthesizing P5 to producing cortisol in response to the stimulation of adrenocorticotropic hormone (ACTH). The increase of fetal cortisol is related to preparing the fetus for extra-uterine life by stimulating different processes necessary for the maturation of organs such as the liver, thyroid gland, lungs, digestive system, bone marrow and cardiovascular system [137]. In addition, cortisol activates the enzymes responsible for the synthesis of PGs which, without the presence of progestogens, increase continuously stimulating the onset of myometrial contractions. In addition, E2 favors the uterine response to PGs and may also promote their synthesis [139].

4.5 Prostaglandins

PGF2α play an important role during delivery by promoting myometrial contractibility, along with oxytocin, and cervical ripening and relaxation (PGE2). Utero-placental tissues are capable of synthesizing PGs and can be found in maternal plasma, fetal plasma and allantoic fluid [140]. However, its bioactivity is controlled by the enzyme 15-hydroxyprostaglandin dehydrogenase (PGDH), which converts the PGs into inactive metabolites, present in the maternal endometrium since approximately 150 days of pregnancy. Since the labile nature of PGs makes it difficult to measure one of these metabolites, 13,14-dihydro-15-keto-prostaglandin F-2α (PGFM) remained at low levels until day 200, then increased to peak pregnancy levels by day 300 and remained at this value until parturition. PGFM uses one of its metabolites as an indicator of its circulating levels, with a term increasingly being described, although it is during the second labor stage when its value increases up to 50 times [141].

4.6 Relaxin

Relaxin is produced by the trophoblastic cells of the placenta and its activity is related to myometrial [137] as well as of the cervix and pelvic ligaments relaxation [142]. Maternal plasma levels increase at the end of gestation and during the second labor stage. After the expulsion of the placenta, it returns to basal values below the detection limit at 36 h, remaining elevated in cases of placental retention [143].

5. HIGH-RISK MARES AND HORMONE SUPPLEMENTATION

5.1 Progesterone

P4 concentrations above 4.0 ng/ml are considered adequate to support early pregnancy. However, when levels are <2.0 ng/ml, P4 supplementation is considered [137]. Several types of P4 products have been used to maintain pregnancies in mares. After oral administration altrenogest is readily absorbed, reaching peak levels after 3–6 h [144]. Altrenogest acts by binding to the P4 receptors but has little effect on endogenous plasma total progestagen concentrations. Specifically, altrenogest is not metabolized to 5α-pregnanes in the horse [128]. For this reason, the only scientific evidence that altrenogest prevents loss pregnancy in mares is during the first trimester, when it prevented abortion induced by repeated administration of PGF2α (cloprostenol) [145]. P4 may exert its effects by interfering with PG production stimulated by proinflammatory cytokines. Daels et al. [146] demonstrated that the rise in endogenous PGF2α concentrations was inhibited by altrenogest treatment. Indeed, when early pregnant mares (21–35 days post-ovulation) were exposed to Salmonella typhimurium endotoxin all mares supplemented with altrenogest until day 70 remained pregnant, whereas 6 out of 7 mares aborted when altrenogest therapy was discontinued on day 50 [147].

Mares with suspected luteal insufficiency can be supplemented with altrenogest (0.044 mg/kg per os once or twice daily) or P4 (150 mg/day IM) starting on day 3 after ovulation and continuing until 100–120 days of pregnancy. Long-acting injectable formulations of P4 and altrenogest are available in some countries [148]. Administration of the GnRH analog, buserelin (40 µg), 10 or 11 days after ovulation has been reported to improve luteal function and reduce early pregnancy loss [149]. Panzani et al. [150] showed that the use of altrenogest improved recipient pregnancy rates compared to untreated controls. A recent clinical study showed a positive effect of altrenogest supplementation on embryonic growth rates between 35 and 45 days after ovulation in Warmblood mares older than 8 years [151]. P4 may need to be supplemented generally in early pregnant mares showing estrus signs, with a history of repeated pregnancy loss in case of endotoxemia and of stressful events. In mares under P4 supplementation continuation of pregnancy has to be monitored regularly, since many will lose their pregnancy despite supplementation of P4 and this will prevent those mares return to estrus [152].

The latter sentence has been checked. It has been reported that the administration of a single dose of 20–40 µg of buserelin between day 9 and day 10 after ovulation increases the number of multiple ovulations and gestation up to 5–10% [153]. Buserelin does not increase circulating P4 levels or preventing the luteolysis, acting independently of CL in the mare [154]. These effects preventing pregnancy loss that operating between day 9 to day 10 and day 13 to day 14 of pregnancy.

In a recent study Köhne et al. [155] reported that hCG administration for induction of ovulation in mares increased progestin concentration in plasma of early pregnancy as well as the embryo size at the time of the start of placentation. Periovulatory treatment of mares with hCG may thus be a valuable tool to enhance conceptus growth during early pregnancy by stimulation of endogenous P4 secretion. However, Biermann et al. [156] report that hCG-treatment of mares on day 5 or day 11 post-ovulation influenced peripheral P4 concentrations due to secondary luteal tissue but did not alter ovarian and uterine blood flow or increase pregnancy rates.

5.2 Progestagens

Several pathological conditions as placentitis, placental separation or fetus as, alteration in umbilical blood flow attributable to a cord pathologic condition stimulates inflammatory and immune responses leading disrupt the endocrine capacity of the FPU and alterations in endocrine profile in plasma maternal attributed to disturbances to the normal synthetic pathway for these pregnanes [126, 157].

Fetal death or imminent fetal expulsión due to uterine torsion, colic, maternal stress, or acute cases of experimentally induced placentitis when the mares abort rapidly (within 7 days of infection) are related with the rapidly declining of P5 and P4 (less than the 95%), consistent with failure of the fetus and feto-placental tissues to produce and metabolize progestagens [158, 159].

In mares with chronic placentitis, placental edema, and placentas with poorly developed or sparse microvilli [159, 160] unusually high concentrations of all the progestagens. This pattern indicates that the fetus and the uteroplacental tissues are metabolically active despite the presence of bacteria or their products. In addition, Shikichi et al. [157] demonstrated that mares with a high concentration of progestins and low concentration of estrogens after day 241 of pregnancy were likely to deliver aborted/dead foals with placentitis. These authors demonstrated elevated and low concentrations of progestins and estrogens in the maternal sera of all cases with placentitis in pregnant mares, respectively.

The mare's exposure to ergopeptine alkaloids from the endophyte fungus found on tall fescue grass (fescue toxicosis), ergot alkaloids inhibit fetal corticotropin-releasing hormone (CRH), inhibiting the normal function of the adrenal gland to produce the cortisol surge and associated changes in pregnane metabolism [137]. In mares with fescue toxicosis, prepartum total plasma progestagen concentrations remain low, their foals have low cortisol concentrations, indicating suppression of fetal adrenocortical activity and P5 production [161].

Recent studies demonstrated that altrenogest, when given in combination with antimicrobials, pentoxifylline and nonsteroidal anti-inflammatory (NSAIDs) drugs to mares with placentitis, decreased the incidence of abortion [162]. In these cases, altrenogest counteracts uterine contractility induced by inflammation of the fetal membranes. In the same way, in bacterial placentitis, a combination of trimethoprim sulfamethoxazole, pentoxifylline and a double dose of altrenogest

(0.088 mg/kg bwt per os s.i.d.) were successful in maintaining pregnancies to term [163], while that untreated control mares aborted. When mares were treated with trimpethoprim sulfamethoxazole and pentoxifylline without altrenogest, only one live foal was born [163, 164]. Despite this, it is not clear what role, if any, altrenogest plays within this multi-treatment approach. However, the mares can still abort while receiving altrenogest treatment in the last trimester of pregnancy.

5.3 Estrogens

In late gestation total estrogen (including E1S, E2, and its metabolites, equilin, and equilenin) may be used for fetal and placental health monitoring. However, it is doubtful that total estrogen concentration can predict fetal death as the fetal gonads are unlikely to respond to fetal stress [157, 165].

Since the production of estrogens requires both contributions by the fetus and placental, reduced concentrations in maternal circulation may indicate or predict a stressed or hypoxic fetus that is not producing the estrogen precursors [165].

Indeed, E2 [166] and E1S [167] concentrations decreased sharply in mares with placental dysfunction and after the induction of abortion. If the fetus is severely compromised or die in the uterus, maternal plasma E1S are baseline because of the absence of the C19 precursors secreted by the fetal gonads. However, pregnancies compromised by equine herpesvirus-1 infection or severe colic can present normal or transiently decreased E1S concentrations [168]. Compared with the adrenal glands, the gonads are unlikely to respond to fetal stress; consequently, so it is doubtful that total estrogen concentrations can predict fetal death. Frequent blood sampling of mares induced to abort with PG between 90 and 150 days of pregnancy indicated that E1S levels did not decline until within 5 h of abortion [145].

In cases of placentitis at gestational ages between 150 and 280 days, Douglas [169] and Shikichi et al. [157] showed hormonal alterations common as elevated progestogens and low estrogens in mares that aborted. Although the decline in E2 associated with placental dysfunction is thought to reflect placental disease per se, Esteller-Vico et al. [170] recommended the estrogen supplementation as a means to reduce the risk of abortion associated with placentitis in mares. Recently, Curcio et al. [171] showed that in addition to basic treatment with trimethoprimsulfamethoxazole and flunixin meglumine, mares with experimentally induced ascending placentitis benefited from E2 cypionate supplementation. Conversely, altrenogest did not appear to make a difference in outcomes.

After fetal death and stress or fetal weakness, androgens and estrogens levels drop rapidly. For better determination of the health state of the fetus, due to the metabolism of both steroids, it is recommended to monitor androgens and estrogens simultaneously [126].

5.4 Relaxin

Relaxin is a useful biomarker to assess placental health and can be monitored in high-risk mares. Ryan et al. [172] reported a positive relationship between circulating levels of relaxin and poor outcomes in high-risk pregnancies. Relaxin is detectable in the blood after the 80th day of pregnancy without any changes until the second stage of labor. In mares with impaired placental function, in cases of placentitis, placental abruption, hydroallantois, and hydramnios relaxin concentrations decrease below 4 ng/mL [143, 172]. Low circulating levels of relaxin have been reported both in pony mares affected by fescue toxicosis associated with placental disease and agalactia and in Thoroughbred mares, with other forms of placental disease or insufficiency [172].

In the case of placental hydrops, the risk of spontaneous rupture of the fetal membranes increases significantly [173]. Relaxin has been explored as a potential marker of treatment success in placentitis due to its level decrease in cases of spontaneously occurring and experimentally induced pregnancy loss [174].

5.5 Prostaglandins

Placentitis is characterized by the production of proinflammatory cytokines (such as IL-6 and IL-8) and PGs [175, 176]. PG release increases uterine contractility and consequently the risk of premature delivery [138]. Proinflammatory cytokines and the PGs of the FPU increases both in response to inflammation/infection, inducing premature activation of the fetal hypothalamic-pituitary-adrenal (HPA) axis [177], accelerating fetal maturation before parturition [138, 178]. The fetal adrenal produces both progestins and, once sufficiently mature, cortisol. Fetal cortisol, in turn, enhances placental and uterine PGs production, further enhancing uterine contractility and resulting in fetal delivery. Since the maturation of the equine fetus occurs later in gestation [137] this implies that placentitis or maternal disease could be devastating to the newborn foal. However, early fetal maturation likely counterbalances premature delivery and may help improve the chances for foal survival [138, 178]. The supplementation with progestin and PG synthetase inhibitor can maintain equine pregnancy in the presence of PGF2 insults [146, 147].

In addition, Esteller-Vico et al. [170] showed that estrogen suppression resulted in a decrease in circulating PGFM, which suggests that estrogens partially regulate PG production during pregnancy since PGFM concentrations were lower but still increased during the last trimester of equine gestation in letrozole-treated mares.

6. CONCISE SUMMARY

Understanding the physiological foundation of the estrous cycle enables comprehension of the interplay between reproductive hormones and the causes or events influencing the cyclicity of mares. These fundamental discoveries have enabled the accurate manipulation of the estrous cycle, the advancement of the reproductive season, and the synchronization of ovulation. A significant advancement in this regard has been achieved through the elucidation of follicular dynamics and the examination of the various structures within the ovaries of mares throughout the year.

Similarly, the proper interplay among the ovary, placenta, and fetus ensures the secretion of appropriate hormone patterns essential for a successful pregnancy. Assessments of progestogens, estrogens, and relaxin, along with other hormones, are valuable for evaluating placental health and embryonic viability. This is primarily attributable to placental diseases or fetal demise.

To modifications of these hormones. Conversely, hormonal diagnosis facilitates the timely identification of pathological problems, enabling the implementation of appropriate treatments to sustain gestation and ensure the development of a live foal. Significant advancements have occurred in recent years regarding the identification and management of high-risk pregnancies.

This understanding significantly enhances professional performance and contributes to improved reproductive outcomes. It is essential to recognize that the continuous generation of fundamental information and its application in equine reproduction will facilitate the enhancement and development of new protocols in reproductive technologies in the future.

REFERENCES

1. Fowden AL, Moore T. Maternal-fetal resource allocation: Co-operation and conflict. Placenta. 2012;33(2):e11-e15. DOI: 10.1016/j.placenta.2012.05.002
2. Napso T, Yong HEY, Lopez-Tello J, Sferruzzi-Perri AN. The role of placental hormones in mediating maternal adaptations to support pregnancy and lactation. Frontiers in Physiology. 2018;9:1091. DOI: 10.3389/ fphys.2018.01091
3. Fowden AL, Giussani DA, Forhead AJ. Intrauterine programming of physiological systems: Causes and consequences. Physiology (Bethesda, Md.). 2006;21:29-37. DOI: 10.1152/ physiol.00050.2005
4. Bergfelt DR. Estrous synchronization. In: Samper JC, editor. Equine Breeding Management and Artificial Insemination. Philadelphia: Saunders Company; 2000. pp. 165-177
5. Ginther OJ, Beg MA, Neves AP, Mattos RC, Petrucci BP, Gastal MO, et al. Miniature ponies: 2. Endocrinology of the estrous cycle. Reproduction, Fertility and Development. 2008;20(3):386-390. DOI: 10.1071/ rd07165
6. Crowell-Davis SL. Sexual behaviour of mares. Hormones and Behavior. 2007;52(1):12-17. DOI: 10.1016/j. yhbeh.2007.03.020
7. Aurich C. Reproductive cycles of horses. Animal Reproduction Science. 2011;124(3-4):220-228. DOI: 10.1016/j. anireprosci.2011.02.005
8. Ginther OJ, Beg MA, Gastal MO, Gastal EL, Baerwald AR, Pierson RA. Systemic concentrations of hormones during development of follicular waves in mares and women: A comparative study. Reproduction. 2005;130:379-388. DOI: 10.1530/rep.1.00757

9. Armstrong DG, Webb R. Ovarian follicular dominance: The role of intraovarian growth factors and novel proteins. Reviews of Reproduction. 1997;2(3):139-146. PMID: 9414477

10. Ginther OJ, Bergfelt DR. Effect of GnRH treatment during the anovulatory season on multiple ovulation rate and on follicular development during the ensuing pregnancy in mares. Reproduction. 1990;88(1):119-126. DOI: 10.1530/jrf.0.0880119

11. Ginther OJ, Beg MA, Bergfelt DR, Donadeu FX, Kot K. Follicle selection in monovular species. Biology of Reproduction. 2001;65(3):638-647. DOI: 10.1095/biolreprod65.3.638

12. Donadeu FX, Ginther OJ. Changes in concentrations of follicular fluid factors during follicle selection in mares. Biology of Reproduction. 2002;66(4):1111-1118. DOI: 10.1095/ biolreprod66.4.1111

13. Ginther OJ, Gastal MO, Gastal EL, Bergfelt DR, Baerwald AR, Pierson RA. Comparative study of the dynamics of follicular waves in mares and women. Biology of Reproduction. 2004;71:1195-1201. DOI: 10.1095/biolreprod.104.031054

14. Ginther OJ. Folliculogenesis during the transitional period and early ovulatory season in mares. Journal of Reproduction and Fertility. 1990;90(1):311-320. DOI: 10.1530/ jrf.0.0900311

15. Irvine CHG, Alexander SL, Mckinnon AO. Reproductive hormone profiles in mares during the autumn transition as determined by collection of jugular blood at 6 h intervals throughout ovulatory and anovulatory cycles. Journal of Reproduction and Fertility. 2000;118:101-109. PMID: 10793631

16. Watson ED, Bae SE, Steele M, Tomassen R, Michele S, Pedersen H, et al. Expression of messenger ribonucleic acid encoding for steroidogenic acute regulatory protein and enzymes, and luteinizing hormone receptor during the spring transitional season in equine follicles. Domestic Animal Endocrinology. 2004;26(3):215-239. DOI: 10.1016/j.domaniend.2003.10.006

17. Ginther OJ. Selection of the dominant follicle in cattle and horses. Animal Reproduction Science. 2000;2(60-61):61-79. PMID: 10844185

18. Gastal EL. Recent advances and new concepts on follicle and endocrine dynamics during the equine periovulatory period. Animal Reproduction. 2009;6(1):144-158. DOI: 10.1111/j.1439-0531.2007.01003.x

19. Satué K, Montesinos P, Gardon JC. Influence of oestrogen and progesterone on circulating neutrophils and monocyte during ovulatory and luteal phase in healthy Spanish Purebred mares. In: Proceeding of XIX Congress of Societa

Italiana Veterinari per Equini (SIVE); 1-3 February 2013; Arezzo, Italy. pp. 383-384

20. Bergfelt DR, Adams GP. Ovulation and corpus luteum development. In: Samper JC, Pycock JF, McKinnon AO, editors. Current Therapy in Equine Reproduction. W.B. Saunders-Elsevier; 2007. pp. 1-13
21. Davies Morel MC, Newcombe JR, Hayward K. Factors affecting preovulatory follicle diameter in the mare: The effect of mare age, season and presence of other ovulatory follicles (multiple ovulation). Theriogenology. 2010;74(7):1241-1247. DOI: 10.1016/j. theriogenology.2010.05.027
22. Gastal EL. Ovulation. Part 1. Follicle development and endocrinology during the periovulatory period. In: AO MK, Squires EL, Vaala WE, Dickson DV, editors. Equine Reproduction. Ames, IA: Wiley-Blackwell; 2011. pp. 2020-2031. ISBN: 978-0-813-81971-6
23. Gastal EL. Ovulation. Part 2: Ultrasonographic morphology of the preovulatory follicle. In: McKinnon AO, Squires EI, Vaala WE, Varner DD, editors. Equine Reproduction. 2nd ed. Vol. 2. Oxford: Blackwell Publishing Ltd; 2011. pp. 2032-2054. ISBN: 978-0-813-81971-6
24. Younqquist RS, Threlfall WR. Current Therapy in Large Animal Theriogenology. 2nd ed. St Louis: Saunders Elsevier; 2007. pp. 47-67
25. Dickson SE, Fraser HM. Inhibition of early luteal angiogenesis by gonadotropin-releasing hormone antagonist treatment in the primate. The Journal of Clinical Endocrinology and Metabolism. 2000;85(6):2339-2344. DOI: 10.1210/jcem.85.6.6621
26. Bergfelt D, Ginther O. Embryo loss following GnRH-induced ovulation in anovulatory mares. Theriogenology. 1992;38(1):33-43. DOI: 10.1016/0093-691x(92)90216-e
27. Daels PF, DeMoraes JJ, Stabenfeldt GH, Hughes JP, Lasley BL. The corpus luteum: Source of oestrogen during early pregnancy in the mare. Journal of Reproduction and Fertility. Supplement. 1991;44:501-508. PMID: 1665517
28. Ginther OJ, editor. Reproductive Biology of the Mare: Basic and Applied Aspects. 2nd ed. Cross Plains, WI: Equiservices Publishing; 1992. pp. 224-226. ISBN: 0964007215
29. Samper JC. Induction of estrus and ovulation: Why some mares respond and others do not. Animal Reproduction Science. 2008;70:445-447. DOI: 10.1016/j. theriogenology.2008.04.040
30. Alexander SL, Irvine CHG. Control of onset of breeding season in the mare and its artificial regulation by progesterone treatment. Journal of Reproduction and Fertility. Supplement. 1991;44:307-318. PMID: 1795275.

31. Medan MS, Nambo Y, Nagamine N, Shinbo H, Watanabe G, Groome N, et al. Plasma concentrations of Ir-inhibin, inhibin A, inhibin pro-αC, FSH, and estradiol-17β during estrous cycle in mares and their relationship with follicular growth. Endocrine. 2004;25(1):7-14. DOI: 10.1385/ ENDO:25:1:07

32. Irvine CHG, Alexander SL. Secretory patterns and rates ofgonadotrophin-releasing hormone, follicle-stimulating hormone, and luteinizing hormone revealed by intensive sampling of pituitary venous blood in the luteal phase mare. Endocrinology. 1993;132:212-218. DOI: 10.1210/endo.132.1.8419124

33. Reichert LE Jr. The functional relationship between FSH and its receptor as studied by synthetic peptide strategies. Molecular and Cellular Endocrinology. 1994;100(1-2):21-27. DOI: 10.1016/0303-7207(94)90273-9

34. Pantke P, Hyland J, Galloway DB, Mclean AA, Hoppen HO. Changes in luteinizing hormone bioactivity associated with gonadotrophin pulses in the cycling mare. Journal of Reproduction and Fertility. Supplement. 1991;44:13-18. PMID: 1795256

35. Honnens A, Weisser S, Welter H, Einspanier R, Bollwein H. Relationships between uterine blood flow, peripheral sex steroids, expression of endometrial estrogen receptors and nitric oxide synthases during the estrous cycle in mares. The Journal of Reproduction and Development. 2011;57(1):43-48. DOI: 10.1262/jrd.10-023t

36. Amer HA, Gamal S, Randa I. Profile of steroid hormones during oestrus and early pregnancy in Arabian mares. Slovenian Veterinary Research. 2008;45(1):25-32. UDC 636.1.082.455:61 2.621.9:637.047:577.175.6

37. Nagy P, Huszenicza G, Reiczigel J, Juhász J, Kulcsár M, Abaváry K, et al. Factors affecting plasma progesterone concentration and the retrospective determination of time of ovulation in cyclic mares. Theriogenology. 2004;61(2-3):203-214. DOI: 10.1016/ s0093-691x(03)00211-5

38. Donadeu FX, Pedersen HG. Follicle development in mares. Reproduction in Domestic Animals. 2008;43(2): 224-231. DOI: 10.1111/j.1439-0531. 2008.01166.x

39. Shand N, Irvine CH, Turner JE, Alexander SL. A detailed study of hormonal profiles in mares at luteolysis. Journal of Reproduction and Fertility. Supplement. 2000;56:271-279. PMID: 20681138

40. Ginther OJ, Beg MA. Hormone concentration changes temporally associated with the hour of transition from preluteolysis to luteolysis in mares. Animal Reproduction. 2011;129(1-2):67-72. DOI: 10.1016/j. anireprosci.2011.09.013

41. Greco GM, Fioratti EG, Segabinazzi LG, Dell'Aqua JA Jr, Crespilho AM, Castro-Chaves MMB, et al. Novel long-acting progesterone protocols used to successfully synchronize donor and recipient mares with satisfactory

pregnancy and pregnancy loss rates. Journal of Equine Veterinary Science. 2016;39:58-61. DOI: 10.1016/j.jevs.2015.07.012

42. Pinto MR, Miragaya MH, Burns P, Douglas R, Neild DM. Strategies for increasing reproductive efficiency in a commercial embryo transfer program with high performance donor mares under training. Journal of Equine Veterinary Science. 2017;54:1-5. DOI: 10.1016/j.jevs.2016.09.004
43. Alexander SL, Irvine CHG. Effect of graded doses of gonadotrophinreleasing hormone on serum LH concentrations in mares in various reproductive states: Comparison with endogenously generated LH pulses. The Journal of Endocrinology. 1986;110: 19-26. DOI: 10.1677/joe.0.1100019
44. Garcia MC, Ginther OJ. Plasma luteinizing hormone concentration in mares treated with gonadotropinreleasing hormone and estradiol.
45. American Journal of Veterinary Research. 1975;36:1581-1584. PMID: 1103666
46. Hyland JH, Wright PJ, Clarke IJ, Carson RS, Langsford DA, Jeffcott LB. Infusion of gonadotropin-releasing hormone (GnRH) induces ovulation and fertile estrus in mares during seasonal anestrous. Journal of Reproduction and Fertility. Supplement. 1987;35:211-220. PMID: 3316638
47. Turner JE, Irvine CHG. The effect of various gonadotropin-releasing hormone regimens on gonadotrophins, follicular growth and ovulation in deeply anestrous mares. Journal of Reproduction and Fertility. Supplement. 1991;44:213-225. PMID: 1839039
48. Minoia P, Mastronardi M. Use of GnRH to induce oestrus in seasonally anoestrus mares. Equine Veterinary Journal. 1987;19:241-242. DOI: 10.1111/j.2042-3306.1987.tb01394.x
49. Lindholm A, Ferris R, Scofield D, Mccue P. Comparison of deslorelin and histrelin for induction of ovulation in mares. Journal of Equine Veterinary Science. 2011;31(5-6):312-313. DOI: 10.1016/j.jevs.2011.03.144
50. Allen WR, Sanderson MW, Greenwood RES, Ellis DR, Crowhurst JS, Simpson DJ, et al. Induction of ovulation in anestrous mares with a slow-release implant of GnRH analogue (ICI 118630). Journal of Reproduction and Fertility. Supplement. 1987;35:469-478. PMID: 2960804
51. Harrison LA, Squires EL, Nett TM, McKinnon AO. Use of gonodotrophinreleasing hormone for hastening ovulation in transitional mares. Journal of Animal Science. 1990;68:690-699. DOI: 10.2527/1990.683690x
52. Mumford EL, Squires EL, Jasko DJ, Nett TM. Use of gonadotropin-releasing hormone, estrogen, or combination to increase releasable pituitary luteinizing

hormone in early transitional mares. Journal of Animal Science. 1994;72:174-177. DOI: 10.2527/1994.721174x

53. Mumford EL, Squires EL, Jochle W, Harrison LA, Nett TM, Trigg TE. Use of deslorelin short-term implants to induce ovulation in cycling mares during three consecutive estrous cycles. Animal Reproduction Science. 1995;39:129-140. DOI: 10.1016/0378-4320(95)01383-B

54. Squires EL, Moran DM, Farlin ME, Jasko DJ, Keefe TJ, Meyers SA, et al. Effect of dose of GnRH analog on ovulation in mares. Theriogenology. 1994;41:757-769. DOI: 10.1016/ 0093-691x(94)90185-l

55. Dascanio J. In: McCue P, editor. Equine Reproductive Procedure. John Wiley & Sons, Inc; 2014. DOI: 10.1002/9781118904398

56. Allen WR, Urwin V, Simpson DJ, Greenwood RES, Crowhurst RC, Ellis DR, et al. Preliminary studies on the use of an oral progestogen to induce oestrus and ovulation in seasonally anoestrous Thoroughbred mares. Equine Veterinary Journal. 1980;12(3):141-145. DOI: 10.1111/j.2042-3306.1980.tb03405.x

57. Webel SK, Squires EL. Control of oestrous cycle in mares with altrenogest. Journal of Reproduction and Fertility. Supplement. 1982;32:193-198.PMID: 6962854

58. Hanlon DW, Firth EC. The reproductive performance of Thoroughbred mares treated with intravaginal progesterone at the start of the breeding season. Theriogenology.2012;77(5):952-958.DOI:10.1016/j.theriogenology.2011.10.001

59. Raz T, Carley S, Card C. Comparison of the effects of eFSH and deslorelin treatment regimes on ovarian stimulation and embryo production of donor mares in early vernal transition. Animal Reproduction Science. 2009;71:1358-1366. DOI: 10.1016/j. theriogenology.2008.09.048

60. Meyers-Brown GA, McCue PM, Niswender KD, Squires EL, DeLuca CA, Bidstrup LA, et al. Superovulation in mares using recombinant equine follicle stimulating hormone: Ovulation rates, embryo retrieval, and hormone profiles. Journal of Equine Veterinary Science. 2010;30(10):560-568. DOI: 10.1016/j. jevs.2010.09.007

61. Meyers-Brown GA, McCue PM, Troedsson MH, Klein C, Zent W, Ferris RA, et al. Induction of ovulation in seasonally anestrous mares under ambient lights using recombinant equine FSH (reFSH). Theriogenology. 2013;80(5):456-462. DOI: 10.1016/j. theriogenology.2013.04.029

62. Meyers-Brown GA, Loud MC, Hyland JC, Roser JF. Deep anestrous mares under natural photoperiod treated with recombinant equine FSH (reFSH) and LH (reLH) have fertile ovulations and become pregnant. Theriogenology. 2017;98:108-115. DOI: 10.1016/j.theriogenology.2017.05.001

63. Havern RL, Whisnant CS, Goodman RL. Hypothalamic sites of catecholamine inhibition of luteinizing hormone in the anestrous Ewe1. Biology of Reproduction. 1991;44(3):476-482. DOI: 10.1095/biolreprod44.3.476

64. Panzani D, Zicchino I, Taras A, Marmorini P, Crisci A, Rota A, et al. Clinical use of dopamine antagonist sulpiride to advance first ovulation in transitional mares. Theriogenology. 2011;75(1):138-143. DOI: 10.1016/j.theriogenology.2010.07.019

65. Mari G, Morganti M, Merlo B, Castagnetti C, Parmeggiani F, Govoni N, et al. Administration of sulpiride or domperidone for advancing the first ovulation in deep anestrous mares. Theriogenology. 2009;71(6):959-965. DOI: 10.1016/j.theriogenology.2008.11.001

66. McCue PM. Clinical cases in equine reproduction. In: Proceedings of the 52nd Annual Convention of the American Association of Equine Practitioners (AAEP); 2-6 December 2006; San Antonio, Texas. Vol. 52. pp. 591-596

67. Thompson DL, Hoffman R, Depew CL. Prolactin administration to seasonally anestrous mares: Reproductive, metabolic, and hairshedding responses. Journal of Animal Science. 1997;75(4):1092-1099. DOI: 10.2527/1997.7541092x

68. Nequin LG, King SS, Johnson AL, Gow GM, Ferreira-Dias GM. Prolactin may play a role in stimulating the equine ovary during the spring reproductive transition. Journal of Equine Veterinary Science. 1993;13:631-635. DOI: 10.1016/ S0737-0806(07)80391-1

69. Yoon M. The estrous cycle and induction of ovulation in mares. Journal of Analytical Science and Technology. 2012;54(3):165-174. DOI: 10.5187/JAST.2012.54.3.165

70. Alexander SL, Irvine CH. Secretion rates and short-term patterns of gonadotrophin-releasing hormone, FSH and LH throughout the periovulatory period in the mare. The Journal of Endocrinology. 1987;114:351-362. DOI: 10.1677/joe.0.1140351

71. Johnson AL. Induction of ovulation in anestrous mares with pulsatile administration of gonadotropinreleasing hormone. American Journal of Veterinary Research. 1986;47:983-986. PMID: 3521408

72. Becker SE, Johnson AL. Effects of gonadotropinreleasing hormone infused in a pulsatile or continuous fashion on serum gonadotropin concentrations and ovulation in the mare. Journal of Animal Science. 1992;70:1208-1215. DOI: 10.2527/1992.7041208x

73. Irvine DS, Downey BR, Parker WG, Sullivan JJ. Duration of oestrus and time of ovulation in mares treated with synthetic Gn-RH (AY-24,031). Journal of Reproduction and Fertility. 1975:279- 283. PMID: 1107542 Duchamp G, Bour B,

74. Combarnous Y, Palmer E. Alternative solutions to hCG induction of ovulation in the mare. Journal of Reproduction and Fertility. Supplement. 1987;35: 221-228. PMID: 3479577

75. Williams GL, Amstalden M, Blodgett GP, Ward JE, Unnerstall DA, Quirk KS. Continuous administration of low dose GnRH in mares. I. Control of persistent anovulation during the ovulatory season. Theriogenology. 2007;68:67-75. DOI: 10.1016/j. theriogenology.2007.03.024

76. Samper JC, Jensen S, Sergenat J. Timing of induction of ovulation in mares treated with ovuplant or chorulon. Journal of Equine Veterinary Science. 2002;22:320-323. DOI: 10.1016/ S0737-0806(02)70080-4

77. Meinert C, Silva JFS, Kroetz L, Klug E, Trigg TE, Hoppen HO, et al. Advancing the time of ovulation in the mare with a short-term implant releasing the GnRH analogue deslorelin. Equine Veterinary Journal. 1993;25:65-68. DOI: 10.1111/j.2042-3306.1993. tb02904.x

78. Farquhar V, McCue P, Vanderwall DK, Squires EL. Efficacy of the GnRH agonist deslorelin acetate for inducing ovulation in mares relative to age of mare and season. Journal of Equine Veterinary Science. 2000;20:8-11. DOI: 10.1016/ S0737-0806(00)80183-5

79. Vanderwall DK, Juergens TD, Woods GL. Reproductive performance of commercial broodmares after induction of ovulation with hCG or Ovuplant™ (deslorelin). Journal of Equine Veterinary Science. 2001;21:539-542. DOI: 10.1016/ S0737-0806(01)70158-X

80. Johnson CA, Thompson DL, Kulinski K, Guitreau AM. Prolonged interovulatory interval and hormonal changes in mares following the use of Ovuplant™ to hasten ovulation. Journal of Equine Veterinary Science. 2000;20:331-336. DOI: 10.1016/ S0737-0806(00)70421-7

81. Farquhar VJ, McCue PM, Nett TM, Squires EL. Effect of deslorelin acetate on gonadotropin secretion and ovarian follicle development in cycling mares. Journal of the American Veterinary Medical Association. 2001;218:749-752. DOI: 10.2460/javma.2001.218.749

82. McCue PM, Farquhar VJ, Carnevale EM, Squires EL. Removal of deslorelin (Ovuplant™) implant 48 h after administration results in normal interovulatory intervals in mares. Theriogenology. 2002;58(5):865-870. DOI: 10.1016/S0093-691X(02)00923-8

83. Stich KL, Wendt KM, Blandchard TL, Brinsko SP. Effects of a new injectable short-term release deslorelin in foal-heat mares. Theriogenology. 2004;62:831-836. DOI: 10.1016/j.theriogenology.2003.12.004

84. McCue PM, Magee C, Gee EK. Comparison of compounded deslorelin and hCG for induction of ovulation in mares. Journal of Equine Veterinary Science. 2007;27:58-61. DOI: 10.1016/j. jevs.2006.12.003

85. Barrier-Battut I, Le Poutre N, Trocherie E, Hecht S, Grandchamp des Raux A, Nicaise JL, et al. Use of buserelin to induce ovulation in the cyclic mare. Theriogenology. 2001;55:1679-1695. DOI: 10.1016/ s0093-691x(01)00512-x

86. Miki W, Oniyama H, Takeda N, Kimura Y, Haneda S, Matsui M, et al. Effects of a single use of the GnRH analog buserelin on the induction of ovulation and endocrine profiles in heavy draft mares. Journal of Equine Science. 2016;27(4):149-156. DOI: 10.1294/jes.27.149

87. Camillo F, Pacini M, Panzani D, Vannozzi I, Rota A, Aria G. Clinical use of twice daily injections of buserelin acetate to induce ovulation in the mare. Veterinary Research Communications. 2004;28(1):169-172. DOI: 10.1023/b:verc.0000045398.62134.e4

88. Newcombe JR, Martinez TA, Peters AR. The effect of the gonadotropin-releasing hormone analog, buserelin, on pregnancy rates in horse and pony mares. Theriogenology. 2001;55:1619-1631. DOI: 10.1016/ s0093-691x(01)00507-6

89. Kanitz W, Schneider F, Hoppen HO, Unger C, Nurmberg G, Becker K. Pregnancy rates, LH and progesterone concentrations in mares treated with GnRH agonist. Animal Reproduction Science. 2007;97:55-62. DOI: 10.1016/j. anireprosci.2005.12.011

90. Cole LA, Kardana A. Discordant results in human chorionic gonadotropin assays. Clinical Chemistry. 1992;38:263-270. PMID: 1371722

91. Kilicarslan MR, Horoz H, Senunver A, Konuk SC, Tek C, Carioglu B. Effect of GnRH and hCG on ovulation and pregnancy in mares. The Veterinary Record. 1996;139:119-120. DOI: 10.1136/vr.139.5.119

92. Wilson C, Downie C, Hughes J. Effects of repeated hCG injections on reproductive efficiency in mares. Journal of Equine Veterinary Science. 1990;10:301-308. DOI: 10.1016/ S0737-0806(06)80015-8

93. Newcombe JR, Wilson MC. The effect of repeated treatment with human chorionic gonadotrophin to induce ovulation in mares. In: Proceedings of the 46th Congress British Equine Veterinary Association (BEVA): 12-15th September 2007; Edinburgh. p. 291

94. Newcombe JR. Human chorionic gonadotrophin. In: McKinnon AO, Squires EL, Vaala WE, Varner DD, editors. Equine Reproduction. United Kingdom: Blackwell Publishing Ltd.; 2011. pp. 1804-1810. ISBN: 978-0-813 81971-6

95. Jablonka-Shariff A, Roser JF, Bousfield GR, Wolfe MW, Sibley LE, Colgin M, et al. Expression and bioactivity of a single chain recombinant equine luteinizing hormone (reLH). Theriogenology. 2007;67:311-320. DOI: 10.1016/j.theriogenology.2006.06.013

96. Yoon MJ, Boime I, Colgin M, Niswender KD, King SS, Alvarenga M, et al. The efficacy of a single chain recombinant equine luteinizing hormone (reLH) in mares: Induction of ovulation, hormone profiles, and inter- ovulatory intervals. Domestic Animal Endocrinology. 2007;33:470-479. DOI: 10.1016/j.domaniend.2007.06.001

97. Goldfarb LG, Cervenakova L, Gajdusek DC. Genetic studies in relation to kuru: An overview. Current Molecular Medicine. 2004;4(4):375-384. DOI: 10.2174/1566524043360627 Chakraborty C, Nandi S,

98. Jana S. Prion disease: A deadly disease for protein misfolding. Current Pharmaceutical Biotechnology. 2005;6(2):167-177. DOI: 10.2174/1389201053642321

99. Zou WQ , Gambetti P. Prion: The chameleon protein. Cellular and Molecular Life Sciences. 2007;64(24):3266-3270. DOI: 10.1007/ s00018-007-7380-8

100. Savage NC, Liptrap RM. Induction of ovulation in cyclic mares by administration of a synthetic prostaglandin, fenprostalene, during oestrus. Journal of Reproduction and Fertility. Supplement. 1987;35:239-243. PMID: 3479578

101. Harrison LA, Squires EL, McKinnon AO. Comparison of hCG, Burserelin and Luprostiol for induction of ovulation in cycling mares.

102. Journal of Equine Veterinary Science. 1991;11:163-166. DOI: 10.1016/ S0737-0806(07)80039-6

103. Jöchle W, Irvine CH, Alexander SL, Newby TJ. Release of LH, FSH and GnRH into pituitary venous blood in mares treated with a PGF analogue, luprostiol, during the transition period. Journal of Reproduction and Fertility. Supplement. 1987;35:261-267. PMID: 3119828

104. Caraty A, Franceschini I. Basic aspects of the control of GnRH and LH secretions by kisspeptin: Potential applications for better control of fertility in females.

105. Reproduction in Domestic Animals. 2008;43(2):172-178. DOI: 10.1111/j.1439-0531.2008.01158.x

106. Clarke H, Dhillo WS, Jayasena CN. Comprehensive review on Kisspeptin and its role in reproductive disorders. Endocrinology and Metabolism. 2015;30(2):124-141. DOI: 10.3803/ EnM.2015.30.2.124

107. Magee C, Foradori CD, Bruemmer JE, Arreguin-Arevalo JA, McCue PM, Handa RJ, et al. Biological and anatomical evidence for kisspeptin regulation of the hypothalamicpituitary-gonadal axis of estrous horse mares. Biomedizinische Technik. 2009;150(6):2813-2821. DOI: 10.1210/ en.2008-1698

108. Ginther OJ. Mobility of the early equine conceptus. Theriogenology. 1983;19(4):603-611. DOI: 10.1016/0093-691x(83)90180-2

109. Ginther OJ. Equine pregnancy: Physical interactions between the uterus and conceptus. In: Proceedings of the 44th Annual Convention of the American Association of Equine Practitioners (AAEP); 6-9 December 1998. Baltimore, Maryland. pp. 73-104

110. Stout TA, Allen WR. Role of prostaglandins in intrauterine migration of the equine conceptus. Reproduction. 2001;121(5):771-775. DOI: 10.1530/ rep.0.1210771

111. Raeside JI, Christie HL, Renaud RL, Waelchli RO, Betteridge KJ. Estrogen metabolism in the equine conceptus and endometrium during early pregnancy in relation to estrogen concentrations in yolk-sac fluid. Biology of Reproduction. 2004;71(4):1120-1127. DOI: 10.1095/ biolreprod.104.028712

112. Raeside JI, Christie HL, Waelchli RO, Betteridge KJ. Biosynthesis of oestrogen by the early equine embryo proper. Reproduction, Fertility, and Development. 2012;24(8):1071-1078. DOI: 10.1071/RD11275

113. Wilsher S, Allen WR. Factors influencing equine chorionic gonadotrophin production in the mare. Equine Veterinary Journal. 2011;43(4):430-438. DOI: 10.1111/j.2042-3306.2010.00309.x

114. Ginther OJ, Santos VG. Natural rescue and resurgence of the equine corpus luteum. Journal of Equine Veterinary Science. 2015;35:1-6. DOI: 10.1016/j. jevs.2014.10.004

115. Legacki EL, Scholtz EL, Ball BA, Stanley SD, Berger T, Conley AJ. The dynamic steroid landscape of equine pregnancy mapped by mass spectrometry. Reproduction. 2016;151(4):421-430. DOI: 10.1530/ REP-15-0547

116. Satué K, Marcilla M, Medica P, Ferlazzo A, Fazio E. Sequential concentrations of placental growth factor and haptoglobin, and their relation to oestrone sulphate and progesterone in pregnant Spanish purebred mare. Theriogenology. 2018;115:77-83. DOI: 10.1016/j. theriogenology.2018.04.033

117. Davies Morel MC. Equine Reproductive Physiology, Breeding and Stud Management. 3rd ed. Wallindorf, UK: CABI; 2008. ISBN: 9781845934507

118. Satué K, Domingo R, Redondo JI. Relationship between progesterone, oestrone sulphate and cortisol and the components of renin angiotensin aldosterone system in Spanish purebred broodmares during pregnancy. Theriogenology. 2011;76(8):1404-1415. DOI: 10.1016/j. theriogenology.2011.06.009

119. Satué K, Marcilla M, Medica P, Ferlazzo A, Fazio E. Testosterone, androstenedione and dehydroepiandrosterone concentrations in pregnant Spanish purebred mare. Theriogenology. 2019;1(123):62-67. DOI: 10.1016/j. theriogenology.2018.09.025

120. Albrecht BA, MacLeod JN, Daels PF. Differential transcription of steroidogenic enzymes in the equine primary corpus luteum during diestrus and early pregnancy. Biology of Reproduction. 1997;56(4):821-829. DOI: 10.1095/ biolreprod56.4.821

121. Daels PF, Chang GC, Hansen B, Mohammed HO. Testosterone secretion during early pregnancy in mares. Theriogenology. 1996;45(6):1211-1219. DOI: 10.1016/0093-691x(96)00076-3

122. Daels PF, Albrecht BA, Mohammed HO. Equine chorionic gonadotropin regulates luteal steroidogenesis in pregnant mares. Biology of Reproduction. 1998;59(5):1062-1068. DOI: 10.1095/ biolreprod59.5.1062

123. Kajihara T, Tanaka K, Oguro T, Tochigi H, Prechapanich J, Uchino S, et al. Androgens modulate the morphological characteristics of human endometrial stromal cells decidualized in vitro. Reproductive Sciences. 2014;21(3):372-380. DOI: 10.1177/1933719113497280

124. Ferraz LES, Vicente WRR, Ramos PRR. Progesterone and estradiol 17-β concentration, and ultrasonic images of the embryonic vesicle during the early pregnancy in Thoroughbred mares. Arquivo Brasileiro de Medicina Veterinária e Zootecnia. 2001;53(4):1-7. DOI: 10.1590/ S0102-09352001000400015

125. Holtan DW, Houghton E, Silver M, Fowden AL, Ousey J, Rossdale PD. Plasma progestagens in the mare, fetus and newborn foal. Journal of Reproduction and Fertility. Supplement. 1991;44: 517-528. PMID: 1795295

126. Han X, Rossdale PD, Ousey J, Holdstock N, Allen WR, Silver M, et al. Localisation of 15-hydroxy prostaglandin dehydrogenase (PGDH) and steroidogenic enzymes in the equine placenta. Equine Veterinary Journal. 1995;27(5):334-339. DOI: 10.1111/ j.2042-3306.1995.tb04067.x

127. Ousey JC, Houghton E, Grainger L, Rossdale PD, Fowden AL. Progestagen profiles during the last trimester of gestation in Thoroughbred mares with normal or compromised pregnancies. Theriogenology. 2005;63(7):1844-1856. DOI: 10.1016/j. theriogenology.2004.08.010

128. Scholtz EL, Krishnan S, Ball BA, Corbin CJ, Moeller BC, Stanley SD, et al. Pregnancy without progesterone in horses defines a second endogenous biopotent progesterone receptor agonist, 5α-dihydroprogesterone. Proceedings of the National Academy of Sciences of the United States of America. 2014;111(9):3365-3370. DOI: 10.1073/pnas.1318163111

129. Conley AJ. Review of the reproductive endocrinology of the pregnant and parturient mare. Theriogenology. 2016;86(1):355-365. DOI: 10.1016/j.theriogenology.2016.04.049

130. Wynn MAA, Esteller-Vico A, Legacki EL, Conley AJ, Loux SC, Stanley SD, et al. A comparison of progesterone assays for determination of peripheral pregnane concentrations in the late pregnant mare. Theriogenology. 2018;106:127-133. DOI: 10.1016/j.theriogenology.2017.10.002

131. Ousey JC, Rossdale PD, Palmer L, Houghton E, Grainger L, Fowden AL. Effects of progesterone administration to mares during late gestation. Theriogenology. 2002;58:793-795. DOI: 10.1016/ S0093-691X(02)00743-4 Ousey JC, Forhead AJ, Rossdale PD, Grainger L, Houghton E, Fowden AL. Ontogeny of uteroplacental progestagen production in pregnant mares during the second half of gestation. Biology of Reproduction. 2003;69(2):540-548. DOI: 10.1095/biolreprod.102.013292

132. Henderson K, Stewart J. A dipstick immunoassay to rapidly measure serum oestrone sulfate concentrations in horses. Reproduction, Fertility, and Development. 2000;12(3-4):183-189. DOI: 10.1071/rd00062

133. Henderson KM, Eayrs K. Pregnancy status determination in mares using a rapid lateral flow test for measuring serum oestrone sulphate. New Zealand Veterinary Journal. 2004;52(4):193-196. DOI: 10.1080/00480169.2004.36428 Fowden AL, Forhead AJ,

134. Ousey JC. The endocrinology of equine parturition. Experimental and Clinical Endocrinology & Diabetes. 2008;116:393-403. DOI: 10.1055/s-2008-1042409

135. Pashen RL, Allen WR. The role of the fetal gonads and placenta in steroid production, maintenance of pregnancy and parturition in the mare. Journal of Reproduction and Fertility.Supplement. 1979;27:499-509. PMID: 289829

136. Hasegawa T, Sato F, Nambo Y, Ishida N. Expression of steroidogenic enzyme genes in the equine fetoplacental unit. Journal of Equine Science. 2001;12(1):25-32. DOI: 10.1294/jes.12.25

137. Canisso IF, Ball BA, Esteller- Vico A, Squires EL, Troedsson MH. Dehydroepiandrosterone sulfate and testosterone concentrations in mares carrying normal pregnancies. In: Proceedings of the Society for Theriogenology Annual Conference; 6-9 August 2014; Portland, OR, USA. p. 383

138. Ousey JC. Endocrinology of pregnancy. In: McKinnon AO, Squires EL, Vaala WE, Varner DD, editors. Equine Reproduction. Hoboken NJ: Wiley-Blackwell; 2011. pp. 2222- 2231. ISBN: 978-0-813-81971-6

139. Ousey JC. Hormone profiles and treatments in the late pregnant mare. The Veterinary Clinics of North America. Equine Practice. 2006;22(3):727-747. DOI: 10.1016/j. cveq.2006.08.004

140. McGlothlin JA, Lester GD, Hansen PJ, Thomas M, Pablo L, Hawkins DL, et al. Alteration in uterine contractility in mares with experimentally induced placentitis. Reproduction. 2004;127(1):57-66. DOI: 10.1530/rep.1.00021

141. Kelleman AA, Act D. Equine pregnancy and clinical applied physiology. In: Proceedings of the 59th Annual Convention of the American Association of Equine Practitioners (AAEP); 7-11 December, 2013. Nashville, Tennessee, USA. pp. 350-358

142. Silver M, Barnes RJ, Comline RS, Fowden AL, Clover L, Mitchell MD. Prostaglandins in maternal and fetal plasma and in allantoic fluid during the second half of gestation in the mare. Journal of Reproduction and Fertility. Supplement. 1979;27:531-539. PMID: 289833

143. Vivrette SL, Kindahl H, Munro CJ, Roser JF, Stabenfeldt GH. Oxytocin release and its relationship to dihydro- 15-keto PGF2alpha and arginine vasopressin release during parturition and to suckling in postpartum mares. Journal of Reproduction and Fertility. 2000;119(2):347-357. DOI: 10.1530/ jrf.0.1190347

144. Bryant-Greenwood GD. Relaxin as a new hormone. Endocrine Reviews. 1992;3(1):62-90. DOI: 10.1210/ edrv-3-1-62

145. Stewart DR, Addiego LA, Pascoe DR, Haluska GJ, Pashen R. Breed differences in circulating equine relaxin. Biology of Reproduction. 1992;46(4):648-652. DOI: 10.1095/ biolreprod46.4.648

146. Machnik M, Hegger I, Kietzmann M, Thevis M, Guddat S, Schänzer W. Pharmacokinetics of altrenogest in horses.Journal of Veterinary Pharmacology and Therapeutics. 2007;30:86-90. DOI: 10.1111/j.1365-2885.2007.00820.x

147. Daels PF, Hussni M, Montavon SME, Stabenfeldt GH, Hughes JP, Odensvik K, et al. Endogenousprostaglandinsecretion during cloprostenol-induced abortion in mares. Animal Reproduction. 1995;40:305-321. DOI: 10.1016/0378-4320(95)01429-2

148. Daels PF, Besognet B, Hansen B, Mohammed H, Odensvik K, Kindahl H. Effect of progesterone on prostaglandin F2 alpha secretion and outcome of pregnancy during cloprostenol-induced abortion in mares. American Journal of Veterinary Research. 1996;57:1331-1337. PMID: 8874729

149. Daels PF, Stabenfeldt GH, Hughes JP, Odensvik K, Kindahl H. Evaluation of progesterone deficiency as a cause of fetal death in mares with experimentally induced endotoxemia. American Journal of Veterinary Research. 1991;52:282-288. PMID: 2012339

150. Vanderwall DK. Early embryonic loss in the mare. Journal of Equine Veterinary Science. 2008;28:691-702. DOI: 10.1016/j.jevs.2008.10.001

151. Pycock J, Newcombe J. The effect of the gonadotrophin-releasing hormone analog, buserelin, administered in diestrus on pregnancy rates and pregnancy failure in mares. Theriogenology. 1996;46:1097-1101. DOI: 10.1016/s0093-691x(96)00274-9

152. Panzani D, Crisci A, Rota A, Camillo F. Effect of day of transfer and treatment administration on the recipient on pregnancy rates after equine embryo transfer.Veterinary Research Communications. 2009;33:113-116. DOI: 10.1007/s11259-009-9303-7

153. Willmann C, Schuler G, Hoffmann B, Parvizi N. Effects of age and altrenogest treatment on conceptus development and secretion of LH, progesterone and eCG in early- pregnant mares. Theriogenology. 2011;75:421-428. DOI: 10.1016/j.theriogenology.2010.05.009

154. Sieme JL, Sielhorst J, Martinsson G, Bollwein H, Thomas S, Burger D. Improving the formation and function of the corpus luteum in the mare. Revista Brasileira de Reprodução Animal. 2015;39:117-120. DOI: 10.5167/ uzh-116508

155. Newcombe JR, Peters AR. The buserelin enigma: How does treatment with this GnRH analogue decrease embryo mortality? Journal of Veterinary Science and Technology. 2014;5:151. DOI: 10.4172/2157-7579.1000151

156. Stout TA, Tremoleda JL, Knaap J, Daels P, Kindahl H, Colenbrander B. Mid-diestrus GnRH-analogue administration does not suppress the luteolytic mechanism in mares. Theriogenology. 2002;58:567-570. DOI: 10.1016/ S0093-691X(02)00860-9

157. Köhne M, Ille N, Erber R, Aurich C. Treatment with human chorionic gonadotrophin before ovulation increases progestin concentration in early equine pregnancies. Animal Reproduction Science. 2014;149:187-193. DOI: 10.1016/j.anireprosci.2014.07.002

158. Biermann J, Klewitz J, Otzen H, Martinsson G, Burger D, Meinecke- Tillmann S, et al. The effect of hCG, administered in diestrus, on luteal, ovarian and uterine blood flow, peripheral progesterone levels and pregnancy rates in mares. Journal of Equine Veterinary Science. 2014;34:166. DOI: 10.1016/j.jevs.2013.10.119

159. Shikichi M, Iwata K, Ito K, Miyakoshi D, Murase H, Sato F, et al. Abnormal pregnancies associated with deviation in progestin and estrogen profiles in late pregnant mares: A diagnostic aid. Theriogenology. 2017;98:75-81. DOI: 10.1016/j. theriogenology.2017.04.024

160. LeBlanc MM, Macpherson M, Sheerin P. Ascending placentitis: What we know about pathophysiology, diagnosis and treatment. In: Proceedings of the Annual Convention of the American Association of Equine Practitioners (AAEP); 4-8 December 2004; Denver, Colorado, USA. pp. 127-143

161. Morris S, Kelleman AA, Stawicki RJ, Hansen PJ, Sheerin PC, Sheerin BR, et al. Transrectal ultrasonography and plasma progestin profiles identifies feto-placental compromise in mares with experimentally induced placentitis. Theriogenology. 2007;67:681-691. DOI: 10.1016/j.theriogenology.2006.05.021

162. Wynn MAA, Ball BA, May J, Esteller-Vico A, Canisso I, Squires E, et al. Changes in maternal pregnane concentrations in mares with experimentally-induced, ascending placentitis. Theriogenology. 2018;122:130-136. DOI: 10.1016/j. theriogenology.2018.09.001

163. Brendemeuhl JP, Williams MA, Boosinger TR, Ruffin DC. Plasma progestagen, trioiodothyronine and cortisol concentrations in postdate gestation foals exposed in utero to the tall fescue endophyte Acremonium coenophialum. Biology of Reproduction. 1995;1:53-59. DOI: 10.1093/biolreprod/52. monograph_series1.53

164. Troedsson MHT, Miller LMJ. Equine placentitis. Pferdeheilkunde. 2016;32(1):49-53. DOI: 10.21836/ PEM20160109

165. Bailey CS, Macpherson ML, Pozor MA, Troedsson MH, Benson SM, Giguere S, et al. Treatment efficacy of trimethoprim sulfamethoxazole, pentoxifylline and altrenogest in experimentally induced equine placentitis. Theriogenology. 2010;74:402-412. DOI: 10.1016/j. theriogenology.2010.02.023

166. Graczyk J, Macpherson ML, Pozor MA, Troedsson MHT, Eichelberger AC, LeBlanc MM, et al. Treatment efficacy of trimethoprim sulfamethoxazole and pentoxifylline in equine placentitis. Animal Reproduction Science. 2006;94:434-435. DOI: 10.1016/j.theriogenology.2010.02.023

167. LeBlanc MM. Ascending placentitis in the mare: An update. Reproduction in Domestic Animals. 2010;45:28-34. DOI: 10.1111/j.1439-0531.2010.01633.x

168. Canisso IF, Ball BA, Esteller- Vico A, Williams NM, Squires EL, Troedsson MH. Changes in maternal androgens and oestrogens in mares with experimentally induced ascending placentitis. Equine Veterinary Journal. 2017;49(2):244-249. DOI: 10.1111/evj.12556

169. Kasman LH, Hughes JP, Stabenfeldt GH, Starr MD, Lasley BL. Estrone sulfate concentrations as an indicator of fetal demise in horses. American Journal of Veterinary Research. 1988;49(2):184-187. PMID: 2831761

170. Santschi EM, LeBlanc MM, Weston PG. Progestagen, oestrone sulphate and cortisol concentrations in pregnant mares during medical and surgical disease. Journal of Reproduction and Fertility. Supplement. 1991;44:627-634. PMID: 1665522

171. Douglas RH. Endocrine diagnostics in the broodmare: What you need to know about progestins and estrogens. In: Annual Meeting for the Society for Theriogenology and American College of Theriogenologists; 4-7 August, 2004; Lexington, KY. pp. 106-115

172. Esteller-Vico A, Ball BA, Troedsson MHT, Squires EL. Endocrine changes, fetal growth, and uterine artery hemodynamics after chronic estrogen suppression during the last trimester of equine pregnancy. Biology of Reproduction. 2017;96:414-423. DOI: 10.1095/biolreprod.116.140533

173. Curcio BR, Canisso IF, Pazinato FM, Borba LA, Feijo LS, Muller V, et al. Estradiol cypionate aided treatment for experimentally induced ascending placentitis in mares. Theriogenology. 2017;102:98-107. DOI: 10.1016/j.theriogenology.2017.03.010

174. Ryan PL, Christiansen DL, Hopper RM, Bagnell CA, Vaala WE, LeBlanc MM. Evaluation of systemic relaxin blood profiles in horses as a means of assessing placental function in high-risk pregnancies and responsiveness to therapeutic strategies. Annals of the New York Academy of Sciences. 2009;1160:169-178. DOI: 10.1111/j.1749-6632.2008.03802.x

175. Christensen BW, Troedsson MHT, Murchie TA, Pozor MA, Macpherson ML, Estrada AH, et al. Management of hydrops amnion in a mare resulting in birth of a live foal. Journal of the American Veterinary Medical Association. 2006;228:1228- 1233. DOI: 10.2460/javma.228.8.1228

176. Klein C. The role of relaxin in mare reproductive physiology: A comparative review with other species. Theriogenology. 2016;86:451-456. DOI: 10.1016/j.theriogenology.2016.04.061

177. LeBlanc MM, Giguere S, Lester GD, Bauer K, Paccamonti L. Relationship between infection, inflammation and premature parturition in mares with experimentally induced placentitis. Equine Veterinary Journal. Supplement. 2012;41:8-14. DOI: 10.1111/j.2042-3306.2011.00502.x

178. Lyle SK. Immunology of infective preterm delivery in the mare. Equine Veterinary Journal. 2014;46:661-668. DOI: 10.1111/evj.12243

179. Lyle SK, Hague M, Lopez MJ, Beehan DP, Staempfil S, Len JA, et al. In vitro production of cortisol by equine fetal adrenal cells in response to ACTH and IL-1b. Animal Reproduction Science. 2010;121:322. DOI: 10.1016/j.anireprosci.2010.04.127

180. Canisso IF, Ball BA, Erol E, Squires EL, Troedsson MHT. Comprehensive review on equine placentitis. In: Proceedings of the 61st Annual Convention of the American Association of Equine Practitioners (AAEP); 5-9 December 2015; Las Vegas, Nevada, USA. pp. 490-509

2 Chapter

COMPREHENDING SOW SEXUAL BEHAVIOR AND THE UTILIZATION OF BOAR PHEROMONE TO ENHANCE SOW REPRODUCTION

1. INTRODUCTION: AN OVERVIEW

In 2018, the global pig population exceeded 700 million, with more than half located in China.The recent proliferation of African Swine Fever (ASF) in China and other regions of Asia has led to a swift drop in the swine population. The migration of breeding animals is restricted in the most pig-dense continent, making the reconstruction of pig populations a difficulty. During outbreaks of diseases like as ASF, when the mobility of breeding animals is curtailed, certain sows must be inseminated without the involvement of adult males. Effective pig breeding is essential for sustaining and replenishing pig populations and the global pork supply.

In cattle herds and poultry flocks, successful breeding often takes place without any adult males. In contrast, most commercial pig farms have adult male pigs (boars) on site to maintain optimum breeding success. Thus, the pig is unique among common food animals in requiring the presence of adult males in commercial production. While some sows will express sexual behaviors without a boar, to get the majority of sows bred, in current commercial production, the male is thought to be required.

In less developed countries, pigs may roam free and are harvested as desired, but these represent a smaller percentage of the world pig inventory over time. Some commercial pigs are kept outdoors in managed systems. The outdoor production system (Figure 1, left) represents a small part of the world's pig herd. Most pigs in the world used for pork production are kept on commercial farms using an indoor sow housing system.

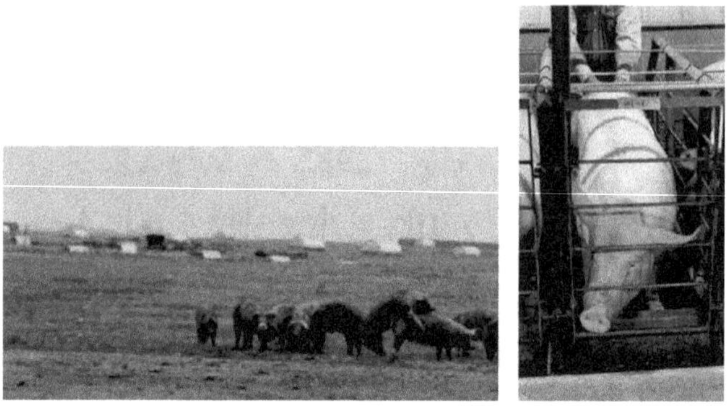

Figure 1. Outdoor systems with natural mating (left) are less common today. Sow in a breeding crate or stall (right). The breeding crate is the most common indoor breeding system. Note that in the outdoor, natural mating system, the sow and boar can fully interact. However, in the breeding crate, a person applies back pressure in the presence of a boar to induce sexual behaviors when a sow is in estrus. If the sow is not in estrus, she will not show sexual behaviors when the person applies pressure to her back.

The most common method of housing the breeding sow is in a crate or pen (Figure 1, right) [2]. The breeding crate is large enough (often 0.6 m × 2.1 m) to accommodate the body of the sow but the breeding crate does not allow the sow to turn around or to express her full repertoire of behaviors. The method of keeping breeding sows (outdoor, indoor in pens or crates) clearly impacts their ability to express natural sexual behaviors and the breeding crate reduces the likelihood of successful mating. Sexual behaviors are best observed in freely-moving sows and boars, but the reality of commercial pork production is that sows are in a breeding crate in which they may have limited fence line contact with an adult male—and this makes training of workers challenging. A better understanding by farm workers of sow and boar sexual behaviors will meaningfully improve reproductive success.

This chapter aims to examine the fundamental behavioral biology of sexual conduct and reproductive efficacy in the domestic pig. This chapter will outline classic literature on the sexual behaviors of sows and boars, and will examine the uses of pheromone technologies as well as the mechanisms via which pheromones might enhance reproductive performance in pig herds. To further our comprehension of porcine sexual behaviors and the influence of boar sexual pheromones on female reproduction, we will also examine the anatomy and physiology of the pig olfactory system.

2. SEXUAL BEHAVIOR IN THE DOMESTIC PIG: EARLY STUDIES AND PREFERRED TERMINOLOGY

While pig farmers have observed sexual behavior for millennia, the earliest scientific description of sow sexual behavior in the scientific literature was in 1941 by Altmann [3]. Altmann was a psychologist at the University of Chicago when animal behavior was developing in the USA. Altmann studied female pig sexual behavior because she used pigs in her conditioning studies, and she wanted to be sure if sows were or were not in heat when she trained them on an operant task. In 1941, she reported several aspects of sow sexual behavior that we know to be true. She said there was a 18–23 day cycle among adult females. She indicated that domestic sows (unlike wild boar) bred year-round, although they often had a "silent heat" in warm weather. She found external signs of estrus to be not reliable indicators of estrus; these included, vaginal mucous, swelling of the vulva and rectal temperature changes. We recently confirmed her observations with quantification of anatomical changes (see below). She indicated behavior and activity were the best methods to determine heat, but a combination of methods increased accuracy.

The next scientist to publish studies in pig sexual behavior was Jean Pierre Signoret from France. His research on sow sexual behavior in the 1960s and early 1970s were summarized in a chapter Signoret co-wrote in Hafez's 1964/1968/1975 editions of the book "The Behaviour of Domestic animals" [4]. The picture of sowboar sexual behavior in that chapter has been widely used to describe pig's sexual behavior. In that picture, he lists sequences of boar-sow behaviors that are shown in Figure 2. The sequence of sexual behaviors between a sow and boar include mutual head sniffing, and then the boar sniffs the sow's rear, he then pushes and may lift the sow from the side, then he sniffs and licks and pushes on the sow's rear. These olfactory and tactile behaviors are accompanied by grunting by the boar and, if the sow is in estrus, she will be silence or she will make soft rhythmic grunts in response (she will squeal if she is not in estrus as a form of objecting to the boar behavior). After touching, smelling and licking her rear, he will mount her and if she is fully in estrus and showing "standing reflex or locked up" behavior, he will copulate with her.

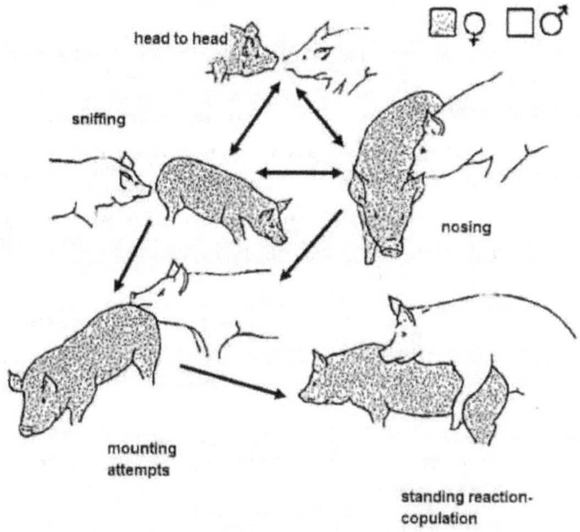

Figure 2.Drawings of sow-boar sexual behaviors from Signoret [4].

We present in Table 1 our definitions of sow sexual behaviors that are observed while a sow is in a breeding crate. Note that because her movements and boar interaction are restricted while in a breeding crate, she will not express the same number of behaviors as in the wild. When the sow expresses intense standing still, we say she is "locked up." A sow can stand still for a few seconds at any time and not be locked up or in estrus. Being locked up is the primary and only reliable sign that a sow is in estrus.

The boar is non-discriminating when deciding which animal or object to mount.

The boar will attempt to mate sows not in estrus and they will mate an object shaped roughly like a sow (e.g., a boar semen collection dummy)—anything shaped like a cylinder that stands still will be mounted by an adult boar.

If the sow is not in full estrus, she will avoid the boar. If she experiences an adult boar while not in heat, then she will vocalize (squeal) and be aggressive towards him to express her objection. In the author's personal observations of feral pigs and outdoor pigs allowed to mate naturally, a sow not in estrus is very aggressive towards adult males. With the matriarchal social structure in nature, the sow is clearly dominant to the boar, except when she is in estrus.

In the period of proestrus, the sow is becoming interested in the boar, but she will still not be willing to stand still for mounting. In this period, she will seek a boar, interact with him and allow for mutual sensory exploration. When these behaviors are observed and the BPT is administered, the sow will not stand still. This period is referred to on the farm as a sow that is coming into estrus but not fully in estrus (proestrus).

Table 1. Definitions of sow sexual behavior when she is in estrus.

Word	Definition
Standing still	Also called standing posture, the sow is motionless for intervals no greater than 10 consecutive seconds
Standing reflex, locked up	When a sow stands still for more than 10 consecutive seconds, usually by applying back pressure. This behavior is exhibited by sows when they see the boar, during the back-pressure test, or when being mounted. Sometimes displayed together with pricked ears and muscle contraction (rigid muscles and in some sow muscle shaking)
Latency to lock up	Time in seconds from application of back pressure until the sow locks up. When a sow is in estrus, latency is usually less than 30 s
Pricked ears	Lifting ears from resting position, usually while sniffing and exhibiting sexual interest. Ears either stand straight up or are obviously higher than resting

Moving	Before and after full estrus, sows will move when back pressure is applied
Sniff	When a boar is near or when they experience a pheromone, they move their rooting disk as they sniff (see videos)
Chomping	When the sow has nose-to-nose contact with a boar, or if they experience the complete pheromone, they will open and close their mouth, and move their tongue in and out while they keep their head level or elevated so they can apply the liquid to their VNO
Vocalization—stress	Sows express a high-pitch squeal when they are objecting to back pressure or a boar. This is a stress vocalization sows make when are not in estrus.
Vocalization—"chatting" or "chanting" with the "boar"	The sow grunts in a low-pitch repeated manner when she sees, smells or hears a boar. This vocalization is not expressed by all sows
We use these and related definitions in our recent work.	

In a breeding crate, the most noticeable sexual behaviors expressed by a sow are locked up and pricked ears (see Table 1 for definition). Stock people that breed sows will be familiar with these sexual behaviors. However, we recognize that there is considerable variation in sexual behaviors within genetic lines and among genetic lines (and breeds). Some individual sows show more extreme sexual behaviors and some show only mild signs of being in estrus. Video in the following link (https://youtu.be/DdgxK1U8ZUo) shows a sow with a strong sexual behavioral response after boar exposure. Video in the following link (https://youtu.be/tspB7RkviBo) shows the same sow that expresses sexual behavior after application of the new boar pheromone [5]. Note the locked up behavior, sniffing and chomping by the sow.

Commercial farms must train workers who perform artificial insemination (AI). Pig breeders must understand sow sexual behavior to achieve success. With training and experience, the AI technician can achieve very high breeding and farrowing rates, but rarely 100% of sows are bred and remain pregnant. Training workers is challenging because sows vary widely in their sexual behaviors. AI workers must be trained with the specific genetic line of pig they are expected to breed. They must understand what normal sexual behavior is for that genetic line and then how to modulate that behavior to achieve high levels of reproductive success. Training is challenging because sows in breeding crates are not able to express the full repertoire of sexual behaviors that they express in an open area and boars are not able to stimulate crated sows through olfactory and tactile senses as they can for penned or pastured pigs.

3. OVERVIEW OF THE ESTRUS CYCLE

3.1 Hormonal changes

The sow estrus cycle is of 18–24 days long [6], with the median and mode of 21 days. Sows are polyestrous animals. This means that with the appropriate nutrition, good health, and the proper environmental conditions, sows will cycle through the year. The sow estrus cycle is only stopped by pregnancy or lactation, and possibly old age. In sows, lactational anestrus is due to the inhibition of the GnRH pulse by the suckling stimulus [7]. Gilts reach puberty at 5 or 6 months old. For sows, the first estrus post-weaning takes place 4–7 days after weaning for most, but not all sows (some have a longer or shorter wean to estrus interval).

During the estrous cycle, sow's hormones change. The hormonal changes mark the different stages of the estrus cycle. The sow estrus cycle is divided in two main phases, follicular and luteal. These phases are further divided into four stages. The follicular phase is divided into proestrus and estrus, while the luteal phase is divided into metestrus and diestrus.

For our discussion, we will assume that the first day of estrus is day 0 of the cycle (Figure 3). The onset of estrus is mainly caused by an increase in estrogens. Sow estrus usually last 40–60 h (from day 0 to day 1–2 of the cycle) [6] but some sows can be on estrus for longer. Sow will only show sexual behaviors and accept the boar during the estrus stage of the cycle. During estrus, estrogen, Follicle stimulating hormone (FSH) and Luteinizing hormone (LH) secretion peaks. During estrus, ovulation is caused by the LH surge. Ovulation occurs 30–40 h after estrus onset [6].

Almost immediately after ovulation, sow will enter the luteal phase. During the metestrus stage of the luteal phase (days 2–5 of the cycle), the follicle tissue will start its development into a corpus luteum. This process is called luteinization [6]. The end of metestrus and the beginning of diestrus is marked by the end of the luteinization process. Diestrus is the longest stage of the estrus cycle. It starts once the corpus luteum is formed and last for 12–15 days after (days 6–17 of the cycle). The corpus luteum will secret progesterone to prepare the uterus for implantation and to maintain pregnancy in case of successful fertilization by the boar or artificial insemination. If the sow is not pregnant, the uterus will start secreting prostaglandin F2 alpha and luteolysis (degradation of the corpus luteus) will start after 15 days post ovulation (proestrus stage) [6]. Proestrus (day 17–21 of the cycle) is characterized by an increase in prostaglandin F2 alpha secretion and the completion of luteolysis. During this phase, progesterone secretion is reduced and estrogen, then LH, and FSH secretion increase. This increase will re-start estrus.

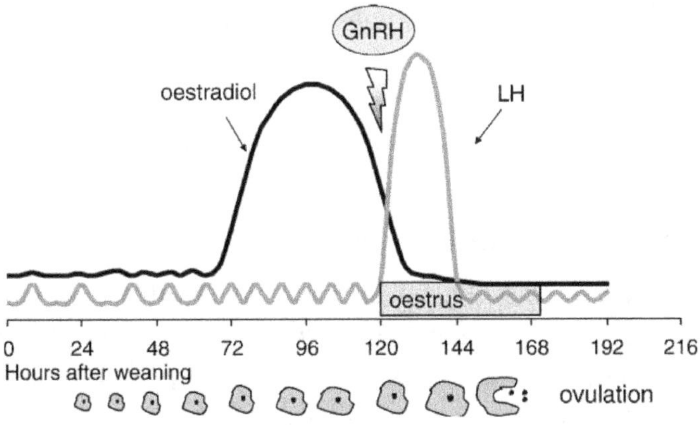

Figure 3. Schematic of the timing of ovulation with associated hormonal and behavioral changes. Weaning is at time zero. From Pedersen [8].

3.2 Anatomical changes (vulva size, color, and temperature)

The introduction of assisted reproductive techniques, such as Artificial Insemination, has shifted the responsibility of estrus detection to humans with the assistance of a live boar. The traditional way to identify if a sow has come into heat and is ready to be breed, is based on the occurrence of sexual behaviors before, during or after the backpressure test (BPT) and by detecting physical changes in sow vulva. Physical changes associated with the onset of estrus are reported to include vulva reddening, increase in vulvar temperature, the presence of sticky mucus, and an increase in vulva size often refer as swelling.

Langendijk et al. [6] found that out of 130 sows only 87% showed an increase in internal vulva redness. In this study, they also found a significant variation on the time vulva reddening occurred. Even when reddening onset varied between individual sows, it always occurred before ovulation. Thus, they suggest that insemination of sows that shows vulva reddening should be delayed until the end of vulva reddening.

The increase in vulva size and infrared temperature observed during estrus have been correlated to the high estrogen levels during estrus. The elevated levels of estrogen increase the vaginal and vulvar blood flow resulting in both an increase in vulva temperature as well as vulva swelling [9]. The literature is contradictory related to vulva features. Sykes et al. [9] and Scolari et al. [10] found that the infrared vulva temperature increased by 1 C° the day of estrus whereas Simoes et al. [11] found that the temperature increase was during the proestrus period.

Un-published studies recently conducted by the authors showed that not all sows will show these physical changes. We carefully measured color, size, surface temperature and vaginal temperature in sows before and during estrus (Table 2).

Sows might show these physical changes at a different stage of the estrus cycle. Because not all sows will show changes in vulva color, temperature, or size during estrus, the onset of these changes varied among individual animals. Vulva physical and thermal changes are not reliable indicators for heat checking for all sows of use on the farm.

3.3 Skeletal and smooth muscle contractions

Myometrial activity before and after estrus is either absent or of low amplitude and frequency [12, 13]. During estrus, sow myometrial electrical activity and contraction frequency and amplitude increase [12]. Myometrial contractions are regulated by progesterone, oxytocin, and estrogen concentrations [14]. High progesterone reduces uterine contractions whereas high oxytocin and estrogen levels increase them [14]. Oxytocin and estrogen secretion increase during estrus and sexual stimulation and arousal, although direct neuromuscular activation could be via the brain and spinal nerves. In vitro studies found that after an estrogen perfusion, there was a significant increase in peristalsis going from the isthmus uteri towards the corpus uteri [15]. Similar results were found with an oxytocin perfusion [15]. Uterine contractions are necessary for the movement of sperm from the uterus to the fallopian tubes. This could explain why seminal oxytocin and estrogen increase uterine contractions [12]. Boar presence induces sow oxytocin release and increases sow's myometrial activity [12]. The effects of each individual boar stimulus (olfactory, tactile, and visual) on oxytocin release are still not clear [12].

Some sows will also show skeletal muscle contraction that one would call shaking during the standing reflex. From our behavioral studies, we estimated that fewer than one in ten sows will show this behavior. Skeletal muscle movement can be easily perceived on sow shoulders, flank, neck and ears.

3.4 Gilt development

To continue the production cycle and swine sustainability, sows need to be replaced by gilts. Breeding farms should target to have an annual replacement rate lower than 50% [16]. In 2012, the average annual replacement rate was 45% [17]. This mean that around 900 gilts are needed per year to replace culled sows in a 2000 sow unit. Usually sows are culled due to low reproductive performance, lameness, or because they were not bred after weaning.

Table 2. Proportion of sows (N = 22) that showed vulva changes before, during, or after the first day of estrus.

Measurement	Day when the change was visible			
	Day before estrus	First day of estrus	Day after first day of estrus	No change
Vulva reddening	31.82%	18.18%	13.64%	36.36%
Vulva IR temperature	4.55%	59.09%	9.09%	27.27%
Vaginal temperature (C°)*	0.00%	15.38%	0.00%	84.61%
Vulva swelling	31.82%	13.64%	0.00%	54.55%
Presence of sticky mucus	40.91%	36.36%	22.73%	0.00%
The percentage figures refer to the % of sows that first show that feature on each day. *n = 13.				

Replacement gilts are selected based on their growth rate, body composition, and their mother's reproductive success [17]. In general, gilts selected as replacement are moved from the growing facility to the gilt development unit (GDU) within the breeding farm when they are around 150 days old. To accelerate the onset of puberty, gilts in the GDU are often exposed to live boars. Gilts can have direct contact with a boar or indirect contact through pen fencing. Usually, groups of vasectomized boars are introduced into gilt's home pen for at least 20 min per day.

Boar should not be housed in the GDU unit since gilts will be habituated the boar olfactory, visual, tactile, and auditory stimuli and this could decrease effective heat detection by farm workers [17].

When boars are introduced into the gilt pen, farm personnel will check gilts for estrus behavior and vulva changes described above. Daily boar exposure will induce estrus in most gilt within 10–20 days [17]. Gilts in heat are then moved to breeding stalls so they can habituate to the new environment and are breed in their second estrus. The term heat-no service (HNS) is commonly used to identify gilts that had their first estrus but were not breed. At the time of first service gilts should weight 135–150 kg and have a back fat of 12–18 mm [16, 17]. After 23 days of boar exposure, gilts that have shown no sign of estrus, can be hormonally treated to induce estrus by use of PG600. Gilts that did not come into heat after 28 days of boar exposure are usually culled from the breeding herd [16]. Gilts can be treated with Altrenogest to synchronize their estrus cycles.

4. SENSORY SYSTEM IMPACTS ON THE ESTRUS CYCLE: THE BOAR EFFECT

4.1 The boar effect

The effect of boar exposure on gilts and sow reproduction has been extensively study across the years. Direct contact with the boar significantly reduces puberty onset in gilts [18–22] and reduce sows weaning to estrus interval. The boar provides sows and gilts with olfactory, tactile, visual, and auditory stimuli that together create a maximum response. Below we discuss the effect of each individual boar stimuli on sow and gilt reproduction.

4.2 Visual, auditory and tactile systems

Pigs have well developed olfactory, tactile, auditory and visual systems. Most of the work on the pig focuses on the pig olfactory sense. Pigs have been used in biomedical research to study the auditory system. The auditory and somatosensory (touch) parts of the brain have been mapped in the pig [23]. The pig auditory system is understudied. In one paper where the auditory, visual and somatosensory regions were mapped in pig reared indoors or outdoors, the authors showed different neuron structures in the outdoor pig in both auditory, visual and somatosensory regions [24]. The auditory neocortex was especially different with diverse housing systems.

Surprisingly few recent studies have been done on the pig visual system. Dudley Klopfer was a psychologist at Washington State University in the 1950s to about 1980. He studied the pig visual system using operant conditioning methods. He found that pigs could see colors. His work was published in a detailed proceedings paper in 1966 [25]. Ewbank [26] and his group put black contact lenses on pigs which made them temporarily blind. Pigs that could not see, had normal fights and formed a dominance hierarchy. In the world, pig do not need their sight to function, even though their eyesight is about the same as humans.

What we can conclude from the limited work on pig senses is that their olfactory system is much more developed than humans (see below) and their auditory, visual and somatosensory systems are at least as developed as humans.

4.3 Olfactory systems

Meese and Baldwin [27] removed the olfactory bulbs in pigs and this did not change their establishment of a dominance order. When pairs of pigs were tested, they fought the same with or without their olfactory bulbs. However, when the group size increased to 3 or 4 pigs, the bulbectomized pigs were at a disadvantage. For reproduction, removal of the olfactory system had large negative effects on reproduction [28].

The boar olfactory stimulus has been widely studied of known mammalian pheromones. During the 1960s, androstenol (5alpha-Androst-16-en-3alpha-ol) and androstenone (5alpha-Androst-16-en-3-one), two steroids secreted by boars' submaxillary salivary glands, were thought to be the boar pheromone. Multiple studies have found that these two steroids have a major role on gilts puberty onset. For instance, puberty age was significantly greater for gilts with their olfactory system inhibited by chemical or mechanical means [29, 30] and for gilts exposed to a sialectomized boar [31]. It is thought that direct contact between boar and sow is necessary to transfer the boar pheromone from boar saliva to the female snout [30]. Although these two steroids are responsible for a significant part of the boar effect on puberty onset, when applied as an individual olfactory stimulus, they were not as effective as the boar [18, 21]. Thus, it was suggested that boar saliva must contain additional analytes that together with androstenol and androstenone are acting as a multicomponent primer pheromone or that other boar stimuli are necessary for the boar pheromone to have a full effect. Recently, it was found that, quinoline was another boar specific salivary molecule (Figure 4) [5, 32]. The mixture of androstenone, androstenol, and quinoline induced more sexual behaviors in weaned sows than the mixture of androstenone and androstenol [5]. This finding might explain the lack of response of sows and prepubertal gilts when exposed to androstenone and androstenol alone.

4.4 Early work on sow and boar preferences and sensory systems

Boars, being a non-discriminating breeder, will investigate sows independent if they are in estrus or not but sows will only be interested in a boar when they are in estrus. When sows are in Proestrus, they will seek a boar. This seeking behavior intensifies when sows are fully in estrus.

Early works showed that sows would only seek the boar when they are in estrus

[33] and that the boar could not detect a sow in estrus. This turned out to be only partially correct. Boars can learn the smell of an estrus sow. It was reported that the boar could not tell an estrus sow from a non-estrus sow [32, 34]. Some boars were found to be able to find an estrus sow while others could not [32, 34]. This could be a learned behavior, or some boars may have better olfactory acuity than other boars. This remains to be determined.

Signoret's classic early research [4] (Table 3) on boar induction of sow sexual behavior is often cited in textbooks and seminars. In his work, he found that the boar odor was the best single stimulus to induce sexual behaviors in estrus sows. He applied back pressure to estrus sows with no odor stimulation and found that 59% of the sows showed standing reflex. If farms found only 59% of the sows that are in heat, they would not be profitable. The goal is to find 100% of the sows in estrus.

With a live boar across a fence, Signoret found that 97% of the sows were detected in estrus. Further, he found that 81% of sows were detected in estrus when they were moved and heat checked in a pen containing the boar odor. This is better than 59%, but not as good as the live boar. Later, when Androstenone was used, Melrose [35] found 78% of the sows in heat—similar to Signoret's finding with the boar odor. Scientists and producers thought at that time that Androstenone was the boar pheromone. However, why would the fence line contact be better than the odor of the boar or Androstenone alone? This is because more than Androstenone (e.g., other molecules) is needed to induce sexual behavior in the sow (see details below).

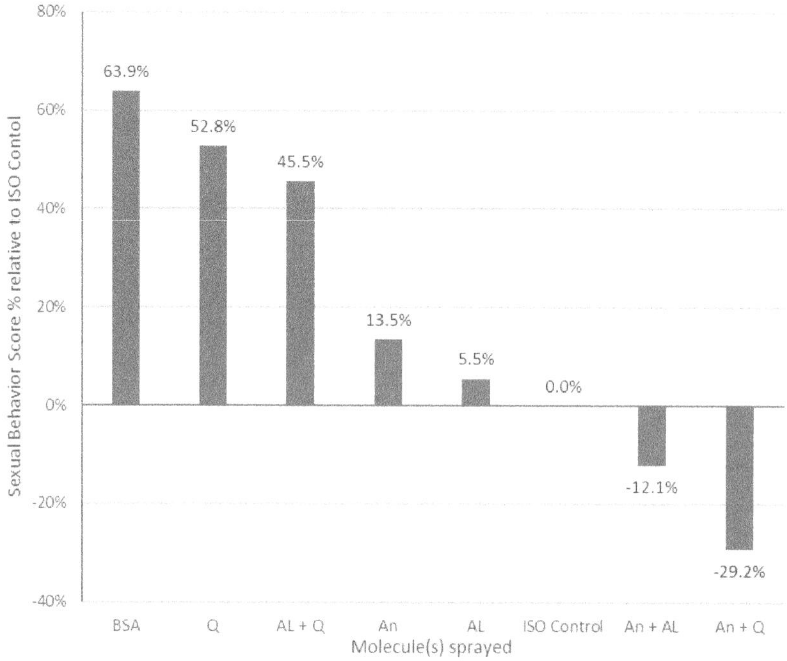

Figure 4. Sow sexual behavioral response to Androstenone (An), Androstenol (AL) and Quinoline (Q) alone or in combination. Note that androstenone increased estrus sow sexual behavior by 13.5% while all three molecules increased sow sexual behavior by over 63%. The N for this study was 947 sows [5].

Table 3. Early research on sensory system impacts on sows showing estrus.

Source	Odor source	Sows showing estrus
Signoret, 1975 [4]	No boar odor	59%
	Boar odor in pen	81%
	Fence-line contact with live boar	97%
Melrose [35]	Androstenone	78%*
Note that Androstenone (*) was not as effective as fence-line contact with a boar.		

5. THE PIG OLFACTORY SYSTEM

The pig is a species with one of the highest numbers of functional olfactory genes [36]. To understand pig pheromone biology, one must understand the different olfactory organs of the pig. Only two of the five olfactory organs described in mammals have been described in the pig. Figure 5. Shows the five olfactory organs described in rats. Of these five organs, only the main olfactory epithelium (MOE) and the vomeronasal organ (VNO) have been described in the pig (Figure 6). The Grueneberg ganglion (GG) is the sensory organ that senses alarm pheromones in mice. Scientist believe that pigs may also have alarm pheromones [39], but they have not been isolated, nor has the GG been found in the pig. Little is known about the septal organ (SO) or the chemical sensory cells of the Trigeminal Nerve in the pig (or in other species). We do believe that the MOE receives molecules in an aerosol, while the VNO receives molecules in liquid form. The GG and SO may also need an aerosol because they are in the nasal airway where aerosols pass as the animal breathers or sniffs.

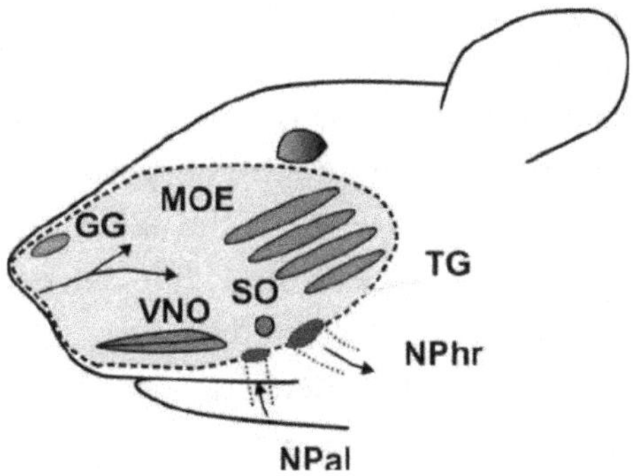

Figure 5. Chemosensory epithelia in the rat nose. GG, Grueneberg ganglion; MOE, main olfactory epithelium; SO, septal organ of Masera; TG, trigeminal system/ nerve; NPal, nasopalatine duct; NPhyr, nasopharyngeal duct. Arrows represent the direction of air flow. From Dauner et al. [37].

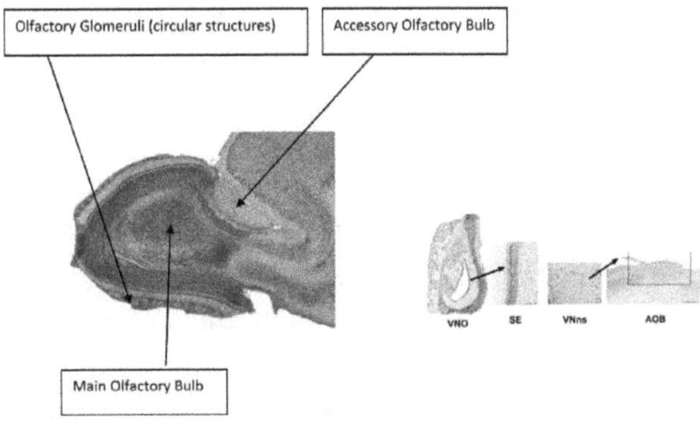

Figure 6. Ignacio Salazar pictures of the pig VNO (right) and the main olfactory bulb (left) with the AOB shown. VNO pictures are from Salazar et al. [38]; olfactory bulb histology is from Salazar, personal communication.

In addition to the olfactory organs, the nasal mucosa contains several olfactory binding proteins (OBPs). Patricia Nagnan-Le Meillour [40] has done the most recent work in pig's OBPs. When the nasal epithelium receives a chemical signal, that signal can bind an olfactory receptor directly, or more commonly for bioactive chemicals, it binds an OBP and it is the OBP odorant complex that activates the olfactory receptors. It is likely that, before pheromone exposure, a small amount of OBPs are present in the olfactory epithelium mucosa.

Pheromone exposure increases OBPs synthesis. Thus, we speculate that a second pheromone exposure 30–60 min after the first exposure could have a large effect on olfactory perception because more OBPs will be present to carry the odorants to the olfactory receptors. However, this still needs to be experimentally demonstrated.

In Figure 6, we show excellent anatomical histological pictures of the pig MOE and the VNO by Salazar [38] (personal communication). He and his laboratory they showed that the MOE and VNO are fully present at birth in piglets.

The VNO is thought to be the olfactory organ in which pheromones are perceived. But we know now that this is not always the case. One of the boar sexual pheromone molecules is sensed by the MOE [41]. The other three molecules may be sensed by the VNO or the MOE or any of the other olfactory organs not yet described in the pig. Our behavioral observations of the sow when she experiences a liquid containing a pheromone show that they chomp (see Table 1). We believe this behavior is analog to the flehmen behavior in other animals and that, by doing this, sows expose the VNO as well as the MOE to the pheromone.

The VNO receives chemical signals from liquids. Some mammals (except humans and some primates) show flehmen (lip curl) behavior when they are drawing liquid chemical signals into the VNO. An example is when the bull licks cow urine and draws it into the VNO. It is likely that more than one olfactory organ is needed to sense complex pheromones that are mixtures of molecules (like the boar pheromone). The pig is not well-known to show Flehman, but they may Flehman when they receive a chemical signal in liquid form.

6. PHEROMONE CONCEPTS

The field of sexual behavior and pheromonal modulation of sexual behaviors have unique terminology. Table 4 provides definitions of key terms used in pheromone biology in its widest sense. This may help the reader navigate this area. The broadest term is Semiochemical in which all chemical communication falls. Sexual pheromones are species specific (the cattle sex pheromone is different than the pig sex pheromone). Certainly, the pig uses chemical communication within and between species, for example, when a pig finds a buried truffle or when a plant drives away insects—these between-species forms of chemical communication are not discussed here. We are mostly concerned with the species-specific boar pheromone that stimulates sow reproductive behavior and performance.

The pheromone concept was first described in insects by Karlson and Luscher in 1959 [42] and at the time, they were primarily referring to insect pheromones. Certainly, semiochemicals are found in most plants and animals. Pheromones were previously referred to as ectohormones. This means a hormone that works outside the animal. But pheromones do not meet the definition of a hormone, although the definitions are similar. Karlson and Luscher [42] used the term pheromone to describe a species-specific molecule that is secreted or excreted from one animal that changes the physiology or behavior of another animal of the same species. The concept was adopted rapidly among invertebrate and vertebrate animal scientists.

Table 4. Definitions of common words in mammalian olfactory communication.

Word	Definition
Pheromone	Substances that are excreted to the outside by an individual and received by a second individual of the same species, in which they release a specific reaction, for example, a definite behavior or a developmental process [42] A chemical substance that is usually produced by an animal and serves especially as a stimulus to other individuals of the same species for one or more behavioral responses [43] A pheromone is an externally secreted signal that sends meaningful information to members of the same species [44]
Kairomone	A chemical substance emitted by one species and especially an insect or plant that has an adaptive benefit (such as a stimulus for oviposition) to another species [45] Kairomones are ligands emitted from one species that generate behavior in another species (such as aversion upon detection by a prey species) [45]
Allomone	A chemical substance secreted externally by certain animals affecting the behavior or physiology of another species detrimentally [46] A chemical that is released by one species that influences the behavior or physiology of a different species. The organism releasing the substance usually benefits. Allomones are a type of semiochemical used in warning [47]
Synomone	An interspecific semiochemical that is beneficial to both interacting organisms [48]
Interomone	An interomone is defined as a semiochemical that acts as pheromone of one species but elicits physiological responses in a different species where the pheromone molecules have not yet been identified [49]
Semiochemical	A chemical substance or mixture released by an organism that affects the behaviors of other individuals (could be between or within species) [50]

Most of the work on mammalian pheromones has been done with rodents. The pig has a highly developed olfactory system (see above), but little work has been done recently on pig pheromones including sexual pheromones. We can learn from work on other species so that we can predict possible pheromones and pheromone effects in the highly-olfactory domestic pig.

An early concept was the bifurcation between priming and releasing pheromones. This dichotomy will be familiar to people who work in pig breeding with gilts and sows. The gilt develops from pre-puberty to post-puberty at around 120– 200 days of age. A pheromone that stimulates the onset of puberty, for example, would be a priming pheromone. Boars certainly cause gilts to have an earlier onset of puberty (see Boar effect above). The molecule(s) that are responsible for priming gilts have not been described, but are likely to be the same as the boar pheromone. Most people might believe at this time that the boar sexual pheromone that causes sexual behavior and stimulates gilt puberty are likely to be the same molecules.

A releasing pheromone is one or more molecules that cause a rapid onset of behavior; sexual behavior in this case. Another releasing pheromone might be one that causes pigs to eat, or piglets to nurse, or pigs to fight, or pigs to stop fighting [39, 51]. None of these releasing pheromone molecule(s), other than the boar pheromone have been described.

What can we learn from other mammalian sexual pheromones? Given that the pig has so many functional receptors, it is likely that if a type of pheromone was described in another mammal that the pig would have a pheromone with a similar effect. Here we summarize the classic reproductive pheromones. Note that each early reproductive pheromone was named after the scientist who first reported the effect.

6.1 The Bruce effect

Hilda Bruce described what has been called the Bruce effect in 1959 [52]—before the concept of pheromone was established. She showed that when a pregnant mouse was exposed to an adult male, preferably a dominant male, that the pregnant mouse lost her pregnancy. The Bruce effect has been replicated by many investigators and what we know is that each male has a specific major histocompability complex (MHC) class 1 protein that is secreted in its urine. The father of the mouse litter has a given MHC protein. If a new male enters the cage with a different MHC protein, the female is likely to lose her pregnancy (not 100% of the time, but at a significant rate). The male MHC protein binds the VNO in the female mice. It makes one wonder if heat checking with a boar during pregnancy might contribute to a lower farrowing rate.

The Bruce effect has not been clearly documented in the pig. Assuming the Bruce effect is found in pigs, one would change the management of the sow herd. On most farms, pregnant sows experience a live, often dominant, boar walking the aisle to see if any bred sows are now in heat (meaning their pregnancy has failed). That live boar would not have the same MHC as the father of the litter because they are commonly bred by artificial insemination. We know that a small (5–10%) percentage of sows lose their pregnancy from breeding until farrowing. Part of this effect could be due to the Bruce effect. To manage this situation, pregnant sows should never experience a live boar that is not the father of her litter or perhaps is not the boar present during breeding. Keeping in mind that the Bruce effect is mediated by MHC proteins and not the boar pheromone, one can use the boar pheromone to check for return to estrus in pregnant sows without inducing the Bruce effect.

6.2 The Vandenbergh effect

John Vandenbergh first described this pheromone in a paper published in 1975 [53]. He showed that female mice have an accelerated onset of puberty when exposed to an adult male mouse or urine from an adult male mouse. The molecule was thought to be a protein, but the actual molecule had not been described.

Pigs clearly show the Vandenberg effect. Gilts will have a delayed onset of puberty if they do not experience an adult boar. With boar exposure, the onset of puberty is accelerated in gilts [54]. The pheromone molecule(s) that are responsible have not been described. One might predict that the boar pheromone that stimulates sow reproductive behavior and performance [5], is the same pheromone that stimulates the accelerated onset of puberty in gilts. However, if these boar pheromone molecules are responsible for the Vandenberg effect in gilts, then the dose and number of applications required to cause the Effect have not yet been determined.

6.3 The Whitten effect

Whitten described the Whitten Effect in a number of papers from 1956, 1957 and 1966 and 1968 [55–58]. The Whitten Effect states that in a group of postpubertal females, the presence of either other cycling adult males will cause the females to synchronize their estrus (or menstrual) cycles. Likewise, adult females tend to synchronize their cycles over time when they are housed together. The Whitten Effect has no valuable application in modern pork production at this time that we can think of; however, production systems change over time and there could be an application in the future. The Whitten Effect takes weeks or months to have its effect. Therefore, we do believe that when gilts approaching puberty are exposed to a boar, that the number or percentage that come into estrus is not evenly distributed over the 21-day cycle, so this may be happening. Boar exposure may partially synchronize a group of gilts first estrus.

7. BENEFITS TO NOT USING A LIVE BOAR

7.1 General benefits

Boars are found on most modern pig farms. They are needed to find sows in estrus when AI is used. Below are reasons to not have boars on the farm. The reasons include cost, safety and disease control.

The boar costs money to buy and they cost money to maintain. Besides the direct cost of the boar, the boar does not live a good life. They are heat checking sows often and rarely if ever breed. They are often housed in a crate or stall individually for their own safety and the safety of other sows and boars.

Boars are dangerous to have on farms. One large farm in the USA reported that they budget $500,000 per year for boar-induced human injuries. The boar can take a single swipe at a person and damage the person severely. If a boar was very aggressive, they could do great damage to a person. While rare, boars sometimes step on people, or bite people or knock them down if a person stands in the way of the boar and his intended direction.

Boars carry disease. While sows move from breeding to gestation to farrowing and back to breeding, the boar resides in the barn for a long time (a year or more). The boar can be a reservoir of disease and continually infect new breeding sows.

When a serious disease (foot and mouth, ASF, etc.) is found in a country, they often limit movement of adults in some or all regions. If the farm cannot get live adult boars, and have no access to pheromones, the breeding rates will be very low.

7.2 Pheromone applications in the field

7.2.1 Sows

Melrose [35] first suggested Androstenone was the boar pheromone. But we and others have observed that this single molecule was not sufficient to elicit the full sexual behavioral response in estrus sows. This led to the project to seek and discover the complete boar pheromone. This was accomplished by using advanced GC-MS technology to identify three unique molecules that are found in boar saliva and not found in sow saliva [59]. If one examines Figure 4, is clear that androstenone alone has only a small effect on sows expressing estrus when they are in fact in heat. But the three molecules together give the largest increase in sow sexual behavior. Furthermore, data we collected recently showed that most sows identified in estrus by a boar, also express estrus behavior to the three-molecule pheromone called BOARBETTER® (BB).

Table 5. Results from McGlone et al. showing that BOARBETTER® caused an increase in pigs born and born alive in parities 1–3 on 12 farms.

Parities	Total born/litter	Born alive/litter
1–3	0.88*	0.73*
4–6	−0.10	−0.23
Overall	0.40*	0.22*
Difference in measures. LSMEANS within a row that differ (P < 0.01) have an *.		

Boar Better (BB) was formulated to include all three molecules in an analog to the natural pheromone. When BB was applied to 12 USA farms in different USA states on nearly 4000 sows, it was discovered that BB increased Farrowing Rate, and litter size born (total or alive). Together, the increase per batch of pigs was significant—over 8% more pigs born per batch. The effect on early parities (1–3) was greater than for older sows that may have maximized their uterine capacity (Table 5). Note that while the overall increase in total pig born per litter was 0.40 more pigs with BB, in parities 1–3, the increase was 0.88 pigs/litter due to BB. This is a remarkable improvement in reproduction that cannot be achieved by any common animal health product on the market.

7.2.2 Gilts

While we believe and hope that BB is also the priming pheromone that accelerated gilt puberty, we do not have solid data to show that this is the case. These studies are underway now. We know cycling gilts can be bred with BB because it is a powerful releasing pheromone. Still, because the live boar can stimulate the onset of puberty, it is likely that BB is also the priming pheromone.

8. FUTURE RESEARCH NEEDS ON FARMS

This area of research is ripe for new discoveries. We know that the pig has a highly developed sense of smell. And we know that pheromones are a major player in the modulation of sexual and other behaviors. The sow releasing pheromone has been discovered and it contains three boar-unique molecules. The primer pheromone that brings gilts into heat has not been identified. It seems likely that the priming pheromone is the same set of molecules that comprise the releasing pheromone. But this must be confirmed through experimentation and practical applications.

We also demonstrate that the novel boar pheromone that was recently discovered induces both sexual behavior in estrus sows and it increases the change of reproductive success in sows. This pheromone is the only known molecule to cause the full effect in behavior and reproduction.

We do not know anything about three olfactory organs that are described in mice, but not yet described in the pig (SO, GG, Trigeminal nerve). Locating these in the pig and documenting how they modulate behavior will be important in the future.

9. CONCISE SUMMARY

This chapter aims to provide the reader with an overview of boar and sow reproduction, olfaction, and pheromones. A comprehensive study of porcine biology is beneficial for those seeking to explore this subject further.

Commercial farm reproductive success metrics indicate that swine reproduction can be enhanced with the use of a synthetic analog of the natural boar pheromone. Breeding rates are likely to improve with a comprehensive understanding of the sow's behavior before, during, and after her estrous cycle, both in housing facilities and free-ranging herds. Additionally, the various stages of estrus must be accurately identified to assess the indicators of a sow in estrus. The animal's anatomy is crucial for pheromones to trigger her "standing reflex" via several olfactory organs, which ascertain her estrus status. The essential aspect is to observe the observable signals indicating that the sow may be in estrus; unreliable markers include perked ears, low, deep grunts, and variations in vulva temperature and color. The primary indicator of estrus in sows is the manifestation of the standing reflex or locked-up behavior. The single behavior that signifies estrus in all sows, excluding those in anestrus, is locking up. Ultimately, the capacity to accurately identify sows in estrus, with or without the presence of a boar, will conserve time, labor, and financial resources. Utilizing the substance BB, which comprises three molecules: Androstenone, Androstanol, and Quinoline, stockpeople may enhance reproductive performance.

REFERENCES

1. Erickson A. China races to corral an outbreak of deadly African swine fever [Internet]. 2019. Available from: https://www.washingtonpost. com/world/ china-races-to-corral-adeadly-outbreak-of-african-swinefever-before-it-spreads/2018/08/29/ defbf39a-aad9-11e8-b1da-ff7faa680710_ story.html [Accessed: 12 November 2019]

2. McGlone J. Gestation stall design and space: Care of pregnant sows in individual gestation housing [Internet]. 2013. Available from: https://porkcdn. s3.amazonaws.com/sites/all/files/doc uments/2013SowHousingWebinars/ Gesatation%20Stall%20Design%20 and%20Space.pdf [Accessed: 12 November 2019]

3. Altmann M. Interrelations of the sex cycle and the behavior of the sow. Journal of Comparative Psychology. 1941;313:481-498

4. Signoret PJ, Balwin BA, Fraser D, ESE H. The behavior of swine. In: ESE H, editor. The Behaviour of Domestic Animals. 1st–3rd ed. Bailliere-Tindale; 1975. pp. 295-329

5. McGlone JJ, Devoraj S, Garcia A. A novel boar mixture induces sow estrus behaviors and reproductive success. Applied Animal Behavior Science. 2019;219:104832. DOI: 10.1016/j. applanim.2019.104832
6. Soede N, Langendijk P, Kemp B. Reproductive cycles in pigs. Animal Reproduction Science. 2011;124:251-258. DOI: 10.1016/j.anireprosci.2011.02.025
7. De Rensis F, Cosgrove J, Foxcroft G. Luteinizing hormone and prolactin responses to naloxone vary with stage of lactation in the sow. Biology of Reproduction. 1993;48(5):970-976. DOI: 10.1095/biolreprod48.5.970
8. Pedersen LJ. Sexual behavior in female pigs. Hormones and Behavior. 2007;52:64-69. DOI: 10.1016/j. yhbeh.2007.03.019
9. Sykes DJ, Couvillion JS, Cromiak A, Bowers S, Schenck E, Crenshaw M, et al. The use of digital infrared thermal imaging to detect estrus in gilts. Theriogenology. 2012;78(1):147-152. DOI: 10.1016/j.theriogenology.2012.01.030
10. Scolari SC, Clark SG, Knox RV, Tamassia MA. Vulvar skin temperature changes significantly during estrus in swine as determined by digital infrared thermography. Journal of Swine Health and Production. 2011;19(3):151-155
11. Simoes VG, Lyazrhi F, Picard- Hagen N, Gayrard V, Martineau G, Waret-Szkuta A. Variations in the vulvar temperature of sows during proestrus and estrus as determined by infrared thermography and its relation to ovulation. Theriogenology. 2014;82(8):1080-1085. DOI: 10.1016/j. theriogenology.2014.07.017
12. Langendijk P, Soede N, Kemp B. Uterine activity, sperm transport, and the role of boar stimuli around insemination in sows. Theriogenology. 2005;63(2):500-513. DOI: 10.1016/j. theriogenology.2004.09.027
13. Langendijk P, Bouwman EG, Soede NM, Taverne MAM, Kemp B. Myometrial activity around estrus in sows: spontaneous activity and effects of estrogens, cloprostenol, seminal plasma and clenbuterol. Theriogenology. 2002;57(5):1563-1577. DOI: 10.1016/S0093-691X(02)00657-X
14. Domino M, Pawlinski B, Gajewska M, Jasinski T, Sady M, Gajewski Z. Uterine EMG activity in the non-pregnant sow during estrous cycle. BMC Veterinary Research. 2018;14(1):176
15. Mueller A, Maltaris T, Siemer J, Binder H, Hoffmann I, Beckmann M, et al. Uterine contractility in response to different prostaglandins: results from extracorporeally perfused non-pregnant swine uteri. Human Reproduction. 2006;21(8):2000-2005. DOI: 10.1093/humrep/del118
16. Williams NH, Patterson J, Foxcroft G. Non-negotiables of gilt development. Advances in Pork Production. 2005;16:281-289

17. Kraeling RR, Webel SK. Current strategies for reproductive management of gilts and sows in North America. Journal of Animal Science and Biotechnology. 2015;6(1):3

18. Booth W. A note on the significance of boar salivary pheromones to the male-effect on puberty attainment in gilts. Animal Science. 1984;39(1):149- 152. DOI: 10.1017/S0003356100027744

19. Deligeorgis SG, Lunney DC, English PR. A note on efficacy of complete v. partial boar exposure on puberty attainment in the gilt. Animal Science. 1984;39(1):145-147. DOI: 10.1017/S0003356100027732

20. Karlbom I. Attainment of puberty in female pigs: Influence of boar stimulation. Animal Reproduction Science. 1982;4(4):313-319. DOI: 10.1016/0378-4320(82)90045-8

21. Pearce GP, Hughes PE. The influence of daily movement of gilts and the environment in which boar exposure occurs on the efficacy of boar-induced precocious puberty in the gilt. Animal Science. 1985;40(1):161-167. DOI: 10.1017/S0003356100031962

22. Pearce GP, Hughes PE. The influence of boar-component stimuli on puberty attainment in the gilt. Animal Science. 1987;44(2):293-302. DOI: 10.1017/S0003356100018663

23. Andrews RJ, Knight RT, Kirby RP. Evoked potential mapping of auditory and somatosensory cortices in the miniature swine. Neuroscience Letters. 1990;114(1):27-31. DOI: 10.1016/0304-3940(90)90423-7

24. Jarvinen MK, Morrow-Tesch J, McGlone JJ, Powley TL. Effects of diverse developmental environments on neuronal morphology in domestic pigs (Sus scrofa). Developmental Brain Research. 1998;107(1):21-31. DOI: 10.1016/S0165-3806(97)00210-1

25. Klopfer FD. Visual learning in swine. In: Bustad LK, editor. Proceedings of Swine in Biomedical Research. Oxfordshire, UK: Oxford University Press; 1966

26. Ewbank R, Meese GB, Cox JE. Individual recognition and the dominance hierarchy in the domestic pig. The role of sight. Animal Behavior. 1974;22:473-474. DOI: 10.1016/ S0003-3472(74)80046-1

27. Meese GB, Baldwin BA. The effects of ablation of the olfactory bulbs on aggressive behaviour in pigs. Applied Animal Ethology. 1975;1:251-262. DOI: 10.1016/0304-3762(75)90018-8

28. Booth WD, Baldwin BA. Changes in oestrus cyclicity following olfactory bublectomy in post-pubertal pigs. Reproduction. 1983;67:143-150. DOI: 10.1530/jrf.0.0670143

29. Kirkwood RN, Forbes JN, Hughes PE. Influence of boar contact on attainment of puberty in gilts after removal of the olfactory bulbs. Reproduction. 1981;61(1):193-196. DOI: 10.1530/jrf.0.0610193

30. Pearce GP, Paterson AM. Physical contact with the boar is required for maximum stimulation of puberty in the gilt because it allows transfer of boar pheromones and not because it induces cortisol release. Animal Reproduction Science. 1992;27(2-3):209-224 10.1016/0378-4320(92)90059-M

31. Pearce GP, Hughes PE, Booth WD. The involvement of boar submaxillary salivary gland secretions in boar- induced precocious puberty attainment in the gilt. Animal Reproduction Science. 1988;16(2):125-134. DOI: 10.1016/0378-4320(88)90032-2

32. May M. Use of solid-phase microextraction to detect semiochemicals in synthetic and biological samples [thesis]. Lubbock: Texas Tech University; 2016

33. Belstra B, Flowers B, See MT, Singleton W. Detection of estrus or heat [Internet]. 2001. Available from: http://porkgateway.org/wp-content/ uploads/2015/07/estrus-or-heat- detection1.pdf [Accessed: 12 November 2019]

34. Baum M, Larriva-Sahd JA. Interactions between the mammalian main and accessory olfactory systems. Frontiers in Neuroanatomy. 2014;8:45. DOI: 10.3389/fnana.2014.00045

35. Melrose DR, Reed HCB, Patterson RLS. Androgen steroids associated with boar odour as an aid to the detection of oestrus in pig artificial insemination. British Veterinary Journal. 1971;127(10):497-502. DOI: 10.1016/ S0007-1935(17)37337-2

36. Brunjes PC, Feldman S, Osterberg SK. The pig olfactory brain: A primer. Chemical Senses. 2016;41(5):415-425. DOI: 10.1093/chemse/bjw016

37. Dauner K, Libmann J, Jerdi S, Frings S, Mohrlen F. Expression patterns of anoctamin 1 and anoctamin 2 chlorine channels in the mammalian nose. Cell and Tissue Research. 2012;347:327-341. DOI: 10.1007/ s00441-012-1324-9

38. Salazar I, Sánchez-Quinteiro P, Lombardero M, Aleman N, de Troconiz PF. The prenatal maturity of the accessory olfactory bulb in pigs. Chemical Senses. 2004;29:3-11. DOI: 10.1093/chemse/bjh001

39. McGlone JJ. Olfactory cues and pig agonistic behavior: Evidence for a submissive pheromone. Physiology and Behavior. 1985;34:195-198. DOI: 10.1016/0031-9384(85)90105-2

40. Meillour NL, Vercoutter-Edouart AS, Hilliou F, Le Danvic C, Levy F. Proteomic analysis of pig (Sus scrofa) olfactory soluble proteome reveals O-linked-N-acetylglucosaminylation of secreted odorant-binding proteins. Frontiers in Endcrinology. 2014;5:202. DOI: 10.3389/fendo.2014.00202

41. Brennan P. Pheromones and mammalian behavior. In: Menini A, editor. The Neurobiology of Olfaction. Florida: CRC Press; 2009. pp. 167-175

42. Karlson M, Luscher M. 'Pheromones': A new term for a class of biologically active substances. Nature. 1959;183:55-56. DOI: 10.1038/183055a0

43. Pheromone; Merriam-Webster dictionary [Internet]. 2019. Available from: https://www.merriam-webster. com/dictionary/pheromone [Accessed: 18 November 2019]

44. Mills DS, Marchant-Forde JN, McGreevy PD. Encyclopedia of Applied Animal Behaviour and Welfare. Wallington Oxfordshire, Eng: CABI; 2010. DOI: 9780851997247

45. Kairomone. Merriam-Webster dictionary [Internet]. 1970. Available from: https://www.merriam-webster. com/dictionary/kairomone [Accessed: 18 November 2019]

46. Allomone definition and meaning. Collins English Dictionary [Internet]. 2019. Available from: https://www.collinsdictionary.com/us/ dictionary/english/ allomone [Accessed: 19 November 2019]

47. Capinera J. Encyclopedia of Entomology. Berlin: Springer; 2008

48. Attractant [Internet]. 2019. Available from: https://en.wikipedia. org/wiki/ Attractant#Synomone [Accessed: 18 November 2019]

49. McGlone JJ, Thompson WG, Guay KA. Case study: The pig pheromone androstenone, acting as an interomone, stops dogs from barking. The Professional Animal Scientist. 2014;30:105-108. DOI: 10.15232/ S1080-7446(15)30091-7

50. Semiochemical [Internet]. 2019. Available from: https://en.wikipedia. org/ wiki/Semiochemical [Accessed: 18 November 2019]

51. McGlone JJ, Curtis SE, Banks EM. Evidence for aggression-modulating pheromones in prepuberal pigs. Behavioral and Neural Biology. 1987;47:27-39. DOI: 10.1016/ s0163-1047(87)90134-8

52. Gangrade BK, Dominic CJ. Studies of the male-originating pheromones involved in the Whitten effect and Bruce effect in mice. Biology of Reproduction. 1984;31(1):89-96. DOI: 10.1095/ biolreprod31.1.89

53. Vandenbergh JG, Whitsett JM, Lombardi JR. Partial isolation of a pheromone accelerating puberty in female mice. Reproduction. 1975;43(3):515-523. DOI: 10.1530/ jrf.0.0430515

54. Kirkwood RN, Hughes PE, Booth WD. The influence of boar- related odours on puberty attainment in gilts. Animal Science. 1983;36(1):131- 136. DOI: 10.1017/ S0003356100040022

55. Whitten WK. Modification of the oestrous cycle of the mouse by external stimuli associated with the male. Journal of Endocrinology. 1956;13(4):399-404. DOI: 10.1677/joe.0.0170307

56. Whitten WK. Effect of exteroceptive factors on the oestrous cycle of mice. Nature. 1957;180(4599):1436. DOI: 10.1038/1801436a0

57. Whitten WK. Pheromones and mammalian reproduction. Advanced Reproductive Physiology. 1966;1:155-177

58. Whitten WK, Bronson FH, Greenstein JA. Estrus-inducing pheromone of male mice: Transport by movement of air. Science. 1968;161(3841):584. DOI: 10.1126/ science.161.3841.584

59. McGlone JJ. Pheromone Composition to Stimulate Reproduction in Female Suids and Methods of Use. US Patent 9480689B1

3 Chapter CHALLENGING PROCESS OF PARTURITION IN DOMESTIC SWINE

1. INTRODUCTION: AN OVERVIEW

In the pig, just as in other mammalian species, the process of parturition includes three phase: opening of the cervix (I), expulsion of the fetuses (II) and expulsion of the placentae (III). In the 1990's, the average duration of farrowing was 1.5.-2 hours [1]. Since 1990, there has been a linear increase in both 1) litter size from about 10 piglets in 1990 to close to 20 piglets in 2019 and 2) duration of farrowing from 1.5–2 hours to 7–8 hours (a conclusion based on 20 studies on duration of farrowing, Figure 1, [2]). While the described tendency is subject to differences between breeds and management (i.e. farrowing crate vs. free farrowing), the overall tendency is rather convincing. The extended duration of farrowing appears an outcome of intensive breeding for prolificacy in the pig [2].

The increasing litter size presents with an immunological challenge for the sow and especially the piglets [2, 3]. The last 20–30% of the fetuses to be born likely miss out on access to good quality colostrum that declines by 50% already by the 6th hour after the birth of the first piglet [4]. On the other hand, they also have less time to suckle colostrum due to decreased window of opportunity for colostrum intake, increased competition for teats and reduced birth weight. This all may show up later in emergence of diseases in the growing phase of piglets/fattening pigs.

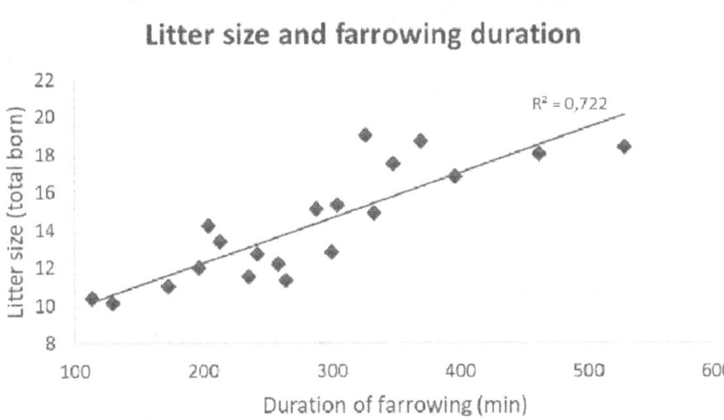

Figure 1. Relationship between litter size and the duration of farrowing in 20 studies from 1992 to 2018 (adapted from Oliviero et al. 2019, reproduction in domestic animals, Wiley-Blackwell).

The metabolic challenge related to hyper-prolific sow production model begins in the growing phase of gilts and goes beyond farrowing and lactation. The sow is supposed to eat enough to meet the requirement of growing litters prior to farrowing, which may cause some of the problems seen at around farrowing [5, 6]. In the early part of lactation, sows with large litters loose more energy while producing milk than what they can consume in their feed, ending up in a negative energy balance (NEB) [7, 8].

The growing litter size and intensity of production as such appear as items for welfare concern for the public. This seems to happen regardless of whether those concerns would be warranted or not. However, this review will tackle those items relating to welfare of the hyper-prolific sow model that we know, based on scientific literature, as having reasons to be addressed.

2. PHYSIOLOGY OF PARTURITION: LOW STATE SYSTEMIC INFLAMMATION INVOLVED (PDS)

Nest building and the phases of farrowing are orchestrated by responding changes in reproductive hormones. It is well established that decline in progesterone and peak in prostaglandin F2alpha triggers nest building behavior while oxytocin rise at the beginning of expulsion phase marks the session of nest building [9].

Prostaglandin F2alpha peak also induces CL regression with a concomitant decline in progesterone, making uterine contractions and parturition possible. Oxytocin is mainly in charge of uterine contractions during the expulsion phase of parturition and letdown of colostrum and milk, while prolactin will promote mammary gland development to the extent that initiation of milk production after parturition will become possible [10–12].

It has also been described in the literature and also shown by our group that allowing the sow to build up a nest prior to farrowing will increase oxytocin release and shorten the duration of farrowing [5, 13]. Other ways of shortening the duration of farrowing include increasing fiber in the feedstuff and encouraging water intake [5, 14]. However, even applying most good management interventions prior to farrowing, duration of farrowing of modern hyperprolific sows is extended four to five hold as described [2, 15, 16]. Prolonged duration of farrowing will mean reduced quality and quantity of colostrum intake by piglets, increased degree of intrapartum hypoxia of fetuses [17], increased rate of retained placentae [18], increased rate of uterine inflammation and post partum dysglactia (PDS) [19] and likely, reduced development of next generation of follicles fertility [3, 17].

Moreover, during the periparturient period, biological mechanisms coordinate the mobilization of body reserves in order to support fetal growth and milk production; insulin concentrations are reduced and the response of hormone-sensitive lipase in adipose tissue (e.g., low insulin, high growth hormone and catecholamines, or high glucocorticoid concentrations) is greater to facilitate lipid mobilization.

This periparturient period is also characterized by a low state of inflammation encompassing an increase in hepatic production of positive acute-phase proteins (APP), and a decrease in the production of negative APP [15, 20]. It has been rather well described in the literature that these responses are mediated by the pro-inflammatory cytokines interleukin (IL)-6, IL-1β, and tumor necrosis factor-α (TNF-α) [15]. Additionally, evidence in the dairy cow indicates that oxidative stress also occurs during this period and is driven by the imbalance between the production of reactive oxygen metabolites (ROM), reactive nitrogen species (RNS), and the neutralizing capacity of antioxidant mechanisms in tissues and blood [21]. The extent and duration of the inflammatory process will determine whether or not the condition is ending up as a clinical disease. However, it is noteworthy, that in the hyper prolific sows lines as those typical of Denmark and Belgium, the incidence of sows contracting a systemic disease postpartum is as high as >30% [15, 22, 23]. Moreover, it is obvious that even in those sows staying healthy as far as clinical symptoms, the inflammatory process is heavily present as indicated by means of those markers described above [15].

Typically, within two to three days post partum, the process of inflammation may develop into endotoxemia, which involves the release of the inflammation markers described. Endotoxemia is associated with clinical symptoms indicating a systemic response to infectious agents such as coliform bacteria – and PDS [24–26]. The condition comes with acute general symptoms such as inappetite, lethargy and fever [25], followed by local symptoms that usually affect either the uterus [19] or the udder [27] or both of them.

After parturition, concomitant with the process of inflammation, the sow undergoes metabolic stress due to loss of body reserves in favor of milk produced for large litters. This change rate is highest during the first 10 days of lactation. One of major mediators of metabolic stress is IGF-1, which is also seen as an indicator for fertility. Low IGF-1 levels indicate inflammation, metabolic stress present and fertility. IGF-1 is also regarded as one of the most important factors driving follicle development [28–30]. The role of extracellular vesicles, although proposed as being key players in follicle development and the cross talk between the mother and the embryo, in this inflammatory process and its effect on follicle development, however, remains less explored [31].

In conclusion, in hyperprolific sows, the physiological process of farrowing is prolonged, making the system vulnerable in terms of increased rate of inflammation and emerging infectious uterine and mammary disease. In fact, recent evidence now shows that even in sows staying without symptoms, there seems to be considerable degree of "silent inflammation" in the body. In an increased proportion of sows, however, post partum disease PDS is detected and hopefully treated. The consequences of inflammation, regardless of clinical symptoms, include reduced quantity and quality of piglet colostrum intake and milk intake during early lactation.

3. CHALLENGES WITH TRANSFER OF IMMUNITY TO PIGLETS

The neonate piglets are born without the protection of immunoglobulins because of the epitheliochorial nature of the porcine placenta, which does not allow transfer of large molecules during the maternal-fetal interface. Neonate piglets must acquire maternal immunoglobulins from ingested colostrum for passive immune protection, before they will adequately produce own immunoglobulins at 3–4 weeks of age [32].

In Europe in the last 30 years there has been a constant increase in number of piglets born, with litter size averagely increasing from 11 to 14 piglets, with some countries reaching an average of 16 piglets [33, 34]. Nowadays, having litters up to 18–20 piglets it is not uncommon when raising hyper-prolific sow lines [18, 34, 35]. Because sows can have averagely an udder with 14–16 teats [36], large litters are challenging to manage during lactation. According to Andersen et al. [37], without balancing of litter size after birth and without any direct help to sow and piglets, a sow is able to wean successfully no more than 10 to 11 piglets. Large litters can also directly affect piglets at birth. The larger is the number of piglets born in a litter, the lower is their average birthweight and the higher is their weight variation within the litter [38–41]. A greater number of piglets born than the available teats at the sow's udder, a lower birthweight and a greater birthweight variation, all increase the piglets' competition for colostrum intake [42]. Similarly, lower birthweight and long farrowing duration are associated with lower piglet vitality at birth, which can delay the access to the udder [43, 44].

The constant presence of maternally secretory IgA (sIgA) in milk guarantees the protection of the intestinal mucosa of piglets. As long as piglets are able to intake sufficient amounts of milk, the sIgA give a localized protection to their intestine, allowing them to develop gradually their own immune response mechanisms [45]. Other immunoglobulins, like IgG are more concentrated into colostrum, with most of colostrum produced before farrowing and right after farrowing [46]. Porcine colostrum contains very high levels of IgG (30-70 g/l) and a mixture of bioactive molecules like growth factors and enzymes. In colostrum, the level of IgG may be four times higher than the level of IgA and IgG in the serum of the sow [2]. Closure of the gut junctions in piglets occurs 24–36 h after their birth, making the absorption of immunoglobulins impossible [32]. Impossibility for piglets to obtain timely a sufficient intake of colostrum is considered the main cause of piglet deaths occurring within the first days after birth [47]. The recommended amount of colostrum needed per piglet is at least 200 g to minimize the mortality and 250 g for good body weight gain [47]. Since the amount of colostrum offered is timely limited by the sow own production, there is a possibility that in large litters some of the piglets may suffer lack of colostrum. Lessard et al. [48] suggested that the genes' expression of immunity and oxidative stress in piglets' intestinal tissue can be affected by birth weight and colostrum intake, with direct effects on the leukocyte populations responsible of innate and cell-mediated immunity of nursing piglets. Piglets born with low weight had a lower amount of intestinal antigen presenting cells and an impaired increase of B cells, when compared to high birth weight piglets [48].

Social stress conditions like competition for colostrum and milk intake, crowding, and regrouping are more common in large litters. These conditions may induce shortand long-term effects in pigs, on their immunity. Psychosocial stress may alterate changes in the reactions of both the innate and adaptive immunity, such as leukocyte distribution, cytokine secretion, lymphocyte proliferation, antibody production and immune responses to viral infection or vaccination [49]. In addition, social stress may induce or promote gastrointestinal (GI) diseases through dysregulation of inflammatory processes and glucocorticoid resistance of lymphocytes [49], cortisol being the main stress-induced glucocorticoid in pigs.

Some studies found an increased association between high pre-weaning mortality and large litters [50, 51], one example is given in Figure 2 for the Netherlands. An explanation to this correlation can be found in prolonged farrowing duration and lower birth weight commonly seen in large litter size [2].

In a recent study performed in Norway they found that, on the first day of life, the level of piglet plasma IgG, was affected negatively by a linear decrease of 0.4 g/L for each piglet born, indicating how prolonged parturition in large litters can impair the uptake of passive immunity of neonate piglets [52]. Several studies report a negative correlation between litter size and piglet birth weight [38–40, 53]. When looking to piglets' individual growth, three different studies consistently found a decline in litter average birth weight, ranging from 35 to 43 g for each additional pig born across three different populations of litters recorded [39, 40, 54]. A lower birth weight can affect negatively colostrum intake, increasing the risk of mortality [55–57]. Piglets serum IgG concentrations increased with increased piglet weight, while piglets from larger litters had lower serum IgG [58]. Similarly, greater amount of colostrum ingested at birth increased the IgG content in serum of piglets at 24 h after birth [59]. Another study found that piglet serum IgG concentration at 24 h, 10 and 20 days of age was positively correlated with colostrum intake and with the serum IgG concentration of the mother, but was not correlated with birth weight

[56]. Increased duration of farrowing in combination with larger competition in the litter, can reduce not only the possibility to intake adequate amount of colostrum, but also retard the time of access to the udder. This is an unfavorable condition considering that colostrum level of immunoglobulins declines fast after the start of parturition [57]. Studies report that a delayed intake, after the birth, of a standard colostrum ration affected negatively the piglets' immunoglobulin absorption and the maturation of their intestinal villi, having possibly long-term harm on their digestion process [60]. A retarded detection of IgG in piglets' serum was reported when the standardized colostrum portion was given only after 12 h from their birth, than in piglets getting it immediately after the birth. The latter piglets had 4.4% more plasma IgG (21.5 vs. 17.1%), probably because of their greater development of intestinal villi [60]. Klobasa et al. [61] found that birth order had an influence on the amount of immunoglobulin absorbed in a population of 600 piglets. The latest piglets born in the litters had the lower IgG level in their plasma, due to the fast decline in colostrum immunoglobulins level from the start of parturition.

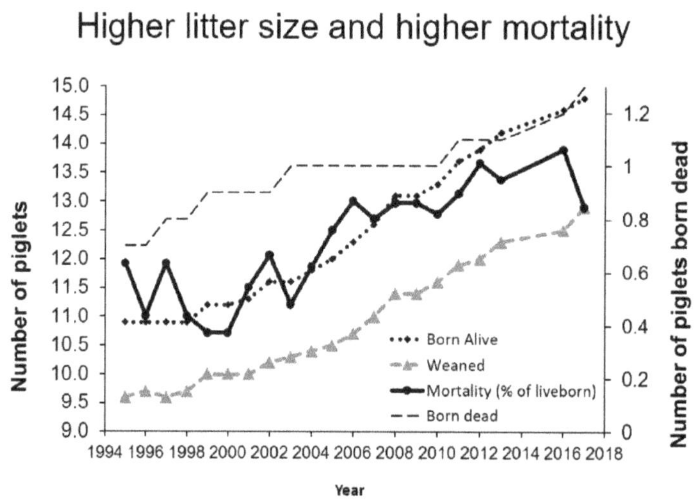

Figure 2. Increased mortality with increased litter size in the Netherlands (adapted from: AgroVision B.V. the Netherlands, 2017).

Correspondingly, another study reported a 4% decrease of plasma IgG concentration in piglets of smaller birth weight, when compared to their bigger siblings [62]. Manjarin et al. [63] indicated the farrowing-to-suckling interval to be fundamental in the acquisition of adequate IgG by piglets. A 4 h delayed intake of colostrum, after the start of parturition, significantly reduced the amount of piglets' plasma proteins 24 hours up to 12 days. It is therefore extremely important to consider also the time of birth of piglets in relation to the start of farrowing, when planning successful strategies to boost colostrum intake in large litters, like for instance split suckling [2].

4.MICROBIOTAINVOLVEMENTDURINGPREGNANCY,PARTURITION AND LACTATION

The composition of gut microbiota constantly shifts over time and it is not constant. In sows, both diversity and abundance of certain microbial population increase with progression of the pregnancy until weaning [64]. Diversified gut microbiota can provide different metabolic capacities and functionality in sows, ensuring the sufficient supply of nutrients for fetal growth and development [64]. In a recent study carried out by Hasan et al. [65], at farrowing, from a phyla level perspective, most gut bacteria were classified in Firmicutes, Bacteroidetes,

Proteobacteria, Actinobacteria, and Candidatus. The Firmicutes represent the most abundant proportion of the total population, followed by Bacteroides. These two phyla accounted for approximately 98% of all bacteria present. These results are in line with the one published by Kim et al. [66], reporting Firmicutes and Bacteroides being 90% of total bacteria present in late pregnancy in the sow gut. However, the findings of the study by Ji et al. [64], reported that Bacteroides increased linearly with the progression of the pregnancy and represented the most dominant (45%) in late pregnancy. Jost et al. [67] reported that Firmicutes exhibited no detectable changes over perinatal period. There are some evidences that gestational body weight gain or increase in the back-fat thickness in the sows, may be associated with an increase in the abundance of Firmicutes or an increase in the Firmicutes to Bacteroides ratio [64, 68]. In terms of phyla, the abundance of Tenericutes, Fibrobacteres, and Cyanobacteria have been shown to increase with the progression of the pregnancy [64]. These phyla have some beneficial effects, for example, Tenericutes increase intestinal cells' integrity and Fibrobacteres are characterized by having the potential to metabolize non-soluble polysaccharides, such as cellulose, hemicellulose or pectin [64]. During late gestation Romboutsia was the dominant genus in sows which is from the phylum Firmicutes, followed by Clostridium sensu stricto, Lactobacillus, Oscillibacter, Intestinimonas, Sporobacter, Christensenella, Barnesiella, Flavonifractor, Terrisporobacter, Acidaminobacter, Lachnospiracea incertae sedis, and Turicibacter, other genera being much less 1% [65].

The changes in the diet can differentiate the composition of the microbiome, and in its potential functionality. Recent studies demonstrate the importance of dietary microbial modulation. Dietary supplementation of hydrolysed yeast [65], resin acid enriched composition [69], probiotics [70] and prebiotics [71, 72] in sow's late gestation diet, significantly changes microbial populations. Different levels and types of protein and fiber in the diet are also modulating the gut microbial population both in gestating sows and in weaning piglets. Fiber has various physicochemical properties, and its supplementation during pregnancy effectively enhances the stability of the gut microbiota population in sow [71, 72]. The most important changes in the gut microbiota composition include a reduction in Proteobacteria and an increase in Ruminococcaceae, Oscillospira, and Eubacterium. Additionally, the genus Eubacterium increases, after dietary soluble fiber supplementation during pregnancy, promoting propionate release, being one of the possible reasons by which dietary fiber increases insulin sensitivity and decrease the general inflammation in sows around farrowing [73]. Those microbiota capable to ferment indigestible carbohydrates, produce short chain fatty acids (SCFA) that can be an important energy source for the sow. Butyrate, in particular, is a gut health-promoting compound that acts as the main energy source for colonocytes and exerts anti-inflammatory properties [74]. The increased production of SCFAs promotes intestinal energy availability, which may contribute to the high energetic demands of hyper-prolific sows for the longer duration of farrowing process; therefore promoting the presence of fiber degrading gut microbiota seems to be favorable for gestating sows. The reduction of pathogenic bacteria in response to dietary supplementation is associated with an increase of beneficial microbiota, which in turn may modify the substrate availability and the physiological conditions of the gastrointestinal tract (e.g. fermentation products, luminal pH and bile acid concentration) [75]. Dietary supplementation of yeast hydrolysate in the pregnancy influenced beneficial and fermentative bacteria (Roseburia, Paraprevotella, Eubacterium), while, some opportunistic pathogens like Desulfovibrio, Escherichia/Shigella and Helicobacter, of the phylum Proteobacteria, were suppressed [65].

Proteobacteria are usually a minority presence within a normal gut microbial community [76]. However, a dysbiotic expansion of facultative anaerobic Proteobacteria are connected with gut inflammation, including irritable bowel syndrome, inflammatory bowel disease in humans [77], and with increased inflammatory responses of women in late pregnancy [78]. Recent studies have proposed that an expansion of Proteobacteria in the gut microbiota community is a potential diagnostic criterion for dysbiosis in gut microbiota and epithelial dysfunction [79, 80]. For instance, Hasan et al. [65] found that some positive sow's productive and physiological performances (high colostrum yield, high colostrum proteins content, high colostrum IgG content, normal blood progesterone level and normal farrowing duration) were positively correlated to the gut bacterial families Lactobacillaceae, Ruminococcaceae and Prevotellaceae, the last two being bacteria able to utilize different plant cell wall polysaccharides. On the contrary, unfavorable productive and physiological performances of the sow (low colostrum yield, low colostrum proteins content, low colostrum IgG content, high level of blood progesterone and long farrowing duration) clustered and were positively correlated with the gut bacterial families Erysipelotrichaceae, Clostridiaceae,

Streptococcaceae, Enterobacteriaceae, Desulfovibrionaceae and Bacteroidaceae, many of these being known pig pathogens bacteria or part of the dysbiotic phylum Proteobacteria.

5. ROBUSTNESS NEEDED, RESILIENCE FAVORED

The climate change requires a brave vision regarding breeding goals in the pig in the future. Buildings housing pigs will need to be energy saving and reducing CO2 emissions in the future. On the other hand, hotter climate will need pigs to be robust and more resilient under heat with less susceptible to becoming stressed under those conditions. Hyper-prolific sows, however, may actually be quite sensitive to heat in comparison to less productive breeds [81].

Consumers appear to asking for improved welfare such as provided by free farrowing /free lactation discussed earlier [34]. Therefore, there appears to be growing demand for cross breeding/genes for these characteristics and traits. Recent developments in reproductive technology may provide tools for international trade of germ cells and embryos in the near future.

6. CONCISE SUMMARY

The parturition process is lengthy and intricate in hyperprolific sows. It elevates the likelihood of uterine contamination, mammary gland inflammation, and retained placenta, hence exacerbating postpartum inflammation and contributing to postpartum dysgalactia (PDS). From the fetal/neonatal perspective, hypoxia may arise due to the prolonged expulsion phase of labor. Furthermore, the quality and quantity of colostrum consumption diminish when the suckling window decreases. During early lactation, metabolic stress is significant due to heightened energy and nutritional demands, exacerbating negative energy balance and potentially impacting the development of subsequent generation follicles and, thus, future piglet generations. The environmental and dietary influences on the gut microbiota of sows and piglets affect gestation, farrowing, and lactation, potentially enhancing the performance of hyperprolific sows and their piglets in extensive litters.

REFERENCES

1. Jackson PGG. Handbook of Veterinary Obstetrics. 2nd ed. London: Saunders; 1995. p. 221-222
2. Oliviero C, Junnikkala S, Peltoniemi O. The challenge of large litters on the immune system of the sow and the piglets. Reprod Dom Anim. 2019;54(Suppl. 3):12-21. DOI: https:// doi.org/10.1111/rda.13463
3. Oliviero C, Kothe S, Heinonen M, Valros A, Peltoniemi O. Prolonged duration of farrowing is associated with subsequent decreased fertility in sows. Theriogenology. 2013;79:1095-1099

4. Le Dividich J, Charneca R, ThomasF. Relationship between birth order, birth weight, colostrum intake, acquisition of passive immunity and pre-weaning mortality of piglets. Spanish Journal of Agricultural Research. 2017;15: e0603. DOI: https://doi.org/10.5424/ sjar/2017152-9921
5. Oliviero C, Heinonen M, Valros A, Halli O, Peltoniemi OAT. Effect of the environment on the physiology of the sow during late pregnancy, farrowing and early lactation. Anim Reprod Sci. 2008;105:365-377
6. Oliviero C, Kokkonen T, Heinonen M, Sankari S, Peltoniemi OAT. Feeding sows a high-fibre diet around farrowing and early lactation: Impact on intestinal activity, energy balance-related parameters and litter performance. Research in Veterinary Science. 2009;86: 314-319
7. Hoving LL, Soede NM, Feitsma H, Kemp B. Lactation weight loss in primiparous sows: consequences for embryo survival and progesterone and relations with metabolic profiles. Reprod Domest Anim. 2012;47:1009-1016
8. Costermans NG, Teerds KJ, Middelkoop A, Roelen BA, Schoevers EJ, van Tol HT, Laurenssen B, Koopmanschap RE, Zhao Y, Blokland M, van Tricht F, Zak L, Keijer J, Kemp B, Soede NM. Consequences of negative energy balance on follicular development and oocyte quality in primiparous sows. Biol Reprod. 2020;102:388-398. DOI: https://doi. org/10.1093/biolre/ioz175
9. Algers B and Uvnäs-Moberg, K. Maternal behavior in pigs. Hormones and Behavior. 2007;52:78-85
10. Taverne MAM and van der Weijden GC. Parturition in Domestic Animals: Targets for Future Research. Reproduction in Domestic Animals. 2008;48:36-42
11. Farmer C. and Quesnel H. Nutritional, hormonal, and environmental effects on colostrum in sows. J Anim Sci. 2009;87:56- 64. http://jas.fass.org/cgi/content/full/87/13_suppl/56
12. Farmer C. Altering prolactin concentrations in sows. Domestic Animal Endocrinology. 2016;56:155- 164. http://dx.doi.org/10.1016/j.domaniend.2015.11.005
13. Castren H, Algers B, de Passille AM, Rushen J, Uvnas-Moberg K. Preparturient variation in progesterone, prolactin, oxytocin and somatostatin in relation to nest-building in sows. Appl Anim Behav Sci. 1993;38:91-102
14. Oliviero C, Heinonen M, Valros A, Peltoniemi O. Environmental and sow-related factors affecting the duration of farrowing. Anim Repro Sci. 2010;119:85-91
15. Kaiser M, Jacobsen S, Haubro- Andersen P, Bækbo P, Cerón J, Dahl J, Escribano D, Jacobson M. Inflammatory markers before and after farrowing in healthy sows and in sows affected with postpartum dysgalactia syndrome. BMC Vet Res. 2018;14:83. Doi.org/10.1186/ s12917-018-1382-7

16. Yun J, Ollila A, Valros A, Larenza Menzies MP, Heinonen M, Oliviero C, Peltoniemi O. Behavioural alterations in piglets after surgical castration: Effects of analgesia and anaesthesia. Research in Veterinary Science. 2019;125:36- 42. https://doi.org/10.1016/j. rvsc.2019.05.009

17. Peltoniemi O, Oliviero C, Yun J, Grahofer A, Björkman S. Management practices to optimize the parturition process in the hyperprolific sow. Journal of Animal Science. 2020;98:96-106

18. Björkman S, Oliviero C, Rajala- Schultz PJ, Soede NM, Peltoniemi OA. The effect of litter size, parity and farrowing duration on placenta expulsion and retention in sows. Theriogenology. 2017;92:36-44

19. Björkman S, Oliviero C, Kauffold J, Soede NM, Peltoniemi OAT. Prolonged parturition and impaired placenta expulsion increase the risk of postpartum metritis and delay uterine involution in sows. Theriogenology. 2018;106:87-92

20. Petersen HH, Nielsen JP, Heegaard PM. Application of acute phase protein measurements in veterinary clinical chemistry. Vet Res. 2004;35:163-187. doi:10.1051/ vetres:2004002

21. Coleman DN, Lopreiato V, Alharthi A, Loor JJ. Amino acids and the regulation of oxidative stress and immune function in dairy cattle. Journal of Animal Science. 2020;98,1:175-193. DOI:10.1093/jas/skaa138

22. Larsen I, Thorup F. The diagnosis of MMA. Proc Int Pig Vet Soc. 2006;52:256

23. Papadopoulos GA, Vanderhaeghe C, Janssens GPJ. Vet J. 2010;184:167-171

24. Bäckström L, Morkoc AC, Connor J, Larson R, Price W. J Am Vet Med Assoc. 1984;185:70-73

25. Peltoniemi OAT, Björkman S and Maes D. Reproduction of group-housed sows. Porcine Health Management. 2016;2:15. DOI: 10.1186/ s40813-016-0033-2

26. Kemper N. Update on postpartum dysgalactia syndrome in sows. Journal of Animal Science. 2020;98:1. DOI: 10.1093/jas/skaa135

27. Farmer C, Maes D, Peltoniemi OAT. The mammary system. In: Zimmerman J, Karriker L, Ramirez A, Schwartz K, Stevenson G, Zhang J, editors. Diseases of swine, 11th ed. USA: Wiley Blackwell, 2019. p. 313-338

28. Han T, Björkman S, Soede NM, Oliviero C, Peltoniemi O. IGF-1 concentration patterns and their relationship with follicle development after weaning in young sows fed different pre-mating diets. Animal. 2020;14:1493-1501. DOI: 10.1017/ S1751731120000063

29. Han T, Björkman S, Soede NM, Oliviero C, Peltoniemi O. Insulin-like growth factor-1 concentrations indicate a rapid metabolic recovery after weaning

of young sows fed different premating diets. Animal. 2020 accepted for publication

30. Han T, Björkman S, Soede NM, Oliviero C, Peltoniemi O. Effect of IGF-1 level at weaning on subsequent luteal developement and progesterone production in primiparous sows. In: Abstract book 11th European Symposium of Porcine Health Management; 22-24 May. Utrecht. The Netherlands: ESPHM; 2019. p. 82-82
31. Almiñana C, Corbin E, Tsikis G, Alcântara-Neto AS, Labas V, Reynaud K, Galio L, Uzbekov R, Garanina AS, Druart X, Mermillod P. Oviduct extracellular vesicles protein content and their role during oviduct–embryo cross-talk. Reproduction. 2017;154:253- 268. DOI: 10.1530/REP-17-0054
32. Rooke JA, Bland IM. The acquisition of passive immunity in the new- born piglet. Production Science. 2002;78:13-23
33. Baumgartner, J. Pig industry in CH, CZ, DE, DK, NL, NO, SE, UK, AT and EU [Internet]. Available from: https:// www.vetmeduni.ac.at/fileadmin/v/tierhaltung/I-Baumgartner_Pig_ industry_in_CH CZ DE DK NL NO SE UK AT_and_EU.pdf [Accessed: 2020-09-15]
34. Kemp B, Da Silva CS, Soede NM. Recent advances in pig reproduction: Focus on impact of genetic selection for female fertility. Reprod Domest Anim. 2018;53:28-36
35. Kobek Thorsen C, Aagaard Schild S, Rangstrup-Christensen L, Bilde T, Juul Pedersen L. The effect of farrowing duration on maternal behavior of hyper-prolific sows in organic outdoor production. Livestock Science. 2017;204:92-97
36. Labroue F, Caugant A, Ligonesche B, Gaudré D. Étude de l'évolution des tétines dápparence douteuse chez la cochette au cours de sa carrier. Journées de la Recherche Porcine en France. 2001;33:145-150
37. Andersen I, Nevdal E, Bøe K. Maternal investment, sibling competition, and offspring survival with increasing litter size and parity in pigs (Sus scrofa). Behavioral Ecology Sociobiology. 2011;65:1159-1167
38. Quesnel H, Brossard L, Valancogne A, Quiniou N. Influence of some sow characteristics on within- litter variation of piglet birth weight. Animal. 2008;2:1842-1849
39. Beaulieu AD, Aalhus JL, Williams NH, Patience JF. Impact of piglet birth weight, birth order, and litter size on subsequent growth performance, carcass quality, muscle composition, and eating quality of pork. Journal of Animal Science. 2010;88:2767-2778

40. Smit M, Spencer J, Almeida F, Patterson J, Chiarini-Garcia H, Dyck M, Foxcroft G. Consequences of a low litter birth weight phenotype for postnatal lean growth performance and neonatal testicular morphology in the pig. Animal. 2013;7:1681-1689. DOI: 10.1017/ S1751731113001249

41. Matheson S, Walling GA, Edwards SA. Genetic selection against intrauterine growth retardation in piglets: a problem at the piglet level with a solution at the sow level. Genetic Selection Evolution. 2018; 50:46

42. Declerck I, Sarrazin S, Dewulf J, Maes D. Sow and piglet factors determining variation of colostrum intake between and within litters. Animal. 2017;11:1336-1343

43. Hoy S, Lutter C, Wähner M, Puppe B. The effect of birth weight on the early postnatal vitality of piglets. Dtsch Tierarztl Wochenschr. 1994;101:393-396

44. Islas-Fabila P, Mota-Rojas D, Martínez-Burnes J, Mora-Medina P, González-Lozano M, Roldan-Santiago P. Physiological and metabolic responses in newborn piglets associated with the birth order. Animal Reproduction Science. 2018;197:247-256

45. Salmon H, Berri M, Gerdts V, Meurens F. Humoral and cellular factors of maternal immunity in swine. Developmental and Comparative Immunology. 2009;33:384-393. doi: 10.1016/j.dci.2008.07.007

46. Theil PK, Lauridsen C, Quesnel H. Neonatal piglet survival: impact of sow nutrition around parturition on fetal glycogen deposition and production and composition of colostrum and transient milk. Animal. 2014;8:1021-1030

47. Quesnel H, Farmer C, Devillers N. Colostrum intake: Influence on piglet performance and factors of variation. Livest Sci. 2012;146:105-114

48. Lessard M, Blais M, Beaudoin F, Deschene K, Lo Verso L, Bissonnette N, Lauzon K, Guay F. Piglet weight gain during the first two weeks of lactation influences the immune system development. Veterinary Immunology and Immunopathology. 2018;206:25-= 34. DOI: https://doi.org/10.1016/j. vetimm.2018.11.005

49. Gimsa U, Tuchscherer M, Kanitz E. Psychosocial Stress and Immunity-What Can We Learn From Pig Studies? Frontiers in Behavioral Neuroscience. 2018;12:64. DOI: 10.3389/ fnbeh.2018.00064

50. Baxter EM, Rutherford KMD, D'Eath RB, Arnott G, Turner SP, Sandøe P, Moustsen PA, Thorup F, Edwards SA and Lawrence AB. The welfare implications of large litter size in the domestic pig II: management factors. Animal Welfare. 2013;22:219-238

51. Rutherford KM, Baxter EM, D'Eath RB, Turner SP, Arnott G, Roehe R, Ask B, Sandøe P, Moustsen VA, Thorup F, Edwards SA, Berg P, Lawrence AB. The welfare implications of large litter size in the domestic pig I: Biological factors. Animal Welfare. 2013;22:199-218

52. Kielland C, Rootwelt V, Reksen O, Framstad T. The association between immunoglobulin G in sow colostrum and piglet plasma. Journal of Animal Science. 2015;93:4453-4462

53. Kapell D, Ashworth CJ, Knap PW, Roehe R. Genetic parameters for piglet survival, litter size and birth weight or its variation within litter in sire and dam lines using Bayesian analysis. Livestock Science. 2011;135:215-224

54. Quiniou N, Dagorn J, Gaudré D. Variation of piglets' birth weight and consequences on subsequent performance. Livest Production Sci. 2002;78:63-70

55. Declerck I, Dewulf J, Sarrazin S, Maes D. Long-term effects of colostrum intake in piglet mortality and performance. J Anim Sci. 2016;94:1633-1643

56. Ferrari C, Sbardella P, Bernardi M, Coutinho M, Vaz I, Wentz I, Bortolozzo F. Effect of birth weight and colostrum intake on mortality and performance of piglets after cross- fostering in sows of different parities. Preventive Veterinary Medicine. 2014;114,259-266

57. Le Dividich J, Charneca R, Thomas F. Relationship between birth order, birth weight, colostrum intake, acquisition of passive immunity and pre-weaning mortality of piglets. Spanish Journal of Agricultural Research. 2017;15:e0603. DOI: https:// doi.org/10.5424/sjar/2017152-9921

58. Nguyen K, Cassar G, Friendship RM, Hodgins D. An investigation of the impacts of induced parturition, birth weight, birth order, litter size, and sow parity on piglet serum concentrations of immunoglobulin G. Journal of Swine Health and Production. 2013;21:139-143

59. Moreira LP, Menegat MB, Barros GP, Bernardi ML, Wentz I, Bortolozzo FP. Effects of colostrum, and protein and energy supplementation on survival and performance of low-birth-weight piglets. Livest Sci. 2017;202:188-193

60. Cabrera R, Lin X, Ashwell M, Moeser A, Odle J. Early postnatal kinetics of colostral immunoglobulin G absorption in fed and fasted piglets and developmental expression of the intestinal immunoglobulin G receptor. Journal of Animal Science. 2013;91:211-218

61. Klobasa F, Werhahn E, Butler JE. Composition of sow milk during lactation. J Anim Sci. 1987;64:1458-1466

62. Cabrera RA, Lin X, Campbell JM, Moeser AJ, Odle J. Influence of birth order, birth weight, colostrum and serum immunoglobulin G on neonatal piglet survival. Journal of Animal Science and Biotechnology. 2012;3:42

63. Manjarin R, Montano YA, Kirkwood RN, Bennet DC, Petrovski KR. Effect of piglet separation from dam at birth on colostrum uptake. Canadian journal of veterinary research. 2018;82:239-242 Ji Y, Li H, Xie P, Li Z, Li H,

64. Yin Y, Blachier F, Kong X. Stages of pregnancy and weaning influence the gut microbiota diversity and function in sows. J Appl Microbiol. 2019;27:867-879. DOI: 10.1111/jam.14344

65. Hasan S, Junnikkala S, Peltoniemi O, Paulin L, Lyyski A, Vuorenmaa J, Oliviero C. Dietary supplementation with yeast hydrolysate in pregnancy influences colostrum yield and gut microbiota of sows and piglets after birth. PLoSONE. 2018;13:e0197586. DOI: https://doi. org/10.1371/journal.pone.0197586

66. Kim HB, Borewicz K, White BA, Singer RS, Sreevatsan S, Tu ZJ, Isaacson RE. Longitudinal investigation of the age-related bacterial diversity in the feces of commercial pigs. Vet Microbiol. 2011;153:124-133

67. Jost T, Lacroix C, Braegger C, Chassard C. Stability of the maternal gut microbiota during late pregnancy and early lactation. Curr Microbiol. 2014;68:419-427

68. Feng ZM, Li TJ, Wu L, Xiao DF, Blachier F, Yin YL. Monosodium L-glutamate and dietary fat differently modify the composition of the intestinal microbiota in growing pigs. Obes Facts. 2015;8:87-100

69. Hasan, S., Saha, S., Junnikkala, S., Orro, T., Peltoniemi, O., Oliviero, C., 2018. Late gestation diet supplementation of resin acid-enriched composition increases sow colostrum immunoglobulin G content, piglet colostrum intake and improve sow gut microbiota. Animal. 2018;27:1-8. DOI: 10.1017/S1751731118003518

70. Menegat M, DeRouchey J, Woodworth J, Dritz S, Tokach M, Goodband R. Effects of Bacillus subtilis C-3102 on sow and progeny performance, fecal consistency, and fecal microbes during gestation, lactation, and nursery periods. Journal of Animal Science. 2019;97:3920-3937. DOI: https://doi.org/10.1093/jas/skz236

71. Tan C, Wei H, Ao J, Long G, Peng J. Inclusion of Konjac Flour in the gestation diet changes the gut microbiota, alleviates oxidative stress, and improves insulin sensitivity in sows. Appl Environ Microbiol. 2016;82:5899-5909

72. Li H, Liu Z, Lyu H, Gu X, Song Z, He X, Fan Z. Effects of dietary inulin during late gestation on sow physiology, farrowing duration and piglet performance. Anim Reprod Sci. 2020;219:106531

73. Xu C, Peng J, Zhang X, Peng J. Inclusion of soluble fiber in the gestation diet changes the gut microbiota, affects plasma propionate and odd-chain fatty acids levels, and improves insulin sensitivity in sows. Int J Mol Sci. 2020;21:635

74. Sassone-Corsi M, Raffatellu M. No vacancy: How beneficial microbes cooperate with immunity to provide colonization resistance to pathogens. J Immunol. 2015;194:4081-4087

75. Liu P, Piao XS, Kim SW, Wang L, Shen YB, Lee HS, Li SY. Effects of chito-oligosaccharide supplementation on the growth performance, nutrient digestibility, intestinal morphology, and fecal shedding of and in weaning pigs. J Anim Sci. 2008;86:2609-2618

76. Eckburg, P. B., Bik, E. M., Bernstein, C. N., Purdom, E., Dethlefsen, L., Sargent, M. Diversity of the human intestinal microbial flora. Science. 2005;308: 1635-1638. DOI: 10.1126/science.1110591

77. Morgan XC, Tickle TL, Sokol H, Gevers D, Devaney KL, Ward DV. Dysfunction of the intestinal microbiome in inflammatory bowel disease and treatment. Genome Biol. 2012;13:79. DOI: 10.1186/ gb-2012-13-9-r79

78. Koren O, Goodrich JK, Cullender TC, Spor A, Laitinen K, Bäckhed HK. Host remodeling of the gut microbiome and metabolic changes during pregnancy. Cell. 2012;150:470- 480. DOI: 10.1016/j.cell.2012.07.008

79. Shin NR, Whon TW, Bae JW. Proteobacteria: microbial signature of dysbiosis in gut microbiota. Trends Biotechnol. 2015;33:496-503. DOI: 10.1016/j. tibtech.2015.06.011

80. Litvak Y, Byndloss MX, Tsolis RM, Bäumler AJ. Dysbiotic Proteobacteria expansion: a microbial signature of epithelial dysfunction. Curr. Opin. Microbiol. 2017;39:1-6. DOI: 10.1016/j. mib.2017.07.003

81. Peltoniemi O, Björkman S, Oropeza- Moe M, Oliviero C.Developments of reproductive management and biotechnology in the pig. Animal Reproduction. 2019;16:524-538. DOI: 10.21451/1984-3143-AR2019-0055

4 Chapter

REPRODUCTION IN SMALL RUMINANTS (GOATS)

1. INTRODUCTION: AN OVERVIEW

The utilization of small ruminants (goats and sheep) has consistently been associated with the advancement of human civilizations, primarily through the consumption of their byproducts, including milk and meat. The current sheep population is over 1 billion, with over 50% concentrated in three countries: China, Australia, and New Zealand. In contrast, the goat population is at roughly 720 million, primarily distributed across Asia, Africa, and South America. Both species exhibit analogous physical features (a pair of nipples), a gestation duration of 150 days, and the occurrence of seasonal anestrus, although they differ in amplitude, depth, and the presence of the male effect. Nonetheless, they exhibit significant disparities in feeding preferences, dietary requirements, and grazing systems, along with variations in the female reproductive tract, among other traits. [1]. Currently the study of reproduction has intensified over the years in the goats and its counterpart that is the buck.

Therefore, in the following topics, the importance of global reproduction of the goat will be discussed, considering that progress has been made today in the application of third generation reproductive techniques and that today they are already consolidated and developed in the bovine species [2].

2. REPRODUCTION IN GOATS

In most areas of the world, goats are mated once yearly in the fall, during their natural mating season, for spring kidding [3–5]. Animals bred at this time are more likely to get pregnant and have multiple kids. A longer breeding season allows for flexibility in breeding and kidding dates to times when the climate is more favorable, and forage is available for the lactating doe. In addition, dates of ethnic/alternative markets should also be considered in the decision about when to breed females. How long the males are kept in with females for mating determines how long kidding will last, but a 40 to 45-day breeding season will guarantee that each doe has had at least two opportunities to come into heat. The male-to-female ratio in this breeding system is approximately 1 male per 30–40 females, but in synchronized breeding, this ratio should be 1 male with 20 or less females.

Likewise, under range conditions, bucks are often maintained with the doe herd throughout the year for continuous breeding. In such a system, proper health management is difficult and only limited supervision can be provided during kidding [1]. Care is also required to routinely remove offspring from the herd to avoid mother/son and father/daughter mating's. Although buck exposure is continuous, kidding under continuous mating will eventually follow seasonal breeding patterns, depending on the location of the farm and the breed of goat used.

However, globally, in intensive milk production systems, the use of basic reproductive techniques has been applied more extensively, for example the estrus synchronization techniques, artificial insemination, (AI), is being used more commonly by goat producers [6]. Artificial insemination makes it possible to obtain or transfer genetic material domestically and internationally. Many goat producers, both meat and dairy, utilize AI to produce animals that are more desired by markets and consumers as well as animals that will do well at local, state and national livestock shows.

2.1 Perspectives and advances in the study of the estrous cycle of the goat

Currently the estrous cycle is being studied from a perspective of hormonal changes according to the ovarian structures that are present during each of the phases that occur (follicular and luteal) [7, 8]. The above is with the objective of evaluating the size of structures and correlating them with hormonal profiles. Considering that by understanding the physiology and anatomy and the perspective of manipulating the oestrus cycle, we can advance or achieve higher gestation rates [9]. It has been stabilized with the application of hormonal products and/or the male effect to have an oestrus presence of 100%. However, pregnancy percentages vary greatly according to a large number of factors (see Figure 1), where each of them affects the final result cross-sectionally, which is pregnancy.

Estrous induction began to develop in goats and sheep for more than 50 years, where injected progesterone began to be used daily, until today with the use of two types of vaginal devices: vaginal sponge and delivery device. Controlled (CIDR), each having its advantages and disadvantages [10, 11]. The response in each of the devices has been accompanied by secondary hormones of intramuscular application that favor the development of the follicles, the synchronization of them for their ovulation and that these become corpus luteum with adequate size and with a sustainable production of progesterone. It is well known that low LH levels during the progestogen synchronization protocol will affect the fate of large follicles.

However, these follicles require LH for their maintenance and development, so they will present atresia and new ovulatory follicles appear that will grow. In long estrous synchronization protocols (above 10 days), when the vaginal devices are removed, they release little progestogen and do not completely suppress LH. With the above, an abnormal follicular development occurs, which become persistent, leading to low fertility and therefore gestation.

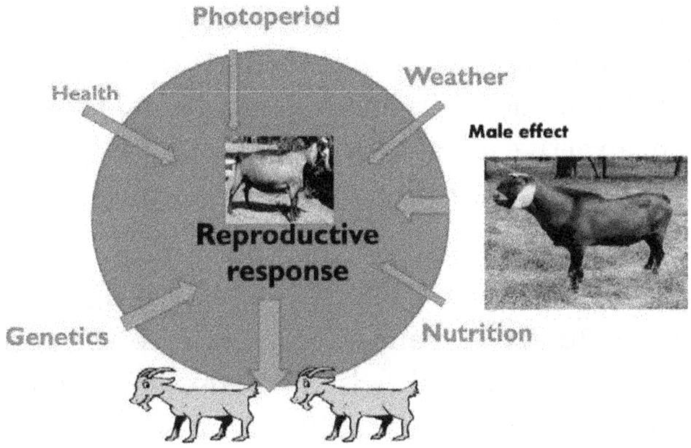

Figure 1. Factors that affect the reproductive response in goats.

2.2 Will it be possible to improve the parameters of presence of estrus and pregnancy using hormones in the coming years?

Changes or results in estrous synchronization programs have been modified over the years depending on the duration of insertion of the sponge or the device in the goat, however, the use of hormones to regulate goat reproduction has been maintained over the years [12, 13], with changes especially in the higher use of nonsteroidal hormones, such as those derived from prostaglandins, gonadotropin-releasing hormones, and hormones of follicular growth and development such as equine chorionic gonadotropin; being the most frequent use in the European community for health reasons. The use of steroid hormones such as progestogens continue to be used globally [14], but under the premise of using short protocols (5 to 7 days). In the present and in future years the use of short protocols of 5–7 days will be used more and more because it has a series of advantages compared to short protocols; these being the decrease in the presence of vaginitis in animals; in the case of CIDR devices, reuse them up to twice more with an effectiveness of up to 90% of estrous in goats. However, the health risk must be considered as it can contaminate bacteria, viruses from one animal to another.

The important thing is to be able to develop vaginal devices with a lower concentration of progesterone and avoid being reused to avoid this type of infection.

On the other hand, the use of estrous synchronization protocols in goats using nonsteroidal hormones in combination with the male effect has been developing more intensively in recent years. For example, the administration of double doses of PGF2α is recommended to synchronize estrous in cycling goats, with an interval of 10–14 days (appointment), which ensures that most does will present the mid luteal phase, when applying the second dose, and that all will respond with the behavior of estrus and ovulation (appointment). However, their response may vary depending on the insemination technique, the dose to be applied and the interval between doses. Besides, it should be considered that only the goat that is cycling with the presence of an active luteal body, would work this protocol. Currently, the male effect is used, so that an estrus occurs, a CL is formed, and the protocol based on prostaglandins is started.

In goats, PGF2α and its analogs are effective luteolytic agents, where very small doses (1.25 mg) of PGF2α are currently required, with the corpus luteum being more sensitive compared to cows. Likewise, responses to low doses of its analogues, such as cloprostenol, have been observed; 125 µg doses have been used in goats, but even a 26 µg dose has been shown to be effective [15, 16]. As in sheep, the age of the corpus luteum and, therefore, the day of the cycle in which PGF2α is administered determines the degree of synchronization obtained and the time required for the heat to appear, the LH peak and the ovulation [17]. Several studies indicate that goats treated on day 6 of the cycle go into heat and show an LH peak much earlier than those treated on day 12 [18, 19].

2.3 Advances and use of the male effect, a case study until today!

The use of the male effect (Figure 2) has been a case study up to nowadays at a global level [20, 21], where different alternatives have been evaluated in order to understand its way of acting under different scenarios of a goat production system and achieve further efficiency in reproduction in the goat [22]. The sudden introduction of the goat increases the release of LH in goats [23], where the first estrus is not silent [24], so the goat effect produces a high degree of estrus synchronization [25]. Also, short cycles of 5–6 days or 10–12 days may appear after introducing the male, in these cases fertility is lower than in normal cycles [26]. Over the years, different scenarios of the male effect have been validated, modified or compared [27]; for example, [28] determined that the male-female ratio does not decrease the ability of sexually active males to induce sexual activity in anovulatory goats, but it does delay the response to the male effect. Likewise, [29] determined that the separation of the goats from the male goats is not necessary as it was thought in previous years to be able to stimulate the sexual activity of goats subjected to the male effect. Followed by another investigation where they verified that the bleating (vocalizations) of the goat were not sufficient to stimulate the presence of estrus and ovulation, therefore, the frequency of pulses of the LH was not increased [30]. Likewise, there are studies where the introduction of estrogenized females when introducing the buck can stimulate the estrous activity of anovulatory goats [31]. Delgadillo et al. [32] reviewing the male effect on goats, mention that in previous years it was mentioned that the male should be in permanent contact with the goats, their studies elucidated that it is not necessary and with a minimum contact of 4–16 hours, percentages of estrus can be reached in goats subjected to the male effect, the same as in groups that are in permanent contact with the males.

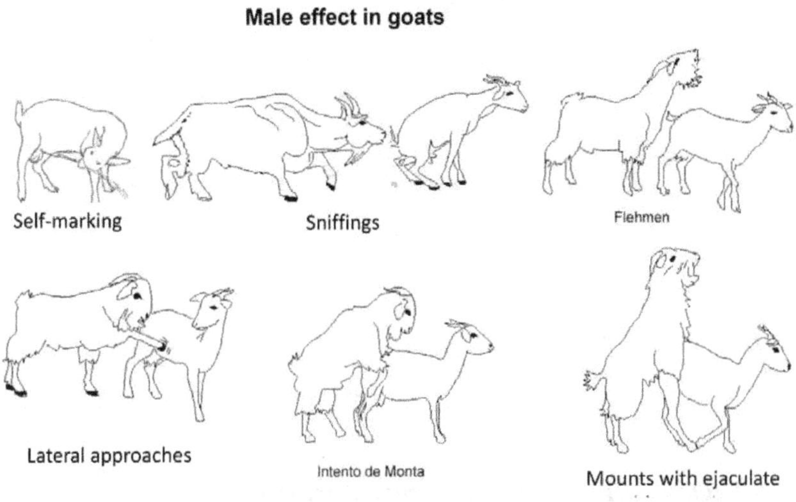

Figure 2. Sequence of sexual behavior in bucks.

However, despite the advantages of using the male effect in goats, even today in large goat populations its use has been limited to continue with the natural breeds according to the time of year. Perhaps the lack of basic infrastructure to install and separate the bucks who are going to have the light programs have made their practical application until today still limited.

2.4 Male social hierarchy and its impact on reproduction

One of the key aspects to improve the performance of the herd is the proper evaluation of the reproductive capacity of the male, performing both a general physical examination, a specific examination of the reproductive system, a seminal quality examination and another of their libido and ability to mount. [33], with the aim of ensuring an adequate selection of males that contribute to improving the efficiency and profitability of the reproductive unit (Figure 3).

Previous studies have evaluated the social hierarchy in rams raised in pairs, identifying that the dominant males exhibit a greater sexual precocity and a greater reproductive capacity compared to the subordinate males. A negative influence on testosterone production has also been reported, due to the stress of the grouping of bucks [34–36].

In goats housed in herds with different densities, the social interactions registered between them were evaluated, as well as the levels of cortisol in blood to determine if the levels of said hormone vary depending on the size of the herd, identifying that the size of the pen and the size of the herd influences the increase in stress due to clustering, negatively impacting the weight gain of the bucks and the productivity of the herd [37, 38].

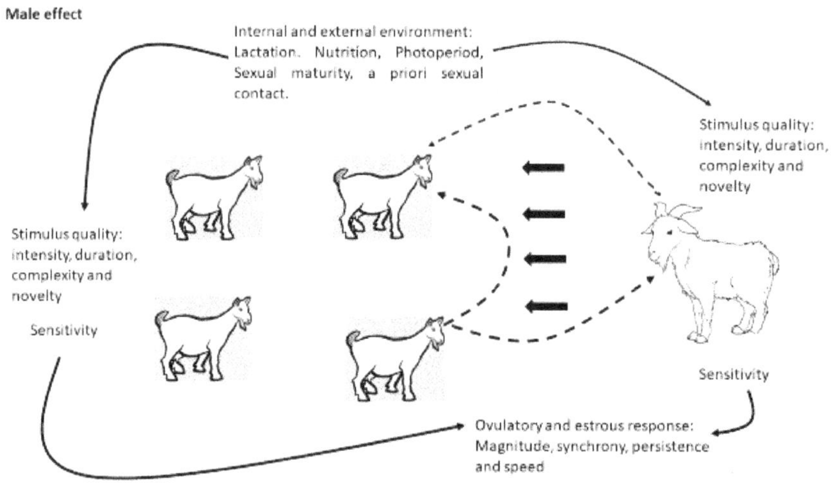

Figure 3. Factors influencing the presentation of the male effect in goats.

Ivasere et al. [39] recorded behavioral changes by intensifying production systems and their effect on productive aspects such as nutrition, reproduction and diseases.

They observed that the social structure is of great importance in the physiological and ethological development in bucks, modifying the frequency of courtship, copulation and the stress level in bucks grouped in herds of different densities. So far there is little information in the literature about the effect of regrouping previously raised male goats in pairs and regarding how serum cortisol and testosterone concentrations, seminal quality and sexual behavior are affected after such grouping.

2.4.1 Cortisol and stress physiology in bucks

Within the management of goats, efforts have been made to develop strategies to improve the quality and efficiency within the herds. At an intensive level, the management carried out ranges from supplying drugs, palpation, semen extraction, and pen cleaning. These management activities, in conjunction with other factors, such as the size of the herd, overcrowding, feeding or the immune system of animals, influence the body's physiological response to various stressful situations [40]. The most common stressors in goat production are mainly those caused by environmental heat and the increase in body temperature, deprivation or lack of access to food or water, as well as modifications in the hierarchical structure of the herd or change of habitat [41].

Among the responses at the physiological level present in male goats in stressful situations is the secretion of glucocorticoids (GC), which exert a negative feedback effect on the hypothalamic-pituitary-gonadal axis, reducing the synthesis of GnRH and together thereby inhibiting the synthesis of gonadotropins and sex steroid hormones [34, 39]. This endocrine mechanism aims to stimulate the body to respond to stressors, such as loss of appetite, suppression of the immune system, energy mobilization, vasoconstriction, and loss of erection and receptive sexual behaviors [42].

2.4.2 Social factors and sexual behavior in males

The grouping of bucks is a widespread practice mainly in stable and mixed management systems around the country [17, 43].

The study of behavior has shown that the establishment of hierarchical ranks and social organization influence sexual behavior that will be exhibited by a male under grouping conditions [44]. This dominance is related in turn to the live weight of the animal and its age, mainly as part of a display of reproductive competition, which guides producers as a key criterion for selecting males [45, 46].

By remaining in coexistence conditions, one of the males tends to monopolize access to the females in estrus in order to ensure their reproductive success, being this considered the dominant male [47], which initiates a display of dominance behaviors, such as competition due to access to food, increased physical activity and hoarding of better resting places, while the subordinate male at the hierarchical level initiates evasive or submissive behaviors and sexual behavior is characterized by opportunistic-type strategies [48]. The dominant male is characterized by having a more aggressive behavior compared to the rest of the males and is also the one with the highest sexual activity [49].

Among the activities carried out mainly by the dominant male, the increase in vocalizations, head movements, tapping, lunges and displacement and protection of the female in heat (tending) from other males stands out [42], thus reaching inhibit the sexual behavior of subordinate males [36].

According to Mainguy et al. [41], the establishment of the dominance position is accentuated with the secondary sexual characteristics, which is also related to the age and body weight of the animal [50], helping to strengthen the male's hierarchical position and social structure within the herd. As they reach sexual maturity, the frequency of mounting with ejaculate, the performance of riding and the production of semen in dominant bucks compared to subordinate's increases [36].

2.4.3 Measurement of sexual behavior in bucks

To determine the potential as a possible male, it is necessary to establish tests that allow the identification and categorization of males according to their score, taking into account comprehensively both their physical characteristics, such as weight, body condition, and sexual behavior [1].

Assessments to determine mount efficiency in bucks typically consist of exposing a male to a female in estrus, for a period of time ranging from 15 to 20 minutes to 1 hour in a pen without distractors [51]. During this period, an observer keeps track of the amount of sexual behavior. They are rapid, practical and inexpensive tests that allow identifying the willingness of the male to serve the female and together with this, discard males with unsuitable profiles within a reproductive program in natural mating in the shortest possible time [52].

In tests of reproductive capacity, motivation is linked to the animal's libido and for this reason some authors recommend the use of more than one female in estrus [49]. Other factors that influence the performance of males in the evaluation of reproductive capacity are the breed of the animal, season of the year, age, the sexual experience they have and the hierarchical position that the male occupies [33].

For the evaluation of sexual behavior in bucks there are different strategies that can be implemented to determine acts of courtship and mating acts. The reaction time test allows us to identify the time it takes for the male to achieve the first mount with ejaculate and thus have an estimate of the libido of the evaluated male [11].

The service ability test is one of the most widely used tests. It consists of placing the male before one or several females in heat for a certain period, usually between 15 to 60 minutes in a pen. During this period an observer counts the number of interactions between the male and the female (s), which can be optionally rated or, only indicate the frequency with which the courtship acts, the mounts or the ejaculations occur as the case may be [42].

Observations may be conducted individually or collectively. Individual observations must occur without the presence of other males, whereas group observations should involve males of comparable ages to ensure test accuracy, aiming to conduct a minimum of three tests to assess service capacity. [25, 53, 54].

REFERENCES

1. Mellado M. Técnicas para el manejo reproductivo de las cabras en agostadero. Tropical and Subtropical Agroecosytem. 2008;9:47-63

2. Grizelj J, Špoljarić B, Dobranić T, Lojkić M, Dávila FS, Samardžija M, et al. Efficiency analysis of standard and day 0 superovulatory protocols in Boer breed goats. Veterinarski arhiv. 2017;87:473-486

3. Abecia JA, Forcada F, González-Bulnes A. Pharmaceutical control of reproduction in sheep and goats. Veterinary Clinics: Food Animal Practice. 2011;27:67-79

4. Dias JCO, Veloso CM, Santos MCDR, Oliveira CTSAMD, Silveira CO, Iglesias E, et al. Seasonal variation in the reproductive activity of male goats raised under tropical climate conditions. Revista Brasileira de Zootecnia. 2017;46:192-201

5. Mendieta ES, Delgadillo JA, Flores JA, Flores MJ, Nandayapa E, Vélez LI, et al. Subtropical goats ovulate in response to the male effect after a prolonged treatment of artificial long days to stimulate their milk yield. Reproduction in Domestic Animals. 2018;53:955-962

6. Arredondo AJG, Gómez AG, Vázquez-Armijo JF, Ledezma-Torres RA, Bernal-Barragán H, Sánchez-Dávila F. Status and implementation of reproductive technologies in goats in emerging countries. African Journal of Biotechnology. 2015;14:719-727

7. Gonzalez-Bulnes A, Menchaca A, Martin GB, Martinez-Ríos P. Seventy years of progestagen treatments for management of the sheep oestrous cycle: Where we are and where we should go. Reproduction, Fertility, and Development. 2020;32:441-452

8. Menchaca A, Neto CDS, Cuadro F. Estrous synchronization treatments in sheep: Brief update. Revista Brasileira de Reproducción Animal. 2017;41:340-344

9. Khan UM, Khan AM, Khan UM, Selamoğlu Z. Effects of seasonal factorsin the goats' reproductive efficiency. Turkish Journal of Agriculture-Food Science and Technology. 2019;7:1937-1940

10. Montes-Quiroz GL, Sánchez-Dávila F, Domínguez-Díaz D, Vázquez-Armijo JF, Grizelj J, Ledezma-Torres RA, et al. Influence of eCG and breed on the number of oocytes collected and the production of in vitro embryos of young goats during the reproductive season. Tropical Animal Health and Production. 2019;51:2521-2527

11. Muñoz GP, Barragán HB, Torres RAL, Morón RU, Dávila FS. Dominancia social sobre comportamiento sexual y calidad seminal en machos cabríos jóvenes criados en parejas durante la estación reproductiva. Revista Academica de Ciencia Animal. 2019;17(Suppl 1): 323-326

12. Brunet AG, Santiago-Moreno J, Toledano-Diaz A, Lopez-Sebastian A. Reproductive seasonality and its control in Spanish sheep and goats. Tropical and Subtropical Agroecosystems. 2011;15:847-870

13. Camacho M. Control of estrous cycle and superovulation in goats [dissertation Ph.D.]. Gottingen, Germany: George August Universitaet; 2020. p. 96
14. Yu XJ, Wang J, Bai YY. Estrous synchronization in ewes: The use of progestogens and prostaglandins. Acta Agriculturae Scandinavica Section A Animal Science. 2018;68:219-230
15. Omontese BO, Rekwot PI, Ate IU, Ayo JO, Kawu MU, Rwuaan JS, et al. An update on oestrus synchronisation of goats in Nigeria. Asian Pacific Journal of Reproduction. 2016;5:96-101
16. Simões J. Recent advances on synchronization of ovulation in goats, out of season, for a more sustainablen production. Asian Pacific Journal of Reproduction. 2015;4:157-165
17. Merlos-Brito M, Martínez-Rojero R, Torres-Hernández R, Mastache LagunasA,Gallegos SánchezJ. Evaluación de características productivas en cabritos Boer x local, Nubia x local y locales en trópico seco de Guerrero, México. Veterinaria México. 2008;33:323-333
18. Meza-Herrera CA, RomeroRodríguez CA, Nevárez-Dominguez A, Flores-Hernández A, Cano-Villegas O, Macías-Cruz U, et al. The Opuntia effect and the reactivation of ovarian function and blood metabolite concentrations of anestrous goats exposed to active males. Animals. 2019;9:1-11
19. Montes-Quiroz GL, Sánchez-Dávila F, Grizelj J, Bernal-Barragán H, Vazquez-Armijo JF, Bosque-González ASD, et al. The reinsertion of controlled internal drug release devices in goats does not increase the pregnancy rate after short oestrus synchronization protocol at the beginning of the breeding season. Journal of Applied Animal Research. 2018;46:714-719
20. Bedos M, Muñoz AL, Orihuela A, Delgadillo JA. The sexual behavior of male goats exposed to long days is as intense as during their breeding season. Applied Animal Behaviour Science. 2016;184:35-40
21. Delgadillo JA, Vélez LI, Flores JA. Continuous light after a long-day treatment is equivalent to melatonin implants to stimulate testosterone secretion in Alpine male goats. Animal. 2016;10:649-654
22. Araya J, Bedos M, Duarte G, Hernández H, Keller M, Chemineau P, et al. Maintaining bucks over 35 days after a male effect improves pregnancy rate in goats. Animal Production Science. 2017;57:2066-2071
23. Espinoza-Flores LA, Andrade-Esparza JD, Hernández H, Zarazaga LA, Abecia JA, Chemineau P, et al. Male effect using photostimulated bucks and nutritional supplementation advance puberty in goats under semi- extensive management. Theriogenology. 2020;143:82-87

24. Zarazaga LA, Gatica MC, Hernández H, Keller M, Chemineau P, Delgadillo JA, et al. The reproductive response to the male effect of 7-or 10-month-old female goats is improved when photostimulated males are used. Animal. 2019;13:1658-1166

25. Madrid-BuryE,González-StagnaroC, Aranguren-Méndez J, Yanez F, Quintero-Moreno A. Sexual behavior of "Criollo Limonero" bulls. Revista Facultad de Agronomáía. 2011;28:505-513

26. Chemineau P, Bodin L, Migaud M, Thiéry JC, Malpaux B. Neuroendocrine and genetic control of seasonal reproduction in sheep and goats. Reproduction in Domestic Animals. 2010;45:42-49

27. Zarazaga LA, Gatica MC, Hernández H, Gallego-Calvo L, Delgadillo JA, Guzmán JL. The isolation of females from males to promote a later male effect is unnecessary if the bucks used are sexually active. Theriogenology. 2017;95:42-47

28. Carrillo E, Véliz FG, Flores JA, Delgadillo JA. El decremento en la proporción macho-hembras no disminuye la capacidad para inducir la actividad estral de cabras anovulatorias. Vol. 45. Técnica Pecuaria en México; 2007. pp. 319-328

29. Véliz-Deras FG, Monroy LV, Cabrera JF, Moreno GD, Massot PP, Malpaux B, et al. La presencia del macho en un grupo de cabras anestricas no impide su respuesta estral a la introducción de un nuevo macho. Veterinaria Mexico. 2004;35:169-178

30. Vielma J, Terrazas A, Véliz FG, Flores JA, Hernandez H, Duarte G, et al. Las vocalizaciones de machos cabríos no estimulan la secreción de la LH ni la ovulación en las cabras anovulatorias. Revista Mexicana de Ciencias Pecuarias. 2008;46:25-36

31. Santiago-Miramontes D, de los Ángeles M, Marcelino-León S, Luna-Orozco JR, Rivas-Muñoz R, Rodríguez-Martínez R, et al. La presencia de hembras estrogenizadas al momento del efecto macho induce la actividad estral de cabras en el semidesierto mexicano. Revista Chapingo Serie Ciencias Forestales y del Ambiente. 2011;17:77-85

32. Delgadillo JA, Gelez H, Ungerfeld R, Hawken PA, Martin GB. The 'male effect' in sheep and goats—Revisiting the dogmas. Behavioural Brain Research. 2009;200:304-314

33. Orihuela A. Ram's sexual behavior. Review. Revista Mexicana de Ciencias Pecuarias. 2014;5:49-89

34. Giriboni J, Lacuesta L, Damián JP, Ungerfeld R. Grouping previously unknown bucks is a stressor with negative effects on reproduction. Tropical Animal Health and Production. 2015;47:317-322

35. Lacuesta L, Ungerfeld R. Sexual performance and stress response of previously unknown rams after grouping them in dyads. Animal Reproduction Science. 2012;134:158-163

36. Sánchez-Dávila F, Barragán HB, del Bosque-González AS, Ungerfeld R. Social dominance affects the development of sexual behaviour but not semen output in yearling bucks. Theriogenology. 2018;110:168-174

37. Kikusui T, Winslow JT, Mori Y. Social buffering: Relief from stress and anxiety. Philosophical Transactions of the Royal Society B. 2006;361:2215-2228

38. Vas J, Chojnacki R, Kjoren M, Lingwa C, Andersen I. Social interactions, cortisol and reproductive success of domestic goats (Capra hircus) subjected to different animal densities during pregnancy. Applied Animal Behavior Science. 2013;147:117-126

39. Iyasere O, James I, Williams T, Daramola J, Lawal K, Oke O, et al. Behavioural and physiological responses of West African Dwarf Goat dams and kids subjected to short-term separation. Tropical and Subtropical Agroecosytem. 2018;51:5-11

40. Solano J, Galindo F, Orihuela A, Galina CS. The effect of social rank on the physiological response during repeated stressful handling in Zebu cattle (Bos indicus). Physiology of Behaviour. 2004;82:679-683

41. Mainguy J, Côté SD, Cardinal E, Houle M. Mating tactics and mate choice in relation to age and social rank in male mountain goats. Journal of Mammalogy. 2008;89:626-635

42. Chenoweth PJ. Sexual behavior of the bull: A review. Journal of Dairy Science. 1983;66:173-179

43. Hernández Z. La caprinocultura en el marco de la ganadería poblana (México): Contribución de la especie caprina y sistemas de producción. Archivos de Zootecnia. 2000;49:341-352

44. Miranda-de la Lama G, Mattielo S. The importance of social behaviour for goat welfare in livestock farming. Small Ruminant Research. 2010;90:1-10

45. Clutton-Brock TH, Huchard E. Social competition and selection in males and females. Philosophical Transactions of the Royal Society B. 2013;368:1-15

46. Clutton-Brock T. Reproductive competition and sexual selection. Philosophical Transactions of the Royal Society B. 2017;372:1-10

47. Ungerfeld R. Managing reproductive seasonality in small ruminants. Archivos Latinoamericanos de Producción Animal. 2016;24:111-116

48. Mainguy K, Côté SD. Age and state-dependent reproductive effortin male mountain goats (Oreamnos americanus). Behavior Ecology Society. 2007;62:935-943

49. Katz LS. Variation in male sexual behavior. Animal Reproduction Science. 2008;105:64-71

50. Pelletier F, Festa-Bianchet M. Sexual selection and social rank in bighorn rams. Animal Behavior. 2006;71:649-655

51. Giriboni J, Lacuesta L, Ungerfeld R. Continuous contact with females in estrus throughout the year enhances testicular activity and improves seminal traits of male goats. Theriogenology. 2017;87:284-289

52. Imwalle DB, Katz LS. Development of sexual behavior over several serving capacity tests in male goats. Applied Animal Behaviour Science. 2004;89:315-319

53. Vejarano OA, Sanabria R, Trujillo G. Diagnostic of bulls reproduction capability from three livestock farms of the upper Magdalena. Revista MVZ Córdoba. 2005;10:648-662

54. Saunders FC, McElligott AG, Safi K, Hayden TJ. Mating tactics of male feral goats (Capra hircus): Risks and benefits. Acta Ethologica. 2005;8:103-110

5

Chapter

INSTRUMENTS AND PROCEDURES FOR ADMINISTERING HYPERPROLIFIC SOWS DURING PARTURITION: ENHANCING PIGLET VIABILITY AND SOWS' REPRODUCTIVE WELL-BEING

1. INTRODUCTION: AN OVERVIEW

1.1 Parturition and birth complications

About 10 years ago, a duration of 300 min was the upper limit for a physiological parturition [1]. Since then, litter size and farrowing duration increased steadily [1]. Nowadays, sows are hyperprolific (average litter size > 16) with an average farrowing duration of longer than 300 min [1–7]. This means that more than half of all parturitions are longer than physiologically. This rapid increase is concerning and leads to a high incidence of dystocia with subsequent negative consequences on piglet survival and sows' fertility and longevity [1–7]. An older survey showed that dystocia was mostly of maternal origin [8], whereas a newer survey identified that dystocia is nowadays almost exclusively due to maternal causes; with uterine inertia being the most common cause [9]. Primary uterine inertia, which is the reduction or complete absence of contractility of the myometrium already at the beginning of parturition, is due to hormonal abnormalities such as increased progesterone, and/or deficiencies of oxytocin and prostaglandin secretion and/or the presence of their receptors. Stress, e.g., caused by the inability of sows to express normal nest-building behavior, is an important cause of primary uterine inertia [10]. Other causes are nutritional factors, e.g., diets low in fiber and high in energy leading to constipation and obesity [11]. Secondary uterine inertia is more common than primary inertia, usually occurring because of a prolonged farrowing particularly associated with a large litter size [12]. Idiopathic dystocia may occur because of the use of prostaglandin F2α and oxytocin to induce or control parturition [12].

Thus, in order to prevent birth complications, the needs of the sow must be fulfilled, stress must be avoided, and nutrition must be optimized. If not, hormonal imbalance will result into weak uterine contraction and subsequently dystocia.

Therefore, active birth management starts before birth in order to prevent this and continues during birth when proper response to hormonal imbalance is needed.

1.2 Colostrum and piglet survival

Sufficient mammary gland development is important for optimal colostrum production and therefore prevention of piglet mortality [13]. Pre-weaning piglet mortality rate was 7.1% (reference value: <11%), when piglets ingested more than 200 g of colostrum, and increased to 43.4% when intake was less than 200 g [14]. Thus, piglets need at least 200 g of good quality (>50 mg IgG/ml) colostrum.

Unfortunately, colostrum yield is highly variable, averaging 3.5 kg and ranging between 1.5 and 6.0 kg [15, 16]. This means that some sows will not produce enough colostrum for their piglets. Further, even though the average yield might be enough for a litter of average size (about 17–18 piglets), it can be difficult for many sows to adequately nurse more than 10–11 piglets without human assistance (such as assisted suckling, cross fostering, movement to a nurse sow, split or suckling assistance) [17]. Thus, factors affecting mammary gland development and colostrum production need to be identified and optimized [13]. One of these factors is the hormonal status of the sow, which can be because of stress, suboptimal feeding, and husbandry during the week(s) before parturition.

Besides the production of a sufficient amount of good quality colostrum, there are further challenges. One of them is the length of the colostral phase. Colostrum is produced only during the first day after the start of parturition. Already after the first 6 h, the IgG content in colostrum is halved [18]. Since large litters can easily extend farrowing beyond 6 h [1], many piglet are born too late in order to get an appropriate amount of good quality colostrum. Therefore, the goal at each parturition is not only to optimize colostrum production by the sow but also the colostrum uptake by neonate piglets. Neonate piglets must acquire a sufficient amount of immunoglobulins from ingested colostrum for energy and passive immune protec tion [19]. The concentration of immunoglobulins in the plasma of piglets shortly after birth correlates positively with their survival rate [20]. Thus, it is necessary to assess colostrum quality and colostrum intake by piglets throughout parturition in order to reduce piglet pre-weaning mortality. This is especially important if mammary gland development is low and/or parturition is prolonged.

1.3 Postpartum dysgalactia syndrome and sows' fertility

PDS is the most important puerperal disease and is characterized by insufficient colostrum and milk production by the sow during the first days of lactation [21]. As consequence, colostrum and milk intake by piglets is reduced, and therefore their mortality increased [21]. Further, PDS negatively affects subsequent reproductive health of the sow [4]. Unspecific symptoms for PDS include fever (>40°C), loss of appetite, and lethargy [21]. Specific symptoms are dysgalactia and vulvar discharge syndrome [21]. Causes of the vulvar discharge syndrome are vaginitis, endometritis, and cystitis [22].

An increasing incidence for PDS of up to 34% was recently reported [23], which is connected with the increase in litter size and farrowing duration [3]. In one study, the percentage of sows with fever during the first 24 h postpartum increased from 40 to 100%, when the farrowing duration increased from less than 2 to more than 4 h [24]. Furthermore, until the third day postpartum, the percentage of sows with reduced appetite was higher in sows with a farrowing duration of more than 4 h than in sows with less than 4 h [24]. In another study, 85.9% of sows with puerperal disease had farrowing durations of more than 6 h, whereas 78.8% of healthy sows completed parturition in less than 3 h [25].

Both prolonged farrowing and PDS share mutual risk factors [11, 21]. Further, both are connected with a decrease in subsequent fertility [4, 5, 26]. Thus, prevention of birth complications and proper birth management will also prevent postpartum disease and therefore optimize subsequent reproductive performance.

2. TOOLS AND PROTOCOLS BEFORE PARTURITION

Proper management of hyperprolific sows in order to optimize piglet survival and sow's reproductive health starts before parturition. The aim is to improve mammary gland development and colostrum production as well as to prevent birth complications and puerperal diseases. In order to do so, optimizing environment, management, and nutrition is highly important. Table 1 provides a checklist for preventive measures.

Factor	Recommendation	Reference
Nutrition		
Constipation score	≥ 2	[11, 21, 41, 83]
Body condition	16 – 20 mm	[11, 21, 38, 57]
Feed intake	Restricted; 18-24 MJ NEa/kg ka	[44-49]
Feeding frequency	≥ 4x/day	[51]
Fiber content in the feed	≥ 7%	[43, 50]
Water intake	≥ 25L/day	[43]
Management		
Ambient temperature	18 – 22 °C	[21, 37, 38]
Drinkers – water flow rate	4L/min	[43]
Hygiene – farrowing unit	Wash, dry& disinfect	[21, 34, 35, 36]
Hygiene – sow	Wash before entering unit	[21, 34, 35, 36]
Moving sows from pregnancy to farrowing unit	5 – 7 days before expected farrowing	[21, 38, 49]
Space allowance	Crates with ≥ 67 cm width; open crate; no crate	[10, 27, 28, 32]
Nestbuilding material	2 kg straw with daily refilling	[10, 27, 28, 32]
Prepartum assessment mammary gland	Number of functional teats and the degree of edema	[52-55]

Table 1. Checklist for prevention of birth complications and puerperal diseases as well as for improving mammary gland development and colostrum production.

2.1 Environment and stress

Modern housing and production systems have promoted the confinement of sows in crates during farrowing. In crates, the sow's movement is severely restricted, and bedding and rooting material is often limited. Consequently, nest-building behavior is reduced or does not occur at all. The lack of space and absence of nest-building materials and behavior are important stressors in sows [27]. This promotes the release of opioids and results into decreased oxytocin secretion and reduced uterine contractility [10, 28]. Thus, the lack of space and bedding material can prolong parturition due to uterine inertia. Considering that a large litter itself can prolong parturition [1, 12], hyperprolific sows need access to space and rooting material in order to prevent birth complications. Allowing the sow to move freely before and during farrowing reduces the duration of farrowing by an average of 100 min, thereby reducing the risk of stillborn piglets and birth of piglets with low vitality [12].

Besides an increase in oxytocin secretion, proper nest-building behavior increases prolactin [29], which is essential for colostrum production. The prepartum decrease in progesterone leads to an increase in prolactin [30]. Delays in progesterone decrease and in prolactin increase relative to the onset of parturition were associated with a strongly reduced yield of colostrum [31]. Thus, as with farrowing duration and prevention of birth complications, studies have found a positive effect of provision of space and nest-building material on oxytocin and prolactin release and therefore colostrum production and maternal nursing behavior [32].

2.2 Management and hygiene

Proper management, especially hygiene, is highly important for the prevention of PDS and therefore piglet mortality and decreased fertility in sows [21]. The current hypothesis is that interactions between endotoxins produced by Gram-negative bacteria in the gut, mammary gland, and/or urogenital tract and alterations in the immune and endocrine functions play a central role in the development of PDS [21]. This is supported by a study where periparturient sows were challenged with lipopolysaccharide (LPS) endotoxin of E. coli, in which sows generated symptoms similar to PDS [33]. E. coli originates from the environment or can already be present in the urogenital tract of prepartum sows or enter during or after parturition. Predominantly, *E. coli* followed by Staphylococcus spp. and Streptococcus spp. are isolated from the urogenital tract in case of cystitis, endometritis, and mastitis [34, 35]. Considering that these are unspecific bacteria originating from feces and environment, it is important to keep hygiene before and during parturition at a high level [36]. Risk factors for PDS are the use of unslatted floor, no washing of sows and no use of disinfectants in the farrowing rooms [36].

Besides hygiene, alterations in the immune and endocrine functions play a central role in the development of PDS [21]. Considering that parturition itself decreases immunity and causes significant inflammatory changes [23], all other factors affecting immunity and endocrinology need to be kept at a minimum level. The most important factor is stress, as described above. Stress needs to be reduced as much as possible. Stress due to restricted space in farrowing crates and lack of nest-building material is discussed above [21]. Other stressors are high ambient temperature and abrupt change from group housing during gestation to restraint in crates a few days before farrowing [37, 38].

2.3 Nutrition and body condition

Nutrition and body condition are important to prepare the sow for farrowing and the production of colostrum and milk. The sow should have an optimal body condition around parturition. Obesity needs to be avoided [11]. The fatter the sow, the longer the duration of parturition. It is possible that the fat deposition stores lipid-soluble steroids such as progesterone. In this case, the prepartum decline in progesterone may be delayed which in turn affects oxytocin receptor activation

[10, 12]. Low concentration of oxytocin receptors will result in weak uterine contractions and colostrum let-down. Higher backfat and progesterone lead also to lower colostrum quality and production [39, 40]. If possible, backfat should be between 16 and 20 mm [11].

Besides body condition, there is a negative correlation between constipation and farrowing duration [11]. The more constipated the sow, the longer the duration of parturition. One reason may be that constipation can cause a physical obstruction to the passage of the piglets [12]. Another reason may be that constipation may result in higher concentrations of LPS. LPS can be absorbed from the gut and affect normal endocrine changes associated with farrowing [41]. A third explanation may be that the discomfort and pain associated with constipation affect hormonal changes associated with parturition [12]. Studies have found that pain releases opioids, which inhibit oxytocin secretion during parturition [28, 42]. Therefore, pain due to prolonged constipation, or any other source of pain, can reduce myometrial contractions and therefore cause birth complications. Constipation can be evaluated using a constipation index [43]. Constipation index should be two or higher, i.e., feces should be present, pellet-shaped, and not dry [11].

In order to prevent constipation and obesity, ad libitum feeding in the last third, especially in the last week, of gestation should be avoided. Restricted feeding supports the birth process, mammary gland development, and colostrum production [44]. There were positive associations between colostrum yield and plasma concentrations of urea, creatinine, and free fatty acids [45]. Further, there was a positive association between backfat loss in the last third of gestation and colostrum yield [46]. These results show that feed restriction with protein and fat mobilization for metabolism has positive effects on colostrum production [30]. Nevertheless, this can probably only be recommended for sows that have reached a good body condition (>18 mm) at the end of gestation. Unfortunately, sows usually receive high-energy concentrated diet low in fiber during late gestation [47]. Such diets can promote obesity and constipation, leading to poor mammary gland development [30], low colostrum quality [48], birth complication [11], and PDS [21, 49]. Late pregnancy diets should contain at least up to 7–10% fiber [43]. A good fiber source can also be provided by offering different types of roughage, e.g., straw or hay, or adding any other feedstuffs with high levels of fiber such as sugar beet pulp [50].

Besides amount and composition of feed, the feeding intervals are important. A short time-lapse between the last meal prior to the onset of the expulsion stage and the onset considerably shortens the duration of farrowing [51]. Farrowing duration, odds for farrowing assistance, and odds for stillbirth were low, intermediate, and high when the time between the last meal and onset of parturition was less than 3, 3–6, and more than 6 h, respectively [51].

2.4 Prepartum assessment of mammary gland

In addition to improving mammary gland development by means of management, environment, and nutrition, the mammary gland needs to be evaluated before each parturition. It is important to assess the number and morphology of functional teats and the degree of edema. The number of functional teats available per piglet is positively associated with piglet survival [52]. If piglets had access to less than one functional teat, mortality increased to more than 14% [52]. If more than one teat was available, mortality was reduced to below 8% [52]. Besides the number of functional teats, also the morphology is important. Piglets tend to suck first from teats that are close to the abdominal midline and have longer inter-teat distances [53]. Thus, a functional teat with short inter-teat distance and/or long distance between teat base and abdominal midline may be unusable for the piglet [54].

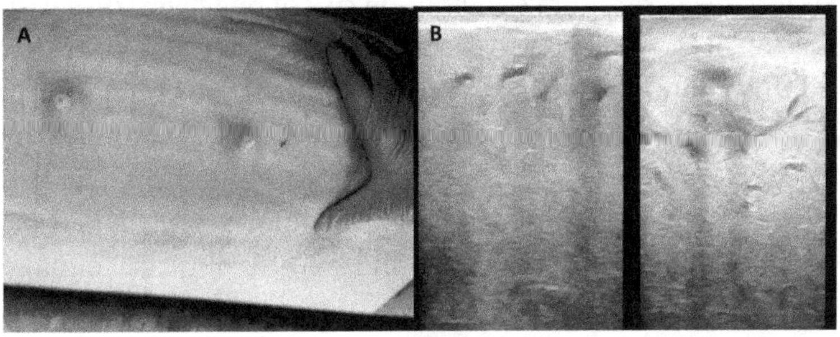

Figure 1. Severe prepartum edema of the mammary gland. Visual inspection (A) reveals dimpled skin with persistent marks of the floor, swollen teats, and indistinguishable gland complexes. Ultrasonographic image (B) shows shadowing, thickened dermal tissue, hyperechoic lobuloalveolar tissue, and enlarged blood vessels, lymphatic ducts, and milk ducts. Images taken by Stefan Björkman.

Furthermore, severe edema of the mammary gland before parturition will have a negative impact on teat accessibility, reduce colostrum quality, and increase the risk of PDS [48, 49]. The degree of mammary gland edema can be graded visually or via ultrasound [48, 49, 55]. At visual inspection, sows with severe udder edema have dimpled skin with persistent marks of the floor (Figure 1A). Further, teats are swollen and mammary glands are indistinct (Figure 1A) [48, 49]. Ultrasound of the mammary glands shows thickened dermal and subdermal tissues, hyperechoic lobuloalveolar tissue with enlarged blood vessels, and severe shadowing (Figure 1B) [48, 49, 55]. Also at the end of lactation, the assessment of the mammary gland, as described above, is crucial and should be used for the decision of removing the sow from the herd.

3. TOOLS AND PROTOCOLS DURING PARTURITION

During parturition, it is important to recognize birth complications and treat accordingly. Further, evaluation of colostrum quality is necessary in order to know whether the sow has good quality colostrum or if piglets need additional colostrum from another sow. Also, the vitality and colostrum uptake of the piglets need to be assessed. Piglets with low vitality and low colostrum uptake are at risk of starving and hypothermia.

Both increase piglet mortality, especially due to crushing by the sow. Tables 2 and 3 provide protocols for diagnosis and treatment of birth complications. Tables 4 and 5 provide guidelines for the assessment of colostrum quality and piglet vitality.

3.1 Diagnosis of birth complications

Appropriate and prompt treatment of a sow with birth complications is important to avoid still or weak-born piglets and to increase piglets' health and survival. This can be achieved through continuous farrowing supervision [56]. Farrowing supervision is also necessary for reducing the risk of puerperal disease [38]. Already before parturition, it is important to spot those sows that may be at risk of dystocia. These sows are usually gilts or old sows (≥6 parity), thin (≤14 mm) or fat (≥23 mm) sows, constipated sows (<2), and sows with history of birth complications and birth of still and weak piglets [11, 57]. These sows need an obstetrical examination if more than 30 min have passed since the last piglet was expelled (Table 2) [12]. This applies also to sows that are restless and have strong abdominal contractions during parturition or to sows with prolonged parturition (>300 min) [12]. Obstetric intervention is usually not indicated before 1–15 h has passed since the last piglet was born in sows without risk for dystocia, which are at the beginning of parturition (<300 min since the expulsion of the first piglet) and show no signs of strong abdominal straining or restlessness [11, 12, 57]. Restlessness can occur if stress and pain are present [58]. For instance, increased stress induces higher frequency of postural changes and longer duration of standing position of sows during the expulsion stage of parturition [58].

Table 2. Risk factors for birth complications. Farrowing supervision should occur every 30 min when sow is at risk. Otherwise, farrowing supervision once an hour.

Factor	Recommendation	Reference
Parity	1, ≥ 6	[57]
Constipation score	< 2	[11]
Body condition	≤ 14 mm, ≥ 23 mm	[11]
Last parturition	Birth complication, birth of dead and weak born piglets	[57]
Current parturition	Prolonged, restlessness, strong abdominal contractions; dead and still born piglets	[12]

Table 3. Guidelines for diagnosis and treatment of birth complications [12, 61–69].

Guideline for diagnosis and treatment of birth complications
Rectalize the sow, remove feces and palpate the birth canal in order to determine whether a piglet is within birth canal
➢ Piglet within birth canal
➢ Wash vulva 3x with warm water & iodine soap, dry with paper towels
➢ Apply rectal glove and plentiful of lubricant
➢ Remove piglet gently by hand
➢ No piglet within birth canal (or any other kind of obstruction)
➢ If at the beginning of parturition: Manual induction of the Ferguson reflex, massaging the udder of the sow, and/or physical exercise
➢ If during or at the end of parturition: Inject oxytocin – low dose of 5 - 10 IU intramuscular

Table 4. Guideline for evaluating colostrum quality (colostrum collected from several anterior teats within 0–3 h from the start of farrowing) using Brix refractometer [70].

Brix %	ELISA IgG (mg/ml) mean ± SEM	IgG quality category
< 20	14.5 ± 1.8	Poor
20-24	43.8 ± 2.3	Borderline
25-29	50.7 ± 2.1	Adequate
≥ 30	78.6 ± 8.4	Very good

Table 5. Behavioral and physiological indicators of low colostrum intake and neonatal mortality.

Indicator	Critical value	Reference
Crown-rump length	< 26 cm	[2, 72]
Body weight	< 1200 g	[2, 72]
Body temperature	< 37 °C	[2, 72, 73]
Skin temperature	< 30 °C	[53, 74]
Meconium staining	Severe	[63]
Latency to moving	> 15 seconds	[2, 63]
Latency to standing	> 5 minutes	[2, 63]
Latency to teat	> 25 minutes	[2, 72]
Latency to suckle	> 30 minutes	[2, 72]

Whenever the abovementioned criteria are fulfilled, an obstetrical examination needs to be performed. An obstetric examination includes palpation and ultrasonography of the birth canal [12, 59]. Palpation of the birth canal should always occur through the rectum and not through the vagina. Vaginal palpation can lead to an increased risk of subsequent dystocia, stillborn piglets, and PDS [3, 7, 12, 57]. Rectal palpation is necessary to determine the exact cause of dystocia before any intervention is undertaken. When no piglet is felt within the birth canal, then the cause of dystocia is uterine inertia [8, 9, 12]. Other causes are, e.g., obstruction of the birth canal due to ventral deviation of the uterine horns or fetal malposition [8, 9, 12]. After these obstructive causes are ruled out, treatment for uterine inertia can be applied [12].

Ultrasonography can be used to determine whether farrowing is over or if the sow has retained piglets [59] or placentae [60] (Figure 2).

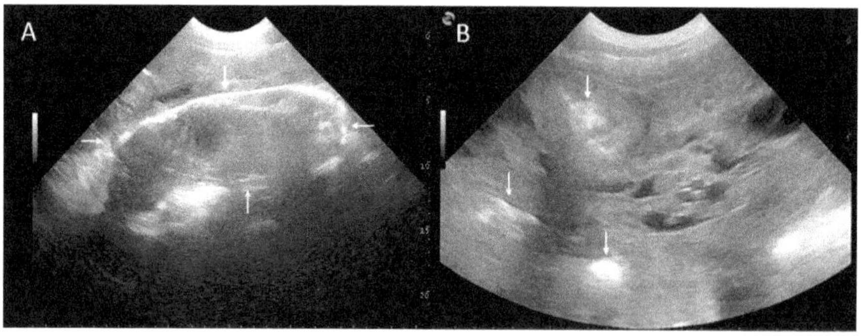

Figure 2. Transabdominal ultrasonographic image of a non-expelled piglet (A; arrows indicate vertical and horizontal dimension) and placentae (B; arrows indicate placentae). Scale bars on right margins in 1 cm steps. Images taken by Alexander Grahofer (A) and Stefan Björkman (B).

3.2 Treatment of birth complications

Oxytocin, an uterotonic agent, is used during farrowing to treat dystocia by provoking uterine contractions [61]. If primary uterine inertia occurs, before administration of any exogenous oxytocin, we recommend trying means of releasing endogenous oxytocin, e.g., manual induction of the Ferguson reflex and massaging the udder of the sow [8]. Furthermore, movement and physical exercise of the sow have positive effects on the farrowing duration, especially if the sow is still at the beginning of the second phase [12]. If that does not help, we recommend waiting for at least 30 min. Often progesterone has not fully declined and oxytocin receptors are not fully expressed [62], which makes oxytocin administration contraindicated. In this case, possible stressors and sources of pain should be investigated, and provision of nest-building material or application of pain medication may be indicated. If the sow is constipated, removing feces from the rectum by hand is beneficial.

Immediate application of exogenous oxytocin is indicated if secondary uterine inertia is diagnosed towards the end of the second phase of parturition [12]. Several studies were conducted to prove the effect of oxytocin on the birth process and piglet survivability and to evaluate the proper dosage of oxytocin in dystotic sows [63–65]. An intramuscular administration of 10 IU of oxytocin did not cause any side effects. However, higher dosages led to an increase in stillborn piglets, changes in the umbilical cord, and higher meconium scoring [63–65]. Furthermore, the improper use of oxytocin can lead to unwanted side effects. These side effects are increased uterine inertia and manual assistance [66, 67] as well as ruptured or damaged umbilical cord [68] and decreased placental blood flow [69]. Hence, we recommend administering oxytocin only restrictively, e.g., 5–10 IU one to two times during parturition [12].

3.3 Colostrum collection and quality assessment

It is possible to easily collect colostrum during parturition due to the almost continuous (every 5–40 min) milk ejections [29]. A brix refractometer can be used for quality assessment. Brix refractometer can be an inexpensive, rapid, and satisfactorily accurate method for estimating IgG concentration on farm [70, 71]. We recommend collecting a colostrum from several anterior teats within 0–3 h from the start of farrowing when the IgG level peaks [70]. If this is done early during parturition, sows with low-quality colostrum can be spotted and more support to her litter, e.g., assisted nursing and split suckling, can be provided. Nevertheless, it is possible to determine colostrum quality at any stage of parturition. This may be indicated if piglets are born late (farrowing duration > 12 h). Differentiation between good and poor IgG content of colostrum is possible interpreting the results with the categories proposed in Table 3. Colostrum with an IgG level of 50 mg IgG/ml is considered of good quality [14]. When Brix values are <20%, they reflect very low levels of IgG, while values from 25% upwards are considered to correspond to good or very good concentration of IgG in colostrum. Results between 20 and 24% are defined as borderline [70]. With borderline results, we suggest taking another sample within 1–2 h to determine whether the development of the estimated IgG content is stable, increasing, or decreasing from the initial value.

Colostrum can also be stored and used later for piglets with low colostrum intake or for litters of sows with low colostrum quality. Colostrum can be stored in a fridge for 1–2 days or in the freezer for 3–6 months. Only sows with high colostrum quantity and quality should be selected. The collected colostrum can be administered to piglets using a feeding bottle with a suitable nipple or using a syringe.

3.4 Assessment of colostrum uptake

Certain behavioral and physiological indicators can be used to identify piglets with low vitality and low colostrum uptake [72]. Piglets with low vitality may need assistance with colostrum uptake in order to prevent starvation, hypothermia, and crushing by the sow [2]. Table 5 provides an overview of these indicators. Besides birth weight and crown-rump length, piglet's survival chance correlates with body temperature, vitality score, rooting response, and latency to teat and suckle [72]. Whenever the following criteria are met, the piglet needs assistance with colostrum uptake: vitality score of less than two (no movements within 15 s of birth), latency to teat and therefore to suckle of more than 30 min, and a body temperature of less than 37oC during the first hour after birth. In order to spot these piglets in time, we suggest looking at them every 30 min during parturition.

However, this may be difficult to implement into practice. It may be helpful to make use of thermal images to overcome these difficulties [53]. Similar to body temperature, skin temperature is linked to birth weight, vitality, and colostrum ingestion and can be used to see whether a piglet has reached the teat and suckled and ingested colostrum within 30 min of birth [73, 74]. As a piglet begins to suck and ingest colostrum, energy and warmth are produced, increasing body and therefore skin temperature [53]. If skin temperature drops below 30oC, the piglet has not been successful [53] and needs to be assisted to suckle and ingest colostrum.

3.5 Assistance of colostrum uptake

It is important to ensure that each piglet in the whole litter has a sufficient intake of good quality colostrum (more than 200 g) within 12–16 h from the beginning of parturition [14, 75]. When possible, piglets with low colostrum uptake should be assisted to suckle, by helping them to attach to the smallest functioning teats. This procedure should be repeated three to four times within the first few hours. Additionally, weakly piglets can be hand-fed with colostrum collected from their own mother or other sows.

Assisted suckling and hand-feeding are appropriate in small or normal size litters where only one or two piglets require help. In large litters or when more piglets require assistance, split suckling is more effective. In order to minimize the sibling competition for colostrum intake, the litter is split into two groups. The heavier and stronger piglets are kept in the creep area or in a separate box, allowing the smaller piglets to suckle for 60–90 min, and then the groups are switched. When separating the piglets, both groups should always have free access to a warm creep area. This can be easily achieved by using a box with an additional heat lamp for the separated group, which leaves the creep area accessible for the remaining group to suckle.

Assisted suckling should be combined with split suckling if some small piglets are still unable to successfully suckle.

Another strategy is to prolong the colostral phase. Piglets ingest colostrum usually until 24 h after the onset of parturition [75]. The composition of colostrum is affected by the status of tight junctions between mammary epithelial cells, and the ability to manipulate mammary tight junctions in the late colostral phase could allow Ig concentrations to be maintained at higher levels for a longer period. Injecting a supraphysiological dose of oxytocin to sows on day 2 of lactation (i.e., between 12 and 20 h after birth of the last piglet) increased the concentrations of IGF-I, IgG, and IgA in milk collected 8h after the injection [76]. The injection of oxytocin in the early postpartum period therefore delayed the occurrence of tightening of mammary tight junctions and prolonged the colostral phase, thereby having beneficial effects on the composition of early milk.

4. TOOLS AND PROTOCOLS AFTER PARTURITION

After parturition, it is important to investigate whether the sow is at risk or suffers from puerperal disease. Sows at risk are, e.g., sows that had constipation or stress, are obese, had a prolonged parturition, experienced birth help, and gave birth to more than one stillborn piglets (Table 6) [3, 21, 35]. These sows need to be checked within 3 days after parturition whether the animals shows general symptoms or other clinical signs of PDS [77, 78]. Underlying causes for PDS can be constipation, endometritis/metritis, cystitis, and mastitis [12, 62]. The underlying cause needs to be diagnosed and immediately treated.

4.1 General symptoms

General symptoms include fever, reduced appetite, lethargy, and vaginal discharge [41]. Body temperature is the most frequently used to evaluate the health status of a sow in the puerperal period [78]. Reference values range from 39 [24] to 40°C [38]. Though body temperature is a sign of inflammation, it can also be affected by several other parameters such as the circadian rhythm [79], parity [79], variation in repeated measurements [80], and positioning of the thermometer in the rectum [81]. Vulvar discharge occurs also in healthy and diseased animals [82, 83] with the highest incidence between days 2 and 4 postpartum [78, 84]. Further, the color, consistency, and quantity of vaginal discharge vary regardless of whether the vaginal discharge is physiological or pathological [85]. The color can vary from clear, whitish, yellowish to reddish (Figure 3). The consistency varies from watery to creamy with lumps, and the amount can be up to 500 ml [85, 86].

Increased volumes of vaginal discharge are associated with endometritis, but otherwise there does not seem to be strong correlations between other characteristics of vaginal discharge and PDS [86].

Table 6. Indicators, based on clinical history and clinical symptoms, for postpartum dysgalactia syndrome.

Indicator	Recommendation	Reference
Body temperature	≥ 40 °C	[24, 38]
Backfat	≥ 20 mm	[21, 35]
Constipation	≤ 1	[21, 35]
Appetite	Diminished; moderate or total anorexia	[21, 24]
Farrowing duration	Prolonged	[3]
Placenta expulsion	Impaired	[3]
Number of dead born piglets	≥ 2	[3]
Birth help	Yes	[3]
Vulvovaginal discharge	Moderate to large amounts	[78, 86]
Milk production	Hypogalactia, dysgalactia, agalactia	[21, 35]

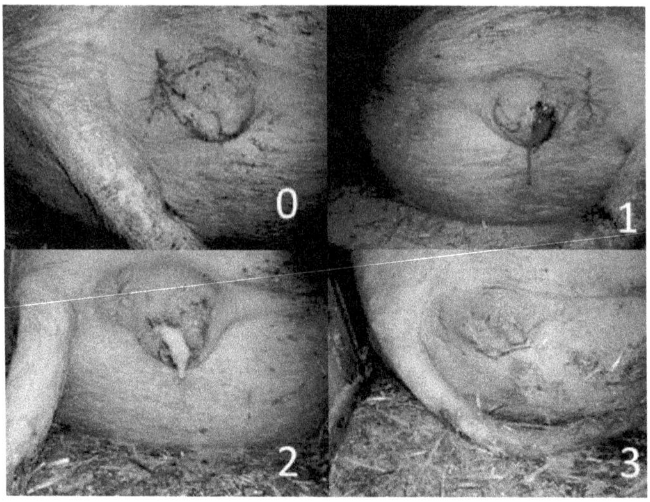

Figure 3. Puerperal vaginal discharge with different colors. 0 = clear, 1 = reddish, 2 = yellowish, and 3 = whitish. The color of vaginal discharge varies regardless of whether the vaginal discharge is physiological or pathological [85]. Increased volumes of vaginal discharge are associated with endometritis. Images taken by Alexander Grahofer.

In conclusion, body temperature, especially under 40.0°C; appetite; and vaginal discharge cannot be used alone and as the single criterion for PDS. Still, body temperature of more than 40.0°C together with other clinical symptoms such as general behavior and feed intake are associated with PDS and require further diagnostics [78, 79]. These symptoms can be normal or associated with an infection of the urogenital tract or the mammary gland and constipation.

4.2 Endometritis

Besides prolonged parturition, obstetrical intervention, and the birth of more than one dead piglet, also retained placentae is a risk factor for endometritis [3]. For both, endometritis and retained placentae, ultrasonography is considered the best tool for diagnosis [3, 59, 78, 87]. Examination of uterine structures currently utilizes three criteria: fluid echogenicity, echotexture, and size [59, 87]. Changes in echotexture are a reflection of changes in the endometrial edema. Increased echotexture and any fluid echogenicity must be considered abnormal and indicative of an exudative inflammation of an acute or acute-chronic type [59, 87]. Fluid echogenicity is often associated with uterine edema and therefore increased echotexture and size of uterine cross-sections [3]. Thus, all criteria, enlarged uterine size, hyperechoic fluid accumulation, and heterogeneous uterine wall, are interconnected and can be used as ultrasonographic parameters to ascertain uterine disorders (Figure 4) [3, 87, 88].

In contrast, chronic endometritis, representing the most common type of uterine inflammation in pigs and most common cause of reproductive failure, cannot be definitively diagnosed by ultrasonography or by any other tool [59, 87]. Therefore, it is essential to recognize acute endometritis in time. This can be done based on the criteria mentioned above, but it must be considered that fluid echogenicity, uterine edema, and increased uterine size during the first few days after parturition may be normal [3, 78, 88]. Furthermore, when interpreting uterine size, the age and parity of the sow as well as the number of postpartum days need to be considered [3, 59, 87].

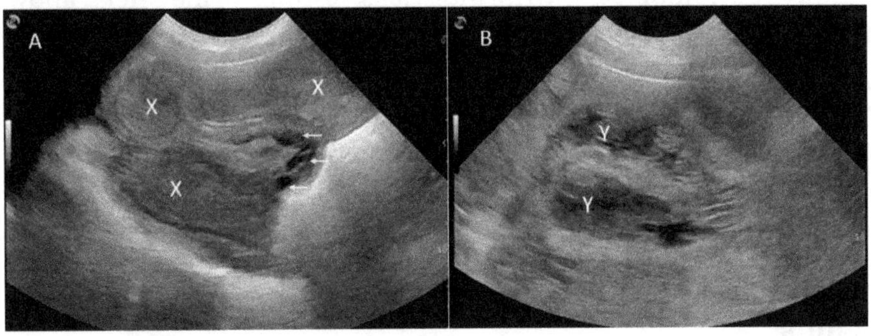

Figure 4. Transabdominal ultrasonographic images of uterine cross-sections (X, Y) of sows assessed 3 days after parturition with enlarged and heterogeneous uterine wall (A) and hyperechoic fluid accumulation (B). Uterine vessels are prominently enlarged (examples marked with arrows). Scale bars on right margins in 1 cm steps. Images taken by Stefan Björkman.

4.3 Cystitis

Ultrasonography can also be used for the diagnosis of cystitis [89, 90]. Still, it is not as reliable as in the diagnosis of acute endometritis. Clear changes in the wall thickness and regularity and the mucosal wall surface are volume dependent [89, 90].

Overall, these measurements seem to be unreliable for diagnosis of cystitis. On the other hand, animals with cystitis have moderate to high amounts of sediment [89, 90]. Unfortunately, half of the sows without cystitis also show moderate to high amounts of sediment, which is mainly caused by the diet [89, 90]. Nevertheless, when none to mild amounts is present, the probability that the sow is suffering from no cystitis is high. When moderate to high amounts of sediment are present, other diagnostic tests need to be applied.

Another diagnostic test is urinalysis. It is preferred to collect spontaneous midstream urine in a transparent tube. The best time for collection is in the morning before feeding. On-farm urinalysis includes macroscopic urine evaluation and urine stix testing. During the macroscopic urine evaluation, the color, odor, and turbidity are evaluated [91, 92]. The color can vary between light yellow and dark yellow, depending on urinary concentration. The color should not be red or brown which indicates hematuria or myoglobinuria. The turbidity of the urine should be clear. Cloudy or turbid appearance indicates the presence of bacteria. The presence of bacteria can also increase ammonia in the urine and cause a putrid odor. Urine turbidity has a sensitivity of 0.74–0.80 and a specificity of 0.50–0.92 and 0.50 [93, 94]. Nevertheless, if urine is physiological, the probability that the sow is suffering from no cystitis is 0.85 [95]. Thus, because of low sensitivities of certain single markers, several markers need to be evaluated together. A macroscopic evaluation should always be combined with urine sticks testing. Urine sticks allow testing for protein, pH, nitrite, blood, and leukocytes. Parameters with low sensitivity are leukocytes, pH, and nitrite [93, 94]. Parameters with good sensitivity are blood and protein [95]. The normal pH is between 5.5 and 8, and an increase above 8 is indicative for the presence of bacteria. On the other hand, many other factors can increase the pH such as feeding, other diseases, and medication. Whenever the majority of these markers indicate cystitis, a urine sample should be sent for bacterial investigation.

4.4 Mastitis

Mammary gland, unlike the urogenital tract, is located outside the body and therefore easily accessible by hand. Thus, the diagnosis of mastitis can be done by palpation of the mammary gland. Mammary glands may appear swollen, firm, and warm [35]. In addition, skin color may be changed.

Other rapid mastitis tests as applied to cows are not available for sows. Diagnosis via cell count is not common and data on thresholds are rare [96]. A threshold of >107 cells per mL was proposed [35]. Further, a milk pH of more than 6.7 was reported [96]. If needed, ultrasonography can be used in the diagnosis. Affected mammary glands provide heterogeneous and hyperechoic images [97].

5. CONCISE SUMMARY

Hyper-prolificacy impairs the sow's performance for parturition, colostrum production, neonatal survival, and fertility. Prevention of birth difficulties, piglet mortality, and puerperal illness is essential. Prior to parturition, it is advisable to permit sows unrestricted movement and to supply nest-building materials such as straw, hay, sawdust, or paper sheets. Altering the sow's late gestation diet to avert constipation and excessive body condition will yield advantageous outcomes. The prompt provision of birth aid during parturition is crucial. The precise etiology of dystocia must be identified and addressed. Excessive oxytocin should be avoided to prevent hyper-stimulation of the uterus. Close attention and support must be provided to underdeveloped piglets, diminutive piglets, and piglets lacking teats. Innovative technology, such Brix refractometers and infrared cameras, facilitate the evaluation of colostrum quality and the condition of newborns. Sows at risk of PDS must be identified and examined within the initial 3 days postpartum. Hungry and vocal piglets exhibiting active nursing behavior indicate PDS. The precise etiology of PDS must be identified for appropriate intervention. Acute endometritis is characterized by copious vaginal discharge and is most accurately detected with ultrasonography. Inspection and palpation of the mammary gland, along with an assessment of the sow's behavior, are the most effective methods for diagnosing mastitis. Cystitis can be detected through macroscopic urine assessment and urine dipstick testing. Urine and vaginal discharge samples may be submitted for bacteriological analysis if necessary. In the absence of indications of mastitis, cystitis, and endometritis, the underlying reason may be constipation.

REFERENCES

1. Oliviero C, Junnikkala S, Peltoniemi OAT. The challenge of large litters on the immune system of the sow and the piglets. Reproduction in Domestic Animals. 2019;54:12-21. DOI: 10.1111/ rda.13463

2. Edwards SA, Baxter EM. Piglet mortality: Causes and prevention. In: Farmer C, editor. The Gestating and Lactating Sow. Wageningen, The Netherlands: Wageningen Academic Publishers; 2015. pp. 169-217. DOI: 10.3920/978-90-8686-803-2_11

3. Björkman S, Oliviero C, Kauffold J, Soede NM, Peltoniemi OAT. Prolonged parturition and impaired placenta expulsion increase the risk of postpartum

metritis and delay uterine involution in sows. Theriogenology. 2018;106:87-92. DOI: 10.1016/j. theriogenology.2017.10.003

4. Hoy S. The impact of puerperal diseases in sows on their fertility and health up to next farrowing. Animal Science. 2016;82(5):701-704. DOI: 10.1079/ASC200670
5. Andersson E, Frössling J, Engblom L, Algers B, Gunnarsson S. Impact of litter size on sow stayability in Swedish commercial piglet producing herds. Acta Veterinaria Scandinavica. 2015;58(1):31. DOI: 10.1186/s13028-016-0213-8
6. Oliviero C. Successful farrowing in sows [thesis]. Helsinki, Finland: Helsinki University Printing House; 2010. ISBN 978-952-92-7637-0
7. Björkman S. Parturition and subsequent uterine health and fertility in sows [thesis]. Helsinki, Finland: Helsinki University Printing House; 2017. ISBN 978-951-51-3666-4
8. Jackson PG. Dystocia in the sow. In: Jackson PG, editor. Handbook of Veterinary Obstetrics. 2nd ed. Edinburgh, UK: Elsevier Ltd; 2004. pp. 129-140
9. Waldmann KH. Schwein. In: Busch W, Schulz J, editors. Geburtshilfe bei Haustieren. 1st ed. Stuttgart, Germany: Enke Verlag; 2008. pp. 461-474
10. Oliviero C, Heinonen M, Valros A, Hälli O, Peltoniemi OAT. Effect of the environment on the physiology of the sow during late pregnancy, farrowing and early lactation. Animal Reproduction Science. 2008;105(3-4):365-377. DOI: 10.1016/j. anireprosci.2007.03.015
11. Oliviero C, Heinonen M, Valros A, Peltoniemi OAT. Environmental and sow-related factors affecting the duration of farrowing. Animal Reproduction science. 2010;119(1-2):85-91. DOI: 10.1016/j.
12. Anireprosci.2009.12.009 Peltoniemi OAT, Björkman S, Oliviero C. Disorders of parturition and the puerperium in the gilt and sow. In: Noakes D, Parkinson T, England G, editors. Veterinary Reproduction and Obstetrics. 10th ed. Edinburgh, UK: Elsevier Ltd; 2018. pp. 315-325
13. Farmer C, Hurley WL. Mammary development. In: Farmer C, editor. The Gestating and Lactating Sow. Wageningen, The Netherlands: Wageningen Academic Publishers; 2015. pp. 193-216. DOI: 10.3920/978-90-8686-803-2_4
14. Devillers N, Le Dividich J, Prunier A. Influence of colostrum intake on piglet survival and immunity. Animal. 2011;5(10):1605-1612. DOI: 10.1017/S175173111100067X
15. Quesnel H. Colostrum production by sows: Variability of colostrum yield and immunoglobulin G concentrations. Animal. 2011;5(10):1546-1553. DOI: 10.1017/S175173111100070X

16. Devillers N, Farmer C, Le Dividich J, Prunier A. Variability of colostrum yield and colostrum intake in pigs. Animal. 2007;1(7):1033-1041. DOI: 10.1017/S175173110700016X

17. Andersen IL, Nævdal E, Bøe KE. Maternal investment, sibling competition, and offspring survival with increasing litter size and parity in pigs (Sus scrofa). Behavioral Ecology and Sociobiology. 2011;65(6):1159-1167. DOI: 10.1007/s00265-010-1128-4

18. Le Dividich J, Rooke JA, Herpin P. Nutritional and immunological importance of colostrum for the newborn pig. The Journal of Agricultural Science. 2005;143(6):469-485. DOI: 10.1017/S0021859605005642

19. Rooke JA, Bland IM. The acquisition of passive immunity in the newborn piglet. Livestock Production Science. 2002;78(1):13-23. DOI: 10.1016/ S0301-6226(02)00182-3

20. Vallet JL, Miles JR, Rempel LA. A simple novel measure of passive transfer of maternal immunoglobulin is predictive of preweaning mortality in piglets. The Veterinary Journal. 2013;195(1):91-97. DOI: 10.1016/j. tvjl.2012.06.009

21. Maes D, Papadopoulos G, Cools A, Janssens GP. Postpartum dysgalactia in sows: Pathophysiology and risk factors. Tierärztliche Praxis Ausgabe G: Großtiere/ Nutztiere. 2010;38(1):15-20

22. Dee SA. Porcine urogenital disease. The Veterinary Clinics of North America. Food Animal Practice. 1992;8(3):641-660. DOI: 10.1016/ s0749-0720(15)30709-x

23. Kaiser M, Jacobsen S, Andersen PH, Bækbo P, Cerón JJ, Dahl J, et al. Hormonal and metabolic indicators before and after farrowing in sows affected with postpartum dysgalactia syndrome. BMC Veterinary Research. 2018;14(1):334. DOI: 10.1186/ s12917-018-1649-z

24. Tummaruk P, Sang-Gassanee K. Effect of farrowing duration, parity number and the type of antiinflammatory drug on postparturient disorders in sows: A clinical study. Tropical Animal Health and Production. 2013;45(4):1071-1077. DOI: 10.1007/ s11250-012-0315-x

25. Bostedt H, Maier G, Herfen K, Hospes R. Clinical examinations of gilts with puerperal septicemia and toxemia. Tierarztliche Praxis. Ausgabe G, Grosstiere/ Nutztiere. 1998;26(6):332-338

26. Oliviero C, Kothe S, Heinonen M, Valros A, Peltoniemi O. Prolonged duration of farrowing is associated with subsequent decreased fertility in sows. Theriogenology. 2013;79(7):1095-1099. DOI: 10.1016/j. theriogenology.2013.02.005

27. Yun J, Valros A. Benefits of prepartum nest-building behaviour on parturition and lactation in sows—A review. Asian-Australasian Journal of Animal Sciences. 2015;28(11):1519- 1524. DOI: 10.5713/ajas.15.0174

28. Douglas AJ, Neumann I, Meeren HK, Leng G, Johnstone LE, Munro G, et al. Central endogenous opioid inhibition of supraoptic oxytocin neurons in pregnant rats. Journal of Neuroscience. 1995;15(7):5049-5057. DOI: 10.1523/JNEUROSCI.15-07-05049.1995

29. Algers B, Uvnäs-Moberg K. Maternal behavior in pigs. Hormones and Behavior. 2007;52(1):78-85. DOI: 10.1016/j.yhbeh.2007.03.022

30. Quesnel H, Farmer C, Theil PK. Colostrum and milk production. In: Farmer C, editor. The Gestating and Lactating Sow. Wageningen, The Netherlands: Wageningen Academic Publishers; 2015. pp. 173-192. DOI: 10.3920/978-90-8686-803-2_8

31. Foisnet A, Farmer C, David C, Quesnel H. Relationships between colostrum production by primiparous sows and sow physiology around parturition. Journal of Animal Science. 2010;88(5):1672-1683. DOI: 10.2527/ jas.2009-2562

32. Yun J, Swan KM, Vienola K, Kim YY, Oliviero C, Peltoniemi OAT, et al. Farrowing environment has an impact on sow metabolic status and piglet colostrum intake in early lactation. Livestock Science. 2014;163:120-125. DOI: 10.1016/j.livsci.2014.02.014

33. Nachreiner RF, Ginther OJ. Induction of agalactia by administration of endotoxin (Escherichia coli) in swine. American Journal of Veterinary Research. 1974;35:619-622

34. Oravainen J, Heinonen M, Tast A, Virolainen JV, Peltoniemi OAT. Vulvar discharge syndrome in loosely housed Finnish pigs: Prevalence and evaluation of vaginoscopy, bacteriology and cytology. Reproduction in Domestic Animals. 2008;43(1):42-47. DOI: 10.1111/j.1439-0531.2007.00852.x

35. Gerjets I, Kemper N. Coliform mastitis in sows: A review. Journal of Swine Health and Production. 2009;17(2):97-105

36. Hultén F, Persson A, Eliasson- Selling L, Heldmer E, Lindberg M, Sjögren U, et al. Evaluation of environmental and management-related risk factors associated with chronic mastitis in sows. American Journal of Veterinary Research. 2004;65(10):1398- 1403. DOI: 10.2460/ajvr.2004.65.1398

37. Quiniou N, Noblet J. Influence of high ambient temperatures on performance of multiparous lactating sows. Journal of Animal Science. 1999;77(8):2124-2134. DOI: 10.2527/1999.7782124x

38. Papadopoulos GA, Vanderhaeghe C, Janssens GP, Dewulf J, Maes DG. Risk factors associated with postpartum dysgalactia syndrome in sows. The Veterinary Journal. 2010;184(2):167- 171. DOI: 10.1016/j.tvjl.2009.01.010

39. Farmer C, Quesnel H. Nutritional, hormonal, and environmental effects on colostrum in sows. Journal of Animal Science. 2009;87(13):56-64. DOI: 10.2527/jas.2008-1203

40. Göransson L. The effect of feed allowance in late pregnancy on the occurrence of agalactia post partum in the sow. Journal of Veterinary Medicine Series A. 1989;36(1-10):505-513. DOI: 10.1111/j.1439-0442.1989.tb00760.x

41. Martineau GP, Smith BB, Doizé B. Pathogenesis, prevention, and treatment of lactational insufficiency in sows. Veterinary Clinics of North America: Food Animal Practice. 1992;8(3):661-684. DOI: 10.1016/ S0749-0720(15)30710-6

42. Leng G, Mansfield S, Bicknell RJ, Brown D, Chapman C, Hollingsworth S, et al. Stress-induced disruption of parturition in the rat may be mediated by endogenous opioids. Journal of Endocrinology. 1987;114(2):247-252. DOI: 10.1677/joe.0.1140247

43. Oliviero C, Kokkonen T, Heinonen M, Sankari S, Peltoniemi OAT. Feeding sows with high fibre diet around farrowing and early lactation: Impact on intestinal activity, energy balance related parameters and litter performance. Research in Veterinary Science. 2009;86(2):314-319. DOI: 10.1016/j.rvsc.2008.07.007

44. Weldon WC, Thulin AJ, MacDougald OA, Johnston LJ, Miller ER, Tucker HA. Effects of increased dietary energy and protein during late gestation on mammary development in gilts. Journal of Animal Science. 1991;69(1):194-200. DOI: 10.2527/ 1991.691194x

45. Loisel F, Farmer C, Ramaekers P, Quesnel H. Colostrum yield and piglet growth during lactation are related to gilt metabolic and hepatic status prepartum. Journal of Animal Science. 2014;92(7):2931-2941. DOI: 10.2527/ jas.2013-7472

46. Decaluwe R, Maes D, Declerck I, Cools A, Wuyts B, De Smet S, et al. Changes in back fat thickness during late gestation predict colostrum yield in sows. Animal. 2013;7(12):1999-2007. DOI: 10.1017/S1751731113001791

47. Einarsson S, Rojkittikhun T. Effects of nutrition on pregnant and lactating sows. Journal of Reproduction and Fertility. 1993;48:229-239

48. Björkman S, Grahofer A, Han T, Oliviero C, Peltoniemi OAT. Severe udder edema as a cause of reduced colostrum quality and milk production in sows—A case report. In: 10th European Symposium of Porcine Health Management; 9-11 May 2018; Barcelona, Spain. pp. 110-111

49. Björkman S, Oliviero C, Hasan SMK, Peltoniemi OAT. Mammary gland edema as a cause of postpartum dysgalactia in the sow—A case report. Reproduction in Domestic Animals. 2017;52:72. DOI: 10.1111/rda.13026

50. Quesnel H, Meunier-Salaun MC, Hamard A, Guillemet R, Etienne M, Farmer C, et al. Dietary fiber for pregnant sows: Influence on sow physiology and performance during lactation. Journal of Animal Science. 2009;87(2):532-543. DOI: 10.2527/ jas.2008-1231

51. Feyera T, Pedersen TF, Krogh U, Foldager L, Theil PK. Impact of sow energy status during farrowing on farrowing kinetics, frequency of stillborn piglets, and farrowing assistance. Journal of Animal Science. 2018;96(6):2320- 2331. DOI: 10.1093/jas/sky141

52. Vasdal G, Andersen IL. A note on teat accessibility and sow parity—Consequences for newborn piglets. Livestock Science. 2012;146(1):91-94. DOI: 10.1016/j.livsci.2012.02.005

53. Alexopoulos JG, Lines DS, Hallett S, Plush KJ. A review of success factors for piglet fostering in lactation. Animals. 2018;8(3):38. DOI: 10.3390/ani8030038

54. Balzani A, Cordell HJ, Edwards SA. Relationship of sow udder morphology with piglet suckling behavior and teat access. Theriogenology. 2016;86(8):1913-1920. DOI: 10.1016/j.theriogenology.2016.06.007

55. Peltoniemi O, Björkman S, Oropeza-Moe M, Oliviero C. Developments of reproductive management and biotechnology in the pig. Animal Reproduction. 2019;16(3):524-538. DOI: 10.21451/1984-3143-ar2019-0055

56. Holyoake PK, Dial GD, Trigg T, King VL. Reducing pig mortality through supervision during the perinatal period. Journal of Animal Science. 1995;73(12):3543-3551. DOI. DOI: 10.2527/1995.73123543x

57. Vanderhaeghe C, Dewulf J, De Vliegher S, Papadopoulos GA, de Kruif A, Maes D. Longitudinal field study to assess sow level risk factors associated with stillborn piglets. Animal Reproduction Science. 2010;120(1-4):78-83. DOI: 10.1016/j. anireprosci.2010.02.010

58. Yun J, Han T, Björkman S, Nystén M, Hasan SMK, Valros A, et al. Factors affecting piglet mortality during the first 24 h after the onset of parturition in large litters: Effects of farrowing housing on behaviour of postpartum sows. Animal. 2019;13(5):1045-1053. DOI: 10.1017/S1751731118002549

59. Kauffold J, Peltoniemi O, Wehrend A, Althouse GC. Principles and clinical uses of real-time ultrasonography in female swine reproduction. Animals. 2019;9(11):950. DOI: 10.1016/j. theriogenology.2006.12.005

60. Björkman S, Oliviero C, Rajala-Schultz PJ, Soede NM, Peltoniemi OAT. The effect of litter size, parity and farrowing duration on placenta expulsion and retention in sows. Theriogenology. 2017;92:36-44. DOI: 10.1016/j.theriogenology.2017.01.003

61. Straw BE, Bush EJ, Dewey CE. Types and doses of injectable medications given to periparturient sows. Journal of the American Veterinary Medical Association. 2000;216(4):510-515. DOI: 10.2460/javma.2000.216.510

62. Taverne MAM, Van Der Weijden GC. Parturition in domestic animals: Targets for future research. Reproduction in Domestic Animals. 2008;43:36-42. DOI: 10.1111/j.1439-0531.2008.01219.x

63. Mota-Rojas D, Martínez-Burnes J, Trujillo-Ortega ME, Alonso-Spilsbury ML, Ramírez-Necoechea R, López A. Effect of oxytocin treatment in sows on umbilical cord morphology, meconium staining, and neonatal mortality of piglets. American Journal of Veterinary Research. 2002;63(11):1571-1574. DOI: 10.2460/ajvr.2002.63.1571

64. Mota-Rojas D, Martínez-Burnes J, Trujillo ME, López A, Rosales AM, Ramírez R, et al. Uterine and fetal asphyxia monitoring in parturient sows treated with oxytocin. Animal Reproduction Science. 2005;86(1-2):131-141. DOI: 10.1016/j.anireprosci.2004.06.004

65. Mota-Rojas D, Villanueva-García D, Velázquez-ArmentaEY,Nava-OcampoAA, Ramírez-Necoechea R, Alonso- Spilsbury M, et al. Influence of time at which oxytocin is administered during labor on uterine activity and perinatal death in pigs. Biological Research. 2007;40(1):55-63. DOI: 10.4067/ S0716-97602007000100006

66. Chantaraprateep P, Prateep P, Lohachit C, Kunavongkrit A, Poomsuwan P. Investigation into the use of prostaglandin F2α (PGF2α:) and oxytocin for the induction of farrowing. Australian Veterinary Journal. 1986;63(8):254-256. DOI: 10.1111/j.1751- 0813.1986.tb02988.x

67. Dial GD, Almond GW, Hilley HD, Repasky RR, Hagan J. Oxytocin precipitation of prostaglandin-induced farrowing in swine: Determination of the optimal dose of oxytocin and optimal interval between prostaglandin F2 alpha and oxytocin. American Journal of Veterinary Research. 1987;48(6):966-970

68. Randall GC. Observations on parturition in the sow. II. Factors influencing stillbirth and perinatal mortality. The Veterinary Record. 1972;90(7):183-186. DOI: 10.1136/ vr.90.7.183

69. Tucker JM, Hauth JC. Intrapartum assessment of fetal well-being. Clinical Obstetrics and Gynecology. 1990;33(3):515-525

70. Hasan SMK, Junnikkala S, Valros A, Peltoniemi OAT, Oliviero C. Validation of Brix refractometer to estimate colostrum immunoglobulin G content and composition in the sow. Animal. 2016;10(10):1728-1733. DOI: 10.1017/S1751731116000896

71. Balzani A, Cordell HJ, Edwards SA. Evaluation of an on-farm method to assess colostrum IgG content in sows. Animal. 2016;10(4):643-648. DOI: 10.1017/S1751731115002451

72. Baxter EM, Jarvis S, D'eath RB, Ross DW, Robson SK, Farish M, et al. Investigating the behavioural and physiological indicators of neonatal survival in pigs. Theriogenology. 2008;69(6):773-783. DOI: 10.1016/j.theriogenology.2007.12.007

73. Santiago PR, Martínez-Burnes J, Mayagoitia AL, Ramírez-Necoechea R, Mota-Rojas D. Relationship of vitality and weight with the temperature of newborn piglets born to sows of different parity. Livestock Science. 2019;220:26-31. DOI: 10.1016/j. livsci.2018.12.011

74. Zhang Z, Zhang H, Liu T. Study on body temperature detection of pig based on infrared technology: A review. Artificial Intelligence in Agriculture. 2019;1:14-26. DOI: 10.1016/j. aiia.2019.02.002

75. Devillers N, Van Milgen J, Prunier A, Le Dividich J. Estimation of colostrum intake in the neonatal pig. Animal Science. 2004;78(2):305-313. DOI: 10.1017/S1357729800054096

76. Farmer C, Lessard M, Knight CH, Quesnel H. Oxytocin injections in the postpartal period affect mammary tight junctions in sows. Journal of Animal Science. 2017;95(8):3532-3539. DOI: 10.2527/jas.2017.1700

77. Björkman S, Han T, Nysten M, Peltoniemi O. Heat detection and insemination of sows with previous puerperal disorders. Reproduction in Domestic Animals. 2019;54:59. DOI: 10.1111/rda.13525

78. Grahofer A, Mäder T, Meile A, Nathues H. Detection and evaluation of puerperal disorders in sows after farrowing. Reproduction in Domestic Animals. 2019;54:59. DOI: 10.1111/ rda.13525

79. Stiehler T, Heuwieser W, Pfuetzner A, Burfeind O. The course of rectal and vaginal temperature in early postpartum sows. Journal of Swine Health and Production. 2015;23(2):72-83

80. Mead J, Bonmarito CL. Reliability of rectal temperatures as an index of internal body temperature. Journal of Applied Physiology. 1949;2(2):97-109. DOI: 10.1152/jappl.1949.2.2.97

81. Rotello LC, Crawford L, Terndrup TE. Comparison of infrared ear thermometer derived and equilibrated rectal temperatures in estimating pulmonary artery temperatures. Critical Care Medicine. 1996;24(9):1501-1506

82. Nachreiner RF, Ginther OJ. Gestational and periparturient periods of sows: Serum chemical, hematologic, and clinical changes during the periparturient period. American Journal of Veterinary Research. 1972;33(11):2233-2238

83. Hermansson I, Einarsson S, Larsson K, Bäckström L. On the agalactia post partum in the sow. A clinical study. Nordisk Veterinaermedicin. 1978;30(11):465-473

84. Madec F, Leon E. Farrowing disorders in the sow: A field study. Journal of Veterinary Medicine Series A. 1992;39(1-10):433-444. DOI: 10.1111/ j.1439-0442.1992.tb00202.x

85. Noakes D. Physiology of the puerperium. In: Noakes D, Parkinson T, England G, editors. Veterinary Reproduction and Obstetrics. 10th ed. Edinburgh, UK: Elsevier Ltd; 2018.pp. 148-156

86. Muirhead MR. Epidemiology and control of vaginal discharges in the sow after service. The Veterinary Record. 1986;119(10):233-235. DOI: 10.1136/ vr.119.10.233

87. Kauffold J, Althouse GC. An update on the use of B-mode ultrasonography in female pig reproduction. Theriogenology. 2007;67(5):901-911. DOI: 10.1016/j. theriogenology.2006.12.005

88. Grahofer A, Meile A, Nathues H. Postpartum uterine involution in free farrowing sows examined by ultrasound. Reproduction in Domestic Animals. 2019;54:93. DOI: 10.1111/rda.13528

89. Kauffold J, Gmeiner K, Sobiraj A, Richter A, Failing K, Wendt M. Ultrasonographic characterization of the urinary bladder in sows with and without urinary tract infection. The Veterinary Journal. 2010;183(1):103-108. DOI: 10.1016/j. tvjl.2008.09.008

90. Gmeiner K. Ultrasonographische Charakterisierung der gesunden und kranken Harnblase bei der Sau [thesis]. Leipzig, Germany: Veterinärmedizinische Fakultät der Universität Leipzig; 2007

91. Grahofer A, Sipos S, Fischer L, Entenfellner F, Sipos W. 6th European Symposium of Porcine Health Management; 7-9 May 2014; Sorrento, Italy. p. 126

92. Kraft W, Dürr UM, Fürll M, Bostedt H, Heinritzi K. Harnapparat. In: Kraft W, Dürr UM, editors. Klinische Labordiagnostik in der Tiermedizin. 6th ed. Stuttgart, Germany: Schattauer; 2005. pp. 186-217

93. Bellino C, Gianella P, Grattarola C, Miniscalco B, Tursi M, Dondo A, et al. Urinary tract infections in sows in Italy: Accuracy of urinalysis and urine

culture against histological findings. Veterinary Record. 2013: vetrec-2012. DOI: 10.1136/ vr.101219

94. Tolstrup LK. Cystitis in sows— Prevalence, diagnosis and reproductive effect [thesis]. Graduate School of Health and Medical Sciences: University of Copenhagen; 2017

95. Becker HA, Kurtz R, Mickwitz G. Chronische Harnwegsinfektionen beim Schwein. Diagnose und Therapie. Praktischer Tierarzt. 1985;12:1006-1011

96. Waldmann KH, Wendt M. Lehrbuch der Schweinekrankheiten. 4th ed. Stuttgart, Germany: Parey Verlag; 2001. p. 608

97. Baer C, Bilkei G. Ultrasonographic and gross pathological findings in the mammary glands of weaned sows having suffered recidiving mastitis metritis agalactia. Reproduction in Domestic Animals. 2005;40(6):544-547. DOI: 10.1111/j.1439-0531.2005.00629.x

6 Chapter THE LIDIA BREED: ADMINISTRATION AND HEALTHCARE

1. INTRODUCTION: AN OVERVIEW

Lidia's cattle breeding remains one of the most authentic sectors of animal production, owing to the unique ethological traits of this breed and the distinctiveness of the production method and the resulting product, specifically animals appropriate for exhibition. [1].

Spain is the first Lidia cattle breeding country and has the most varied and important genetic heritage of this breed [2] that is also present in Portugal, southern France, and much of South America such as Mexico, Colombia, Venezuela, Peru, and Ecuador [3].

Lidia cattle sector represents in Spain a socioeconomic activity of considerable importance, with a total turnover of approximately 1.5 billion euros per year, which does not only affect entrepreneurs, ranchers, and bullfighters, but also more than 200,000 jobs that depend directly or indirectly on the bullfighting activities [4], which constitute the second mass spectacle of Spain and Portugal [5]. Lidia cattle, the second pure breed in the bovine census in Spain [6], are considered the greatest exponent of an extensive breeding system, due to their ethological characteristics, the need for wide spaces, and the difficulty in handling that it presents [7]. In turn, it is a breed of great rusticity, able to adapt and take advantage of all types of terrain, including those of extreme weather conditions [8]. Many farms are located in territories of high landscape value such as natural parks, playing an important role in maintaining biodiversity and contributing to the conservation of the ecosystem [9].

The characteristics of a Lidia standard farm are an average size of 253 mother cows and a total number of heads of 748 animals, including animals of other breeds or those belonging to other species, necessaries for livestock's handling, with an annual replacement rate of 12% [10]. However, after the economic crisis of 2008, most livestock farms have decreased the number of heads. Nevertheless, the livestock internal distribution remains stable. For a Lidia cattle farm of 100 mother cows, the ideal average internal scheme, considering the different types of animals classified by sex and age, could be the one presented in Table 1 [11].

Table 1. Internal distribution of a standard Lidia farm considering the different types of animals classified by sex and age [11].

Sires	3
Cows	100
Calf male <1 year	40
Males 1–2 years	38
Males 2–3 years	36
Males 3–4 years	35
Bulls 4–6 years	34
Calf female <1 year	40
Heifers 1–2 years	36
Heifers 2–3 years	20
Halters	12

The standard farm has a number of hectares ranging from 586 to 721, of which 92% of the land is used as pastures [12].

2. FEED MANAGEMENT

Today, the farming system of the Lidia breed continues to be, mainly, an extensive management system that has gradually adapted to new grazing techniques and food supplementation in times of natural grass decline, such as winter and summer, in dry climates [13]. The extension of the farms is still remarkable, but of much less spacious than that of several decades ago and in terms of quality, the brave cattle have been relegated to less productive and more stepped mountain farms in favor of agriculture or other more profitable species, such as the Iberian pig in Spain and Portugal [7]. In Mexico, most farms are located in the central part of the country, with a dry climate similar to Spain, carrying out similar feeding management. On the other hand, Lidia cattle in Colombia, Venezuela, Ecuador, and Peru are in territories with a tropical climate, whose diet is based on natural grass with a concentrated supplementation during the last stage of preparing the males for the show [14].

2.1 Cow feeding

The Lidia cow is a very rustic animal, of few requirements, since its small size also dictated its nutritional needs. Even so, adequate feeding is essential to obtain a good fertility rate, avoiding abortions and perinatal mortality, and, after a good lactation, wean the calf in an optimal state [7, 15]. Currently, the use of natural resources is maximized, preferably by grazing and the supplementation of hay or silage, and if necessary, concentrated food is used at a rate of 2–4 kg/day, depending on the richness of the grass and forage [16, 17].

2.2 Feeding of young animals

During the first 3–4 months, calves are fed exclusively with cow's milk and develop optimal growth, as long as it comes from a well-fed cow that produces milk of adequate quality and quantity.

After weaning, and when the animals are between 9 and 10 months old, they are usually supplemented in times of shortage of grass with rations whose fundamental components are fibrous products (beet and citrus pulps, dehydrated or henified alfalfa, and cereal straw), industrial by-products (gluten-feed, wheat bran, soy cake, and beet molasses), and common products in the composition of concentrates of other types of farm animals (corn, barley, wheat, and sunflower meal).

Galvanized iron feeders are frequently used, 5 m long by 40 cm wide approximately, which allow to guarantee half a meter of free space per animal, avoiding hierarchy problems, present in any group of this breed, which could result in some type of undernourishment particularly important in this stage of development.

Likewise, several water points distributed along the fenced space must be installed, arranged around the feeder area, to favor the movement of animals across different areas and to avoid their concentration in one point.

When the animals are around 23 months of age, they are slowly provided, during 4 weeks of adaptation, an increasing proportion of the ration designed for adult animals of 3 and 4 years, in order to adapt them to the finishing feeding diet composition.

Livestock facilities used for these animals have similar characteristics to the ones described for young animals, although in case of using individual feeders, the number of feeders is usually 10% greater than the number of animals to be fed [18]. Also, the different water points are often installed at a greater separation distance from the feeders (at least 500 m), to facilitate a better distribution throughout the land surface. As in previous phases, a supplementation is necessary, which as an example could be based on the addition of 0.5 kg of alfalfa hay to the total supplementation established in the previous phase, thus leaving 2.5 kg of alfalfa hay added to 0.5 kg of concentrate per animal per day [15].

2.3 Bull feeding (4–5 years)

The feeding systems described during the 1980s based on a final bait are still in force today. Although each farmer has its own feeding methodology, depending on the availability of grass and other types of food on the farm, the possibility of growing the forage or concentrate on the farm itself or the use of agricultural byproducts such as citrus pulp or some derived from the olive oil industry.

This final bait is carried out in fenced areas of small size, frequently without grass, with a daily supply of rations of high energy concentration and high digestibility [19]. This last feeding stage is called "pre-lidia bait" or "finishing," and it can vary between 5 and 12 months and usually begins during the winter [20], adapting the amount of ration supplied to the bulls at the date on which they have to fight.

The average fenced area used for these bulls is usually around 60 hectares per farm, and the average number of animals per enclosure is 20 (which is equivalent to a density of 3 hectares per bull), although each farm distributes its animals in a way different. The average daily gain (GMD) is approximately 450 g/day (Figure 1), which means that in this period, the bulls gain about 150 kg of weight, 30% of their final body weight, considering a standard bull of 500 kg of weight at 4 years of age [7].

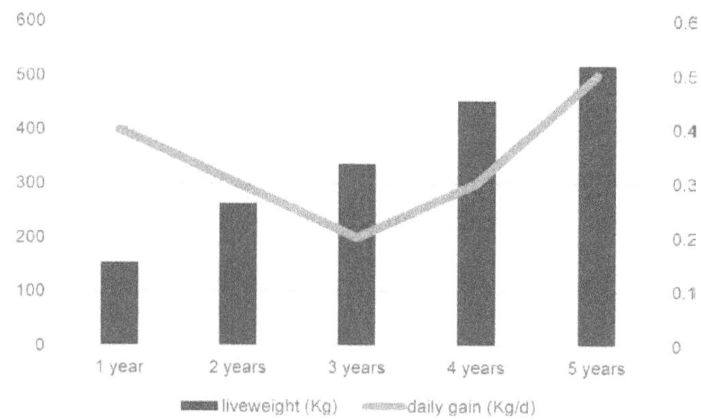

Figure 1. Lidia bull growth estimation [9].

The use of long feeders is common, especially in southern Spain, compared to the classic individual and small feeder used in farms located on the center of Spain (Figure 2). The distribution of food is done during the morning and the afternoon in most of the farms [21].

There is a critical point in the strategy of feeding management, due to the overfeeding carried out during the last year, prior to the fight, which causes an overload of weight in the bone structure, added to the state of obesity that causes a lack of strength and mobility of the animal that limits its behavior in the arena and, therefore, the show itself.

The problem lies in the overfeeding to which it is subjected in the final phase of its growth during variable periods of time (from 8 to 12 months) that generates a series of pathologies and inconveniences that negatively influence its productive aptitude: the behavior in the ring.

Several studies have been carried out on the effect of intensive bait on rumen physiology of Lidia cattle [16, 20, 22–31], and all of them point to ruminal acidosis, a primary pathology that predisposes the appearance of secondary lesions such as liver abscesses, gastrointestinal ulcers, ruminal parakeratosis, laminitis, anthill, and so on. Later we will address this pathology more widely.

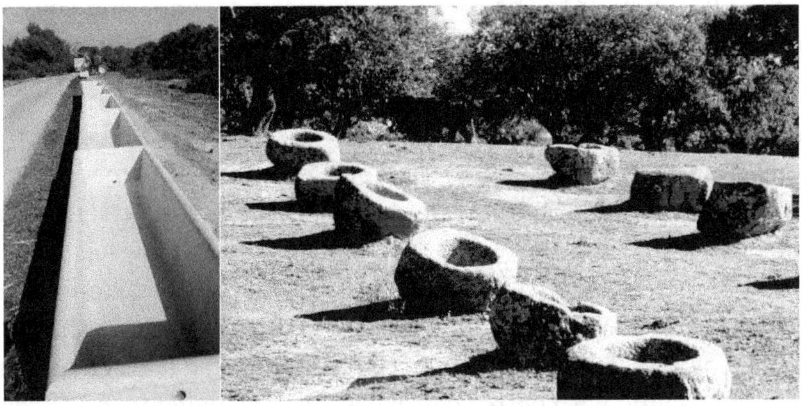

Figure 2. Long feeder and single feeders.

3. REPRODUCTIVE MANAGEMENT

Lidia females reach puberty at approximately 12 months of age but must reach the two-third of adult body weight before becoming pregnant [7] at approximately 2 years of age, and the productive lifespan time lasts for 8–10 years with a calvinggestation interval of 2–4 months [32].

Lidia bulls begin to show sexual activity from 6 months of age reaching puberty at 10–12 months, having been necessary to separate them from females before 1-year olds [7]. At 2 or 3 years, the selected sires are tested with a small group of females, but they are not profusely used until their female offspring are tested, and the quality of their genetic is proved, once this happens, they could be 15 years contributing its genetic flow in natural mating to the cattle ranch [32].

At present, in the majority of Lidia farms, the reproductive handling is very traditional with natural mating of one sire and 30–40 cows during several months. The outstanding difference with the past management is that now the fertility is greater due to a better cow's body condition that allows them to perform a successful gestation and lactation every year [33] (Figures 3 and 4).

In Europe, the duration of the mating period in Lidia cattle is similar to that of other extensive bovine breeds, being able to reach up to 8 months (autumn–spring) in livestock farms with longer periods, but its duration is often shorter, from the end of winter to the beginning of summer (March–July), since at this time, the best results are obtained in heat of the cows and fertility, due to both photoperiod and feeding reasons. In countries as Colombia without reproductive stations, the cycle is continuous.

There are relevant anatomical differences in the reproductive system of the female of the Lidia cattle: the cervix is longer in length than other bovine breeds; they present a uterine body very short, and it seems as nonexistent during transrectal palpation [34]. It is similar to the bipartite uterus in rodents, and the ovary has a very small size compared to other breeds of similar size presenting at the oviduct level the largest infundibulum that surrounds much of the ovary [35].

At the same time, there are hormonal differences because the Lidia cow reaches puberty earlier and has a shorter gestation period than other breeds: 286 days [36]. The natural mating should last long enough to guarantee a good fertility rate, with a minimum recommended period of 3–4 months (each cow has at least three opportunities to get pregnant), but there are farmers who extend it more, and there are even systems with continuous natural mating, more common in tropical countries like Colombia. Short mating periods have the advantage of being able to concentrate the calving with better control of herd management and feeding. It is done more in larger herds, in large areas, where lactation is adapted to times of pasture abundance.

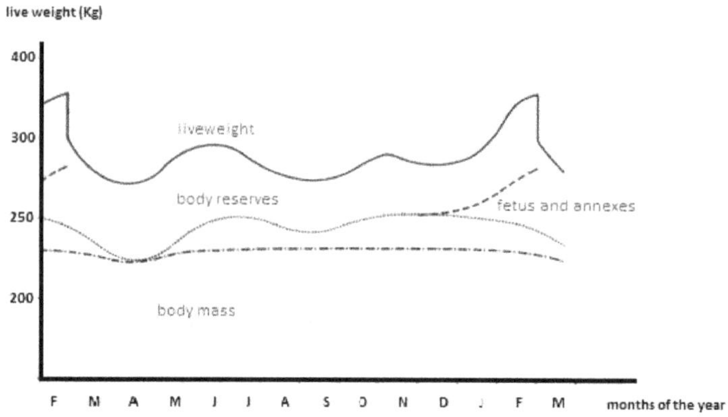

Figure 3. Live weight variation of a Lidia cow [23].

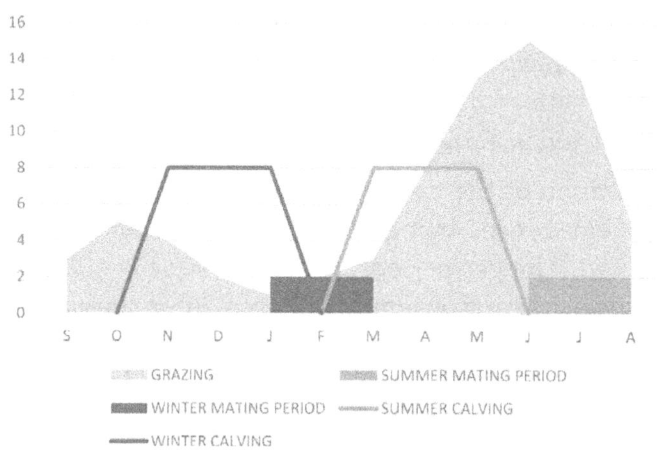

Figure 4. Calving and natural mating management based on grazing availability in seasonal countries.

The utilization of techniques for semen collection and conservation for artificial insemination (AI) began to be used three decades ago in Lidia bulls. Later, embryo-transfer from high genetic merit Lidia cows to dairy cattle and cloning of one sire to preserve the excellent genetic quality was achieved. These reproductive methods, used to improve the productive characteristic of dairy and beef cattle, could be useful future tools to increase the genetic progress in Lidia cattle behavior selection [37].

There are immense advantages in using cryopreservation, due to semen dilution and conservation during medium and large periods, increasing the possibilities to use it for decades through AI when the behavioral results of their offspring are well known. There is also the possibility to extract post-mortem semen from the epididymis after the fight in the bulls of extraordinary behavior [38]. In this way, each farmer begins to have his own semen bank of his own sires and bulls. In turn, this would allow the exchange of semen between breeders, to refresh the blood of their livestock, being easy to transport to farms located in the countries of America. Among the advantages of this technique are avoid risks of contagions of potential pathologies, allowing the reproduction of animals of different sizes because natural mating is not necessary, and also is not necessary to move the male, allows the collection of semen in extreme situations, and, above all, enables the possibility to use some improving individuals of a contrasted character in a large number of females [39].

The biggest problems are due to the handling difficulties of these animals due to the untidy nature of this breed. Insemination implies added high-risk management both for animals and for people that seriously conditions, from a technical and economic point of view, its generalization in the Lidia cattle [37]. The introduction of other reproductive techniques such as early pregnancy diagnosis allows to discover and treat uterine pathologies, helping to detect nonpregnant cows that could be resynchronized or intended for natural mating and reducing calving pregnancy intervals. Reproduction control does not necessarily imply the hormonal treatment of all animals nor their subsequent insemination because it is possible to use mixed models in which the natural mating and AI are used in a complementary way [40].

Once the AI technique will be established, the next step will be to adapt an embryo transfer program to this type of cattle. Currently, it is used to preserve the valuable genetic material of small farms and to increase the reproductive efficiency of some females. In recent years, this technique has contributed to the formation of germplasm banks as genetic reserve in cases of farms with severe health problems or encastes1 in danger of extinction [35].

At the same time, the use sexed semen to obtain a greater number of males than females could create an opportunity, considering the superior economic value of those. However, its use could jeopardize the process of selection and breeding of the farms due to the fact that reducing the numbers of females could be a risk if the proper and strict selection pressure is not applied.

Regarding cloning, there are many questions about its efficacy in general and in Lidia cattle in particular. It is not known, for example, if a cloned animal can develop and interact normally with its peers in a highly hierarchical and of great rivalry environment. A cloned individual may have a poor development of the immune or cardiovascular system, and it is not known whether the libido and fertility of a future cloned breeder will be normal. At the moment, it is known that it ages quicker and has a shorter productive lifespan [41]. A cloned bull must also be tested, and in the event that his quality would be acceptable, it will be also necessary to test its offspring to see if it is able to convey his characters.

The cloning of a sire, with the aim of collect semen, may be important in the case of some farms with few breeding males or if it is an individual of outstanding genetic merit and advanced age [42]. In any case, a clone might not have the same ethological characteristics as the animal from which it proceeds, since the behavior is the consequence of its genetic background, the environment in which it develops [33] its ontogenesis or sequential development.

4. SELECTION

Traditionally, three types of selection are made: genealogical, morphological, and functional [32]. In relation to the first, the farmer systematically records information, in his own books, the lines, or families that form the basis of the genetic heritage of his livestock, as well as the results of the offspring of each generation.

This information is used to choose future breeding animals. In addition, each farm defines its morphological preferences, depending on the type it belongs to or the priorities of the owner. The selection criteria are usually higher for males than those used for females. They focus, fundamentally, on aspects related to external appearance, neck musculature conformation, bone structure and development, and so on [43]. And finally, the functional selection consists in measuring the brave character of each animal, although each farmer understands the meaning of this term in a very subjective way. A series of tests are carried out on both females and males to assess their bravery [32].

In the case of females, animals of 1, 2, or 3 years are evaluated. The test is practiced in the tienta,2 under the direction of the farmer and with the participation of professional bullfighters, trying to discover the functional performance of each animal. The behavior of each individual in each phase of the test is assessed using the horse and with the muleta. There are different parameters (prompt response, attack, fixity, mobility, nobility, fierceness, aggressiveness, repetition, and so on) that are evaluated by the farmer, to achieve a final note for each animal and, subsequently, keep the best females as breeders [44].

In the test of males, animals of 2–4 years of age are chosen, initially selecting the specimens that have obtained the best results in the genealogical and morphological tests. They are tested in a small bullring, and if the animal does not respond properly, the test is interrupted, and the bull is withdrawn and will be destined for normal fighting. Those animals initially selected, after testing the behavior of their offspring, will become part of the livestock as a sire or will be discarded, losing their value for a standard fight since they have developed sense during the test fight [32].

There is another circumstantial and sporadic form of sire selection, performed by fans and not by the farmer, which is the case of indulto.3 It occurs in the context of a bullfight where many influential factors could alter the true criteria by which a bull must be selected. Therefore, it is the breeder who will decide, later, if the animal should be used for reproductive purpose or not.

Currently, another type of selection, genetics, has been introduced by livestock associations, which has become increasingly important [9]. It consists of identifying the individuals carrying the most beneficial genes for the interest characters and using them as breeding animals to transmit them to their descendants. The way to evaluate whether or not the phenotype of an animal is a good reflection of the genes of which it is a carrier (genetic value or merit) is based on calculating the heritability of that character [45].

The capacity to transfer behavioral characters is very slow because it is limited by the production of a calf per year, at the most, as well as the complexity to accurately and quickly assess the ethological response of its products in the show [46].

According to Cañón et al. [2], many of the behavioral characters manifested by the Lidia bull, such as mobility, repetition, nobility, rhythm, and fierceness, despite its complexity and subjective assessments, if scored with enough rigor, can manifest high heritability (>0.35) that makes them susceptible to be selected in one way or another, at the choice of the farm's owner.

A very precise selection of the best individuals entails the maintenance of a population with high consanguinity; therefore, controlling it is an always necessary activity in a Lidia cattle ranch, preserving the necessary genetic variability within it. In general, in Lidia farms, the level of consanguinity does not seem to be very high: 0.12 and 0.13 [47]. Even so, it is possible to find bulls with a consanguinity coefficient of 0.25 [48]. However, regulated mating strategies should be followed, to avoid mating animals with common ancestors, establishing a shortor mediumterm conservation program. However, we must be aware of the difficulties involved in the conservation of some minority genetic lines, cattle ranches, or "encastes" [48], because the smaller a population is and the greater the imbalance between the sexes the more difficult it is to preserve their genetic characteristics, complicating the task of avoiding mating between related animals.

Finally, the incorporation of the computer methods to control the productive data of the animals allows organization and best valuation of each reproductive potential. With the information reduced to informative schemes, the results can be checked immediately, which make it possible to know, through the corresponding analysis of the offspring, the racing power of the father or mother [45, 49–51].

5. MAIN PATHOLOGIES

The most frequent diseases of Lidia cattle, which also affect extensive cattle, are parasitic processes (coccidiosis, ostertagiosis, dictyocaulosis, and sarcosporidiosis), infectious processes (clostridiosis, anthrax, paratuberculosis, tuberculosis, actinomycosis, actinobacillosis, and pyobacillosis), poisonings (aflatoxicosis, ochratoxicosis, aluminum phosphide, and lead poisoning), and deficiency processes as poliencefalomalacia [52].

In addition, the extensive nature of this animal production system predisposes him to suffer from eye problems such as infectious keratoconjunctivitis and horn wounds due to fights between animals [53]. The latter represents a very important chapter in the economies of Lidia farming assuming losses of traumatic etiology ranging from 3 to 15% of male adult individual. Most of them require surgical treatment; some of the interventions are simple, and others are more complicated, but all have in common the septic character of the traumatic focus [54].

The gorings have an etiology closely related to the age of the bulls, strength, and encaste, with an increase in frequency of incidence in 4-year-old bulls with a weight of 500 kg, and the wounds occur with a greater probability in the head and extremity regions. They are caused by external violence in which the surface of the traumatic agent is wide. We can find open or closed wounds. The closed wounds, even when not seen to affect external skin tissues, can cause internal muscular or vascular lesions. Hematomas or serous effusions (blood and lymphatic exudates) of difficult reabsorption due to their large size appear, and they require intervention. They evolve to contamination and abscess formation [55].

The treatment of all types of wounds should be focused on controlling, primarily, the bleeding, either by suturing damaged vessels or by hemostatic parenteral treatments, then preventing or controlling the infection, disinfecting and cleaning the affected area, and finally achieving the rapid healing, usually by second attempt, and is always suggested to leave a drain at the trauma point even if it is small [56].

Another pathology that has been observed with a high incidence in the Lidia breed is osteochondrosis [57]. It is a degenerative process of the joint surfaces, widely described in horses and in bait cattle of other breeds, with few studies in fighting bulls to know if it could influence the mobility of the animal during the show [27].

5.1 Ruminal acidosis (RA)

RA is a metabolic disease that settles in the rumen and is produced by the ruminal fermentation of large amounts of nonfibrous carbohydrates, such as starch and sugars, which lead to the production of high amounts of volatile fatty acids (VFAs) and lactate, which accumulate in the rumen and cause an abnormal reduction in rumen pH [58]. Ruminal epithelial cells, not protected by mucus, are vulnerable to chemical acid damage [59], and this decrease in ruminal pH together with high concentrations of VFAs causes ruminitis, erosions, and ulcerations of the ruminal epithelium. In turn, abnormal thickening of the stratum corneum of the mucosa occurs due to accumulation of corneal cells with perturbations in their keratinization resulting in hyper and parakeratosis, observing partially pigmented ruminal mucous membranes [60, 61].

Among the works carried out on the feeding management of the Lidia bull, the one carried out by Bartolomé [26] stands out because he observes 66.2% of the animals studied with ruminal pH values compatible with RA, of which 41.5% chronically (pH = 6.2–5.6) according to the classification of González et al. [62]. In addition, 70.7% of animals presented parakeratosis in the mucosa, and in 26.9% of bulls sampled, liver lesions were detected. In the same line, Lomillos et al. [27] reported a 43% reduction in the length of the ruminal papilla of bulls subjected to the finishing bait, added to an increase in the thickness of their mucosa, which approximately doubled the value obtained in the group of animals considered control, and maintained in pure extensive regime (Figures 5 and 6).

In this context, the decrease in rumen pH predisposes the epithelium to become fragile and loses its ability to act as a barrier between the ruminal environment and the blood, which predisposes the appearance of continuity solutions, which allow the passage of microorganisms toward the bloodstream and the consequent risk of suffering sepsis for the animal [60]. Among others, Fusobacterium necrophorum and Corynebacterium pyogenes, are bacteria often carried to the liver through the portal vein, and there they begin infection and abscess formation, which compromise their metabolic capacity [5]. From the liver, they can go to the peritoneum, generating peritonitis, and sometimes they can go to the lung, heart valves, kidneys, joints, and so on [63]. In this sense, García et al. [12] recorded abscesses at the liver level in 4% of the studied bulls and hepatic-diaphragmatic adhesions in 21% of cases that extended to the pulmonary pleura, confirming, after culture, Fusobacterium necrophorum as the main causative agent of lesions.

At the same time, the intense finishing feeding management based on the use of high amounts of carbohydrates is a predisposing cause of hoof lesions such as the lameness by diffuse aseptic pododermatitis observed in the animals as an excessive growth of the hoof [60] widely described in Lidia cattle [25, 29] and detected with a prevalence of 28% in the fought animals [12].

According to Nocek [64], the relationship between RA and laminitis seems to be associated with hemodynamic alterations of peripheral microcirculation.

During acidosis, as a consequence of the decrease in ruminal pH, a process of bacteriolysis takes place in the rumen, releasing vasoactive substances (histamine and endotoxins), which are absorbed through the damaged rumen wall and cause vasoconstriction and dilation, which destroy microcirculation at the level of synovial joints and chorionic tissue of the hoof [65, 66]. The combination of high concentrations of histamine in areas of terminal circulation [67], the increase in digital blood flow and high blood osmolarity induce an increase in blood pressure inside the animal's hoof, producing a serum exudate, which results in edema, internal hemorrhages from thrombosis, and finally, the expansion of the chorion, causes intense pain [60, 64]. The disease presents with signs of lameness, excessive growth of the hooves, and the appearance of dark lines or bands on the surface

of the hooves, a consequence of the ischemia generated by vascular damage and edema [68]. At present, lameness is treated with anti-inflammatories, and the hoof overgrowth is usually remedied in livestock by a functional cut of the hoof, using the cattle crush facilities to immobilize the animal.

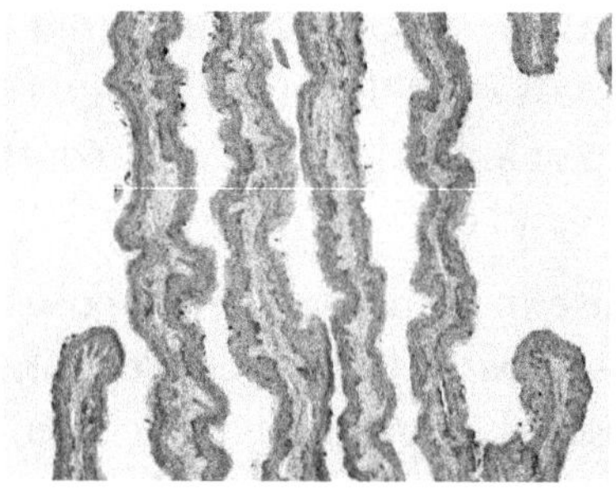

Figure 5. Normal papilla of extensive animal.

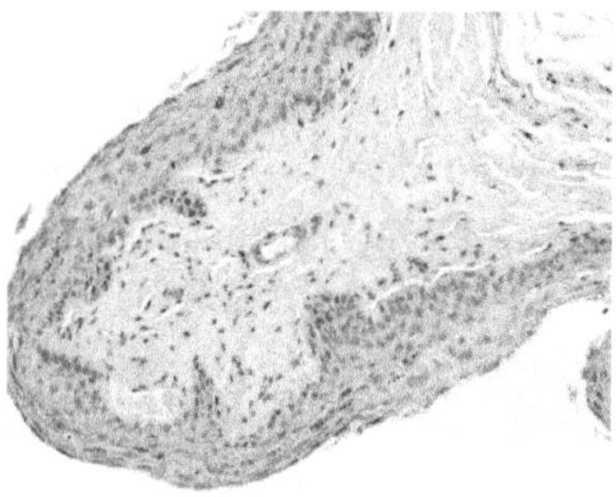

Figure 6. Thickened and shortened papilla of finished bulls [27].

It seems clear that the RA generated after the intensive bait and the pathological processes to which it predisposes or directly causes, affects the performance of the bull in the arena in the form of physical decline of the animal that hinders its ethological and physical performance [12, 20, 26, 69]. Therefore, it is of great importance to explore possible solutions or prevention strategies by designing a new food management.

To control the process, in principle, it would be enough to reduce the amount of nonfibrous carbohydrates provided with the diet, but this measure would lead to a decrease in the rations' energy level, with the consequent delay in the fattening of the bull and the consequent economic losses.

In the case of the final bull bait, improved rationing and feeding management could have a considerable impact on rumen pH stability. Adapting the ruminal environment by slowly and gradually changing from one forage feed ration to another concentrate would stimulate the development of the rumen papillae and the growth of the lactic acid transforming flora [5], in such a way so that a greater amount is metabolized and the mucosa of the rumen can absorb a greater amount of generated VFAs. This adaptation of the mucosa to concentrated rations takes approximately 4–6 weeks [64] and changes in microflora about 3 weeks [70].

The adoption of the mixed total ration type feeding system, better known as "unifeed" carriage (Figure 7), widely used in dairy cattle, ensures a balanced consumption of concentrate and forage, which is a very important advantage. In this way, it is possible to increase the energy density of the rations by reducing the risk of digestive problems [71]. In fact, in recent years, this type of food management has begun to be incorporated into the Lidia farms, mainly in farms located in the south of the peninsula, later extending through Madrid and Salamanca [72].

In this sense, the contribution of compensated and high fiber rations through the use of "unifeed" mixer cart during the bull bait does not generate a pH decrease below the physiological limits, as shown in Graph 1 that describes the pH ruminal of bulls fed following this pattern of food management for a month [31]. However, it is not clear that this handling is the solution to the RA of the bull since the use of these mixing machines during the entire bait period, which usually lasts between and 9 months, can generate lesions in the morphology of the papilla ruminal (decrease in length and thickening of the mucosa) similar to those found in animals fed through traditional feeding management. In addition, the feeding time generates a negative effect on the severity of the lesions, with the animals fed for more than 6 months being the ones with the greatest lesions at the level of the rumen mucosa [27].

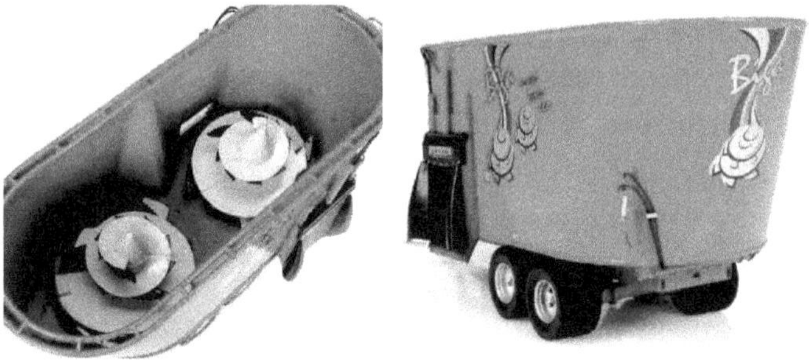

Figure 7. Small format "unifeed" mixer truck, adapted to Lidia cattle (BIGA).

Another strategy to prevent RA is the use of additives both chemical and microbial. Among the first are buffer substances such as bicarbonate, alkalizing agents such as magnesium oxide, or adjuvants such as bentonite, which can help fight RA because it absorbs part of the volatile fatty acids at the ruminal level [5, 65, 73, 74]. The most commonly used microbial additives to combat RA are yeast extracts and live yeasts.

These microorganisms help maintain ruminal pH by stimulating the growth of cellulolytic bacteria and lactic acid users, preventing their accumulation in the rumen [75].

5.2 Falling syndrome

Muscle weakness syndrome, which involves motor incoordination and transient loss of standing and balance, all encompassed under the common term of "falling syndrome," has been worrying different authors for almost a century [76]. The frequency with which this problem occurs in the arena had not become worrisome until the beginning of the last century, from the being of 1930 when the manifestation of the problem became general and the falls were more frequent and alarming [77], reaching incidence percentages in the most critical decades close to 99% [78] or 98% [26] of the sampled animals. It affects both males and females and specimens of all ages: bulls, calves, and cows [79, 80]. It is observed in individuals of different livestock farms, regardless of their weight, the category of the arena where they fought, the distance from its farm of origin [77], and, additionally, within the same livestock, the incidence of this problem can be very diverse.

Despite recent research work done in this regard, the falling syndrome of the brave bull is an issue in which consensus is not yet perceived. The theories that have come to light in order to explain the etiology of the syndrome have been very numerous and varied, without any of them providing definitive conclusions to date. The simplest attributes the problem to physical reasons such as transport trauma and intentional fraud, while others, more complex, consider that the origin of the syndrome is genetic, due to the inheritance of a gene that determines the fall [81].

However, given the appearance of the problem in cattle ranches whose original genetic distance is very wide, it is logical to assume that the appearance of this syndrome must be influenced by the action of the environment, within which food management, in addition to other factors, such as the health status of the livestock itself would play a very important role.

Nowadays, in view of the different studies carried out, it is possible to think that the falling syndrome is a multicausal problem, where we can observe some predisposing causes, such as the genetic endowment, the characteristics of the transport, the physical demands of the fight, the effect of the puya and the banderillas, the lack of functional gymnastics, nutritional deficiencies, and other more determinants, such as the possible pathological, circulatory, nervous, metabolic, endocrine, genetic, or ethological causes [76].

On the other hand, the bull is by nature a sedentary animal. In the last year of life, he is transferred to small enclosures where his chances of exercising naturally are limited and the energetic components in his diet are increased. Although cattle are not considered an athletic species, the bull is subjected to tremendous exercise in the arena, lasting approximately 20 min, maintaining a physical and metabolic effort of great intensity to which it is not accustomed [82]. These circumstances mean a lack of physical condition for the show.

This muscle weakness, manifested in the falling syndrome, is projected in various acute muscle injuries associated with intense physical exercise and in chronic muscle injuries that may result from nutrient deficiencies of selenium and vitamin E [83]. On the other hand, Aceña et al. [84] demostrated the existence of a reduction in glycogen stored and very high concentrations of lactic acid in the muscles at the end of the fight, results that indicate the existence of muscle fatigue due to physical exercise in an anaerobic situationss. Similarly, a high correlation has been observed between the main parameters indicative of metabolic acidosis (HCO -, lactate, and low blood pH) and respiratory acidosis (PCO2) with the falling syndrome [69].

Therefore, it is essential to subject the animals to a physical preparation and adaptation to the fight. In fact, in recent years, the number of farmers who seek to achieve adequate physical condition in their animals has increased, through an empirical training program along a running track or by moving them in the same enclosure where they normally live.

There are few studies on the effect of training on the physiology of the bull [85–87]; however, we can state that training potentially increases athletic performance, as can be deduced from muscular and blood metabolic adaptations [88, 89]. It has been observed that training favors the β-oxidative metabolic pathway of fatty acids (oxidative metabolism) prevailing over the glycolytic pathway, requiring a protocol of at least 6 months to increase its antioxidant capacity [89, 90].

In addition, this training would increase the muscle mass of the animal favoring physical performance [91]. To train, and for the result to be effective, great care of the diet should be taken into account since, in the finishing phase of the bulls, it is intended that the animal's body weight increases and that the training will serve to increase muscles and adapt the cardiovascular system to an aerobic exercise. With this training management, it is being pursued that the bull endures the fight better, increasing its mobility while achieving greater lung capacity and, therefore, a greater chance of recovery, after efforts made in the first moments of fight.

With training, physical capacity is enhanced, stimulating the body's level of work above normal. These animals have a great capacity for adaptation and although at the beginning of the training they show signs of fatigue and body loss, this is followed by a phase of recovery/adaptation and maintenance of body weight.

A basic training program would consist of three sessions per week, within a total period of 5–6 months, depending on the date scheduled for the fight. A group of animals, with a variable number of bulls, around 12, are forced to move for approximately 3 km, accompanied by horsemen.

It usually begins with a weekly session, increasing the pace until reaching 3 sessions/week in the second month. The intensity is progressive, each session begins with the first minute to the step, to warm the animals, increasing the pace until they are trotted or lightly galloped, to return to the initial point in a progressive cooling. The orography of the land is usually flat, but there are farmers who prefer to exercise the cattle on sloping terrain to increase the intensity of the session. This training is interrupted approximately 15 days before the fight [92].

Each breeder has been carrying out a particular training protocol, adapted to their availability of time and cowboys, the number of animals they intend to prepare, and the date of their fight. Generally, a more intense preparation is usually carried out with bulls whose destiny is first or second category arena. In turn, the orographic characteristics of the farm, its distribution of fenced areas, and its extension will have an important influence on the programmed exercise.

5.3 Health management

Considering the high economic value of the Lidia breed animals, the number of farmers who establish a health management program in their livestock as a control system against infectious or parasitic diseases, and to increase fertility and pregnancy rates as well as to decrease mortality rates in new-born calves, is rising in recent years.

Problems related to infectious and contagious diseases represent the main source of economic losses. The pathogens that have tropism for the reproductive, respiratory, or digestive system stand out. Therefore, reproductive and respiratory alterations and neonatal diarrhea are the main problems we find in these cattle [93].

Currently, there are several emerging diseases that could affect these animals during the last decade such as blue tongue, foot and mouth disease, or bovine spongiform encephalopathy, which have joined those that already have an eradication program in our country (brucellosis and tuberculosis), which require periodic official livestock checking on farms (Order DES/6/2011). On many occasions, the health problem itself is linked to a cumbersome legislation that hinders the transit of animals through the various communities of the national territory and between intracommunity countries such as Spain, France, and Portugal (Royal Decree 186/2011).

The official campaigns of eradication of brucellosis and tuberculosis are based on hard controls of the herds and on the application of a legal regulation on these aspects that makes, in certain cases, the movement of animals from the infected cattle ranches, including sales for bullfighting, impossible [94]. It is essential to consider the peculiar factors of this cattle production system. One of them is the level of consanguinity within some farms with a very small number of individuals, which works against disease resistance. It is also necessary to consider the complexity of handling these animals, which coexist in extensive systems with species of different sanitary categories (hunting and/or wild) that could be reservoir for numerous diseases.

In addition, cross-reactions with paratuberculosis (a widespread disease in the Spanish countryside) compromise the reliability of diagnostic analytical tests, posing serious problems when addressing eradication plans [95]. The fight against diseases, both endemic (tuberculosis and brucellosis) and emerging (bluetongue), to achieve eradication and control, will be one of the workhorses for the Lidia sector. This should not entail, in any case, any risk to the maintenance of the diversity of encastes and genetic lines that characterize this breed. Important and unique farms for their genealogy are being decimated by this cause, to the point of endangering the survival of certain encastes.

6. SHEATHED OF HORNS

One of the most valued and delicate body parts of the bull is its horns. They suffer a risk of deterioration, mainly in the last year of life, as a result of potential fights, friction, contacts, or blows with the ground, with trees, fencing, feeders, or the walls of the handling facilities [96]. Therefore, to protect the horns during the last year of animal live, a fiberglass bandage is placed on the horns, easy to handle, porous and that hardens quickly by polymerization with water, providing good consistency (Figure 8). The technique consists of immobilizing the animal in the restraining facilities and wrapping the horn with this bandage to protect it from any aggression or friction. The distal part of the horn is reinforced in many cases with metal tubes or similar hard materials, in order to reduce the wear of the apical zone [97, 98].

The horn is increased in thickness by the sheath, and the end of the horn is blunt, which decreases the effect of the lesions of horns between animals by 90% and, in addition, improves their handling for vaccinations, deworming, and other treatments, due to the risks of deterioration of the defenses when the animals pass through the handling facilities minimized [99]. In spite of the obvious advantages of the sheathing mentioned above, and the answer to many questions about the influence of this management practice on the structure and corneal anatomy and the ethological performance of the animal in the arena provided by Alonso et al. [100], there is still some controversy about its usefulness.

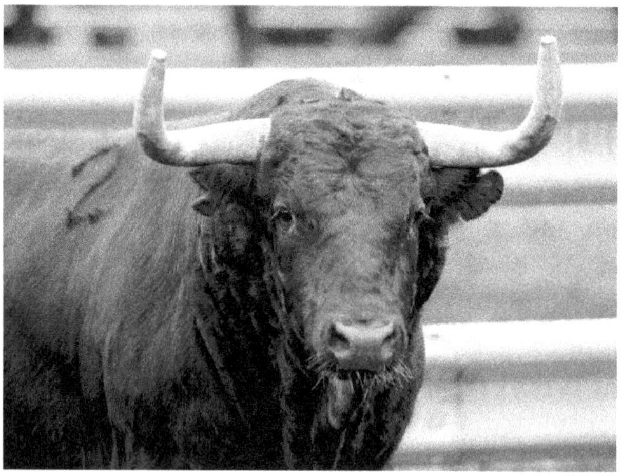

Figure 8. Lidia bull with protected horns.

7. CONCISE SUMMARY

Lidia cattle production exhibits distinct characteristics that necessitate farmers and veterinarians to possess information regarding the specificities of these animals and their management. The Lidia production business has evolved since its inception by leveraging contemporary technical advancements. The feeding system, selection criteria, and reproduction processes have been altered, necessitating the modernization of medical and management practices.

Nevertheless, challenges arise in breeding due to the animals' temperament, which complicates handling, and their susceptibility to diseases that significantly impact their health, including ruminal acidosis, falling syndrome, and various health issues common among extensive bovine cattle.

FOOTNOTES

1. encastes = specific genetic lines in Lidia cattle breed.
2. tienta = selection test applied mainly to female Lidia animals where a bullfighting show is played on livestock farm.

3. indulto = situation when a bull that has been excellent in the fight and is not sacrificed to be incorporated into his home field as a study.

REFERENCES

4. Sañudo C. Manual de diferenciación racial. Zaragoza: Merial; 2008
5. Cañón J, Tupac-Yupanqui I, GarcíaAtance MA, Cortés O, García D, Fernández J, et al. Genetic variation within the Lidia bovine breed. Animal Genetics. 2008;39:439-445
6. Rodríguez A. Prototipos raciales del vacuno de lidia. Madrid: Ministerio de Agricultura, Pesca y Alimentación; 2002. 211 pp
7. Rodríguez L. Estudio socioeconómico de los ganaderos de Lidia de Castilla y León. In: Junta de Castilla y León. Valladolid: ITACYL; 2007
8. Cerrato-Sánchez M, Calsamiglia S. Acidosis ruminal y estrategias de prevención en vacuno lechero. Producción Animal. 2006;220:66-76
9. ARCA. Ministerio de Medio Ambiente y Medio Rural y Marino. Sistema Nacional de Información de Razas (ARCA). 2020
10. Purroy A, Azpilicueta G, Alzón M. La alimentación en el ganado de lidia. In: Libro de ponencias de las III Jornadas sobre Ganado de Lidia, Universidad Pública de Navarr; 21 y 22 de febrero; Pamplona, Españaa; 2003. pp. 123-148
11. Sánchez A, Mora H, Frías J, Balbas JÁ. Geografía del Toro de Lidia. Madrid: Ministerio de Agricultura; 1980
12. García IR, Mazzucchelli F, Parrilla G, Pizarro M. Bases de alimentación del ganado bravo en situaciones de escasez o fincas poco productivas. Cría y Salud. 2011;35:54-51
13. Purroy A, Grijalba M. Estudio técnico-económico de las ganaderías de toros de Lidia. In: Libro de las VI Jornadas sobre Ganado de Lidia. Pamplona; 2006. pp. 33-62
14. Cruz J. El toro de lidia en la biología, en la zootecnia y en la cultura. Valladolid: Junta de Castilla y León, Consejería de Agricultura y Ganaderia; 1991. 198 pp
15. García JJ, Posado R, Hernández R, Vicente A, Olmedo S, Rodríguez L. Estudio socioeconómico de los ganaderos de lidia de Castilla y León. Valladolid, España: Instituto Tecnológico Agrario de Castilla y León; 2007. 78 pp
16. Daza A. Producción de vacuno de carne en la dehesa. In: Monografía Bovis, n° 87. Madrid, España: Luzán; 1999. 100 pp
17. Bouet C. Nuevas estrategias de producción del ganado de lidia mexicano. Sistema de producción y unidad de producción. In: Garza HN, Colin JP, editors.

Sistemas de Producción y Desarrollo Agrícola. Francia: Pierre Milleville; 1993. pp. 279-283

18. Jimeno V, Mazzuchelli F, Parrila G, García I. Gestión de la alimentación del ganado de lidia. Del nacimiento a utrero. Mundo Ganadero. 2005;177:52-56
19. Carbonell A, Gómez A. La alimentación del toro de lidia. Aplicación en la ganadería de Jaralta. In: Colección: Ganadería—Serie Alimentación Animal. España: Consejería de Agricultura y Pesca de la Junta de Andalucía; 2001. 78 pp
20. Carmona A. Técnicas modernas en la alimentación del toro de lidia. In: I Congreso Mundial Taurino de Veterinaria, 1, 2 y 3 de diciembre; Zaragoza, España. 1994. pp. 47-58
21. Purroy A, Mendizábal JA. Manejo de la alimentación en el ganado de lidia. In: Zootecnia, Bases de Producción Animal: Producciones Equinas y de Ganado de Lidia. Tomo XI; 1996. pp. 281-294
22. Domecq B. Lidia del toro en la plaza. La ficha del ganadero. Revista 6Toros6. 2009;706:18-21
23. Lomillos JM. Aplicación de nuevas tecnologías a la caracterización, cría y manejo de ganado vacuno de lidia [tesis doctoral]. Universidad de León; 2012
24. Lomillos JM, Alonso ME. Revisión de la alimentación de la raza de lidia y caracterización de las principales patologías asociadas al cebo del toro en la actualidad. ITEA Informacion Tecnica Economica Agraria. 2019;115(4):376-398
25. Alonso-Vaz F. La alimentación y su influencia en las caídas de los toros. In: Libro de Actas del IV Congreso Mundial Taurino de Veterinaria; 28 Noviembre 2002; Salamanca, España. 2002. pp. 53-61
26. Caballero JR. Análisis de la evolución del crecimiento del toro de lidia en la fase de acabado. In: Libro de Actas del V Congreso Mundial de Veterinaria Taurina 1 al 30 de Septiembre Valladolid, España. 2005. pp. 106-109
27. Compan H, Arriola J. Acidosis ruminal en el toro de lidia (III). Revista Toro Bravo. 1998;15:30-33
28. Arriola J. Acidosis ruminal en el Toro de Lidia (I). Toro Bravo. 1998;13:30-33
29. Bartolomé DJ, Posado R, García JJ, Alonso ME, Gaudioso VR. Acidosis ruminal en el toro bravo. Albéitar. 2011;148:14-16
30. Lomillos JM, Alonso ME, González JR, Gaudioso VR. Effect of feeding management on the structure of the Lidia bull ruminal mucosa Revista Científica. FCV-LUZ. 2017;5(22):310-318
31. Rodríguez-Medina PL. La alimentación del ganado de Lidia. In: I Symposium del Toro de Lidia. Zafra; 1993

32. Gómez-Peinado A. Acidosis ruminal y su incidencia en la lidia. In: Purroy A, Buxadé C, editors. II Jornadas sobre ganado de Lidia. Pamplona: Universidad Pública de Navarra; 2001. pp. 137-148 (333)

33. Jimeno V, Majano MA, Mazzucheli F, Mirat F. Patologías nutritivas en la terminación del toro de lidia. In: VI Symposium del Toro de Lidia. Zafra; 2003. pp. 51-61

34. García JJ, Posado R, Zúñiga J, Tabernero de Paz M, Bodas R. Monitoring rumen environment in finishing Lidia bulls. Revista MVZ Córdoba. 2016;21(2):5355-5366

35. Gaudioso V, Riol A. Selección y reproducción en el ganado de Lidia. In: Producciones equinas y de Ganado de Lidia, Cap. XVII. Zootecnia, bases de producción animal. Madrid: Mundiprensa; 1996

36. Purroy A. Nuevas técnicas reproductivas para la mejora del carácter bravura. In: Purroy A, Buxadé C, editors. VI Jornadas sobre ganado de Lidia. Pamplona: Universidad Pública de Navarra. 2008. pp. 27-42

37. Correia P, Baron E, Pavani K, Lima JP, Lopes S, Nunes H, et al. Morphometric characterization of Lidia cow (Bos taurus) reproductive apparatus. Spanish Journal of Agricultural Research. 2018;16(3):1-4. DOI: 10.5424/sjar/2018163-12833

38. Gómez A. Programa de transferencia de embriones en la ganadería de lidia. In: Tomo I, editor. Manual de reproducción y genética del Toro de Lidia. Valladolid: ITACYL; 2008

39. Caballero JR, González M. Influencia de diversos factores sobre la duración de la gestación en vacas bravas. Archivos de Zootecnia. 1997;46:81-84

40. Lira F, Quevedo L. Problemática de las técnicas reproductivas en el ganad bovino. In: V Congreso Mundial Taurino de Veterinaria; Valladolid. 2005. pp. 38-44

41. Quevedo L. Extracción de semen y evacuación seminal al semental de Lidia. In: Manual de reproducción y genética del Toro de Lidia. Tomo I. Valladolid: ITACYL. 2008. pp. 28-41

42. Barga R. El Toro de Lidia. Madrid: Alianza Editorial; 1995

43. Blanco FJ. Protocolos de sincronización e inseminación artificial en ganadería de lidia. In: Tomo I, editor. Manual de reproducción y genética del Toro de Lidia. Valladolid: ITACYL; 2008. pp. 74-83

44. Seva J. La clonación, ventajas e inconvenientes. In: IV Encuentro de aulas taurinas de Veterinaria; Murcia. 2011

45. Serrano A. Últimos avances y retos en biotecnología y sus aplicaciones al toro de Lidia. In: IX Symposium del Toro de Lidia; Zafra. 2009. pp. 25-36
46. Cabrera R. Trapío y casta Del toro Del siglo XXI. In: XX Jornadas técnicas de la Asociación de Veterinarios Taurinos. Santander. 2012
47. García JMN. These: Développement et validation d´une nouvelle méthode quantitative et objective d´evaluation du comportement et des dépenses énergétiques du taureau Brave au cours de la corrida: Applications á l´etude de La faiblesse dês taureaux lors de La corrida. Toulouse: Université Paul-Sabatier de Toulouse; 2008
48. González E, Duran CV, Domínguez JF. Heredabilidad y repetibilidad de la nota de tienta y la nota de lidia en una ganadería de reses bravas. Archivos de Zootecnia. 1994;43:225-237
49. Cañón J. Mejora genética en el Ganado de Lidia: métodos deselección. In: Tomo I, editor. Manual de reproducción y genética del Toro de Lidia. Valladolid: ITACYL; 2008. pp. 69-73, 183
50. Rodero A, Alonso F, García J. Consanguinidad en el toro de lidia. Archivos de Zootecnia. 1985;34(130):225-234
51. Alfonso L. Nuevas perspectivas de la mejora genética del ganado de Lidia. In: Purroy A, Buxadé C, editors. I Jornadas sobre ganado de Lidia. Pamplona: Universidad Pública de Navarra; 1999. pp. 111-124, 195
52. Almenara-Barrios J, García R. Assessment scale for behaviour in bullfighting cattle (EBL 10). Reliability and validity. Archivos de Zootecnia. 2011;60:215-224
53. Sánchez JM, Riol JA, Eguren VG, Gaudioso VR. Metodología de obtención de un programa informático para la valoración del toro durante la lidia. Acta Veterinaria. 1990;4:17-26
54. Sánchez JM, Riol JA, Eguren VG, Gaudioso VR. Comportamiento del toro de lidia frente al caballo y muleta: Aspectos aplicativos a la selección de la raza. Archivos de Zootecnia. 1990;39(144):165-174
55. Méndez A. Patología y Patología Clínica en el Toro de Lidia Español. Facultad de Veterinaria, Universidad de Córdoba: Publicación Cátedra de Taurología; 2007
56. Carceller H. Patologías oculares. Tratamiento médico y quirúrgico. In: Manual de patología médica y quirúrgica del toro de lidia. Junta de Castilla y León: Instituto Tecnológico Agrario de Castilla y León; 2007. Capítulo 7, p. 56
57. Gómez-Peinado A. Patologías quirúrgicas más frecuentes y su resolución. In: Manual de patología médica y quirúrgica del toro de lidia, Capítulo 4. Junta de Castilla y León: Instituto Tecnológico Agrario de Castilla y León; 2007. p. 40

58. Blanco J. Actualización en anestesia del ganado bravo. Tratamiento médico y quirúrgico. In: Manual de patología médica y quirúrgica del toro de lidia. Junta de Castilla y León: Instituto Tecnológico Agrario de Castilla y León; 2007. Capítulo I. p. 8
59. Prieto JL. Guía De Campo Del Toro De Lidia. Almuzara; 2005. 137 pp
60. Martínez Arteaga P. Lesiones anatómicas producidas en el toro por los trebejos empleados en la lidia. Zacatecas, México: Hispano Mex Publicaciones A.C; 2003
61. Sauvant D, Meschy F, Mertens D. Les composantes de l'acidose ruminale et les effets acidogènes des rations. Inra. Productions Animales. 1999;12(1):49-60
62. McDonald P. Nutrición Animal. Zaragoza, España: Acribia; 2006. 604 pp
63. Owens FN, Secrist DS, Hill WJ, Gill DR. Acidosis in cattle: A review. Journal Animal Science. 1998;76:275-286
64. Gentile A, Rademarcher G, Klee W. Acidosi ruminale fermentativa nel vitello lactante. Objettivi & Documenti Veterinari. 1997;12:63-75
65. González LA, Manteca X, CalsamigliaS,Schwartzkopf-GensweinKS, Ferret A. Ruminal acidosis in feedlot cattle: Interplay between feed ingredients, rumen function and feeding behavior (a review). Animal Feed Science and Technology. 2012;172(1-2):66-79
66. Kleen JL, Hooijer GA, Rehage J, Noordhizen JPTM. Subacute ruminal acidosis (SARA): A review. Journal of Veterinary Science. 2003;50:406-410
67. Nocek JE. Bovine acidosis: Implications on laminitis. Journal of Dairy Science. 1997;80:1005-1028
68. Bach A. Trastornos ruminales en vacuno lechero: un enfoque práctico. Producción Animal. 2003;191:13-33
69. Enemark JMD, Jorgensen RJ. Rumen acidosis with special emphasis on diagnostic aspects of subclinical rumen acidosis: A review. Veterinarija ir Zotechnika. 2002;20(42):16-29
70. Viñas L. Acidosis crónica-latente (subclínica o subliminal y subaguda) y meteorismos ruminales de génesis alimentaria en los terneros de cebo en cría intensiva. Madrid, España: Elanco Sanidad Animal; 1996. 62 pp
71. Radostits OM, Gay CC, Blood DC, Hinchcliff KW. Veterinary Medicine: A Textbook of the Diseases of Cattle, Sheep, Pig, Goats and Horses. London, England: WB Saunders Company; 2000
72. Escalera F. Indicadores sanguíneos y su relación con el síndrome de caída en el toro bravo durante la lidia [tesis doctoral]. Universidad de León; 2011

73. Nordlund KV, Garret EF, Oetzel GR. Herd-based rumenocentesis: A clinical approach to the diagnosis of subacute rumen acidosis. Compendium on Continuing Education for the Practising Veterinarian. 1995;17:48-56

74. Roquet J. Alimentación de terneros sin monensina. Aspectos prácticos. Buiatría Española. 2005;10(1):33-43

75. Lomillos JM, Alonso ME, Gaudioso V. Análisis de la evolución del manejo en las explotaciones de toro de lidia. Desafíos del sector. ITEA. 2013;109(1):49-68

76. Calsamiglia S, Ferret A. Fisiología ruminal relacionada con la patología digestiva: acidosis y meteorismo. Producción Animal. 2003;192:2-23

77. Vázquez P, Pereira V, Hernández J, Castillo C, Méndez J, López-Alonso M, et al. Acidosis crónica en terneros: nuevas pautas de prevención. Producción Animal. 2005;216:4-15

78. Waldrip HM, Martin SA. Effects of an Aspergillus oryzae fermentation extract and other factors on lactate utilization by the ruminal bacterium Megasphaera elsdenii. Journal of Animal Science. 1993;71:2770-2776

79. Alonso ME, Sánchez JM, Riol JA, Gutiérrez P, Gaudioso VR. Estudio de la manifestación del síndrome de caída en el Toro de Lidia. Manifestación e incidencia. ITEA. 1995;91(2):81-92

80. Ministerio del Interior. Datos de temporadas 2001-2019. In: Página Web del Ministerio del Interior. 2019. Available from: http://www.interior.gob.es/

81. Gaudioso V, Alonso ME. Aproximación al síndrome de la caída. In: I Congreso Mundial Taurino de Veterinaria. Zaragoza. 1994. pp. 81-82

82. Castejón FJ. Incoordinación motora y caída del ganado bravo durante la lidia. Boletín Informativo SYVA. 1985;Febrero:40-44

83. Domecq A. El Toro Bravo. Madrid: Espasa; 1998

84. Montaner LJ. Heredity of falling condition in Lidia cattle [master's thesis]. Department of Veterinary Pathology, Kansas State University; 1991

85. Castro MJ, Sánchez JM, Riol JA, Alonso ME, Gaudioso VR. Evaluación de la reacción de estrés en animales de raza de lidia ante diferentes prácticas habituales de manejo. Revista ITEA. 1994;90(2):104-111

86. García-Belenguer S, Purroy A, González JM, Gascón M. Efecto de la complementación con selenio y vitamina E sobre la adaptación de vacas bravas al estrés físico de la tienta. ITEA. 1992;88(3):205-211

87. Aceña MC, García-Belenguer S, Gascón M, Purroy A. Modifications hematologiques et musculaires pendant la corrida chez le taureau de combat.

In: Diméglio F, éd. Biomécanique de la tauromachie 1992-1995. 1995. pp. 185-193

88. Agüera EI, Muñoz A, Castejón FM, Essén-Gustavsson B. Skeletal muscle fibre characteristics in young and old bulls and metabolic response after a bullfight. Journal of Veterinary Medicine. 2001;48:313-319

89. Agüera EI, Rubio MA, Vivo R, Escribano BM, Muñóz A, Villafuerte JL, et al. Adaptaciones fisiológicas a la lidia en el Toro Bravo. Parámetro plasmáticos y musculares. Veterinaria México. 1998;29(4):399-403

90. Picard B, Santé-Lhoutellier V, Aameslant C, Micol D, Boissy A, Hocquette JF, et al. Caractéristiques physiologiques de taureaux de la race Brave à l'issue de la corrida. Revue de Médice Vétérinaire. 2006;157(5):293-301

91. Agüera E. Manejo para la mejora del rendimiento físico del Toro de Lidia: pautas de entrenamiento. In: Tomo I, editor. Manual de reproducción y genética del Toro de Lidia. Valladolid: ITACYL; 2008. pp. 100-109, 83

92. Escribano BM, Tunez I, Requena F, Rubio MD, de Miguel R, Montilla P, et al. Effects of an aerobic training program on oxidative stress biomarkers in bulls. Veterinarni Medicina. 2010;55(9):422-428

93. Requena F, Rubio MD,= Escribano BM, Santisteban R, Tovar P, Agüera EI. Determinación de la ruta metabólica muscular en toros de Lidia entrenados. In: IX Symposium del Toro de Lidia; Zafra. 2009. pp. 165-166

94. Rivero JL, Ruz MC, Serrano A, Diz AM, Galisteo AM. Efecto del entrenamiento y desentrenamiento sobre la proporción de los tipos de fibras musculares em diferentes razas de caballos. Avances en Ciencias Veterinarias. 1993;8:110-118

95. Requena F. Evaluación de la capacidad física del toro de Lidia con el entrenamiento [tesis doctoral]. Universidad de Córdoba; 2012

96. San Miguel JM. Programa sanitario para una explotación de vacuno de lidia. In: Manual de patología médica y quirúrgica del toro de lidia, Tomo II. Junta de Castilla y León: Instituto Tecnológico Agrario de Castilla y León; 2008. pp. 44-67

97. Perea A. Balance de la situación epizootiológica en la cabaña de Lidia. In: VII Simposium del Toro de Lidia. Zafra. 2005. pp. 185-198

98. Sanes JM, Seva JI, Pallarés FJ. Coinfección natural de tuberculosis y paratuberculosis en ganaderías de Lidia. In: VII Congreso Mundial Taurino de Veterinaria. Cáceres. 2011. pp. 13-22

99. Aparicio JB, Peña F, Barona LF. Estudio de las encornaduras del Toro de Lidia. Junta de Andalucía: Córdoba; 2000

100. Pizarro M, Horcajada J, Ortuño S, Fernández C. Utilización de fundas en cuernos. Posible modificación de la estructura y consistencia. In: VI Congreso Mundial Taurino de Veterinaria. Murcia. 2008. pp. 179-182

101. Pizarro M, Carceller H, Alonso R, Horcajada J, Hebrero C. Utilización de fundas en cuernos. Colocación e incidencia en el reconocimiento y comportamiento. In: VI Congreso Mundial Taurino de Veterinaria. Murcia. 2008. pp. 175-178

102. Lira F. Avances en el cuidado y protección de las defensas del Toro de Lidia. In: Manual de patología médica y quirúrgica del toro de lidia, Tomo II. Junta de Castilla y León: Instituto Tecnológico Agrario de Castilla y León; 2008. pp. 28-43

103. Alonso ME, Lomillos JM, González JR. La cornamenta del toro de lidia análisis de su integridad y efecto del enfundado. León: EOLAS Ediciones; 2016

7 Chapter

INDUCTION AND SYNCHRONIZATION OF ESTRUS

1. INTRODUCTION: AN OVERVIEW

Since prehistoric times, animals have been an integral component of human existence. As time has progressed, reliance on domesticated animals has intensified. Currently, human society is inconceivable without the animal products we utilize daily. A substantial global cattle population is helping to the attainment of food security. The predicted surge in human population, anticipated to reach approximately 9.7 billion by 2050, has escalated the need for animal products. Research efforts are focused on increasing animal production.

The primary obstacles to this objective include various diseases and the limited availability of animal feed, particularly in underdeveloped or emerging nations. Among various diseases, issues related to animal reproductive have consistently been a significant concern for animal producers. Female animals with reproductive issues are unable to conceive and produce children. Moreover, it primarily precludes milk production. The major reproductive issues include anestrus, repeat breeding, delayed estrus, different infections, etc. Among them the problem of anestrus has an incidence rate of 2.13–67.11% in the bovine population of a country like India which is the largest producer of milk [1]. Anestrus is a condition when there is absence of regular reproductive cyclicity in the female animal.

Consequently, the animal becomes unproductive and causes a huge economical loss to the farmers or producers. So, it is very much important to address this problem with much care. Already, there are several established as well as developing methodologies which can induce estrus in anestrus animals. It encompasses practices like administration of hormone to the use of biostimulation. Besides inducing estrus, some technologies can also synchronize it according to the need. The synchronization of estrus can facilitate management procedures and enhance advanced technologies such as embryo transfer, in vitro fertilization, and cloning. This chapter will address the regular estrus cycle, the anestrus issue, and the approaches devised by researchers for the induction and synchronization of estrus..

2. ESTRUS CYCLE OF DOMESTIC ANIMALS

Estrus cycle can be defined as the rhythmic changes that occur in the reproductive system of a female animal starting from one estrus phase to another. The normal duration of estrus cycle is 21 days in cow, sow, and mare, 17 days in ewe, and 20 days in doe. The domestic animals can exhibit a single estrus cycle or more than one estrus cycle in a year. The canine species show only one cycle in its breeding season; hence they can be called the monestrous. Other species which come into estrus twice or more are termed polyestrous animals. Among them some species have estrus cycles in a particular season and defined as seasonal polyestrous. It includes goats, sheep, and horses. On the other hand, cattle undergo estrus throughout the year. The seasonal polyestrous animals are greatly regulated by the photoperiod of the season for their reproductive activity.

The estrus cycle can be grossly divided into two phases, that is, follicular phase and luteal phase. The main event occurring in follicular phase is the development of the ovarian follicles, whereas in luteal phase there is formation and growth of the corpus luteum (CL). The follicular phase is again consisting of proestrus and estrus. The proestrus lasts for 3–4 days and the estrus phase only for 12–18 hours. FSH (follicle-stimulating hormone) is the principal hormone controlling the follicular phase. It causes enlargement of the follicles, increase in estrogen secretion from the granulosa cells of the ovary, and increase in the vascularity of the female reproductive tract. After the proestrus phase, there is a rapid increase in the luteinizing hormone (LH) level known as LH surge. This surge is responsible for the ovulation of the matured graafian follicle. In cattle, ovulation generally occurs 12 hours after the end of the estrus. At estrus phase, the animal shows the signs of estrus or heat. It includes mucous discharge from the vagina, restlessness, frequent micturition, bellowing, swelling of the vulva, etc. The animal tries to mount other animals and also stands to be mounted by other animals called as standing heat. After the estrus phase, the ruptured follicle starts to convert into corpus luteum and the animal enters into luteal phase. This phase is also divided into metestrus and diestrus. The duration of metestrus is 3–4 days, whereas diestrus can last from 10 to 14 days. In metestrus the estrogen level starts decreasing and progesterone increases. Though ovulation occurs in metestrus phase in cattle, it happens in the last portion of estrus phase in other domestic species like sheep, goat, horse, etc. The uterine contraction subsides and endometrial glands start growing in metestrus. The progesterone level continues increasing in diestrus and achieves a peak on 13–14 days after estrus phase. Afterward the size of the corpus luteum also starts decreasing, and the follicle grows if the animal is not pregnant. In the case of pregnant animals, the CL does not regress and secrete progesterone throughout the gestation period. If the animal is not conceived, the CL is destroyed after the end of this phase, and the animal enters into the follicular phase.

FSH and LH are the two gonadotropins majorly responsible for the events in estrus cycle. These are secreted from the anterior pituitary upon the stimulation of gonadotropin-releasing hormone (GnRH). GnRH that resides on the top of hypothalamo-pituitary-gonadal (HPG) axis controls the reproductive activities of the animals. The FSH and LH eventually act on the gonads and secrete sex steroids like estrogen and progesterone in female and testosterone in male. Estrogen and testosterone help in the development of secondary sexual characters in females and males, respectively. The secretion of GnRH depends upon different internal and external signals. For example, leptin secreted from the adipose tissue and melatonin from the pineal gland have a clear effect on the GnRH release. It is also stimulated by kisspeptin, a neuropeptide secreted from preoptic and arcuate nucleus of hypothalamus. So, any physiological or pathological condition which disturbs the release of GnRH can affect the normal reproductive behavior of the animals. The overall hormonal balance is very much essential for maintaining estrus cyclicity.

3. ANESTRUS AND ITS TYPES

Anestrus is the lack of estrus or heat syndromes in female animals. It can be observed in heifers as well as cow. A good number of post-parturient cows show anestrus. Anestrus can be caused by different reasons and can be classified into different ways. Kumar et al. [1] have divided anestrus into two major parts based on the causes, that is, physiological anestrus and pathological causes of anestrus (Figure 1).

Physiological anestrus can be either ovulatory or anovulatory. Ovulatory anestrus is seen during gestation period of the animal. Anovulatory anestrus can be prepubertal, lactational, or postpartum. The animals before coming into puberty show follicular growth, but they cannot mature. Due to the action of FSH, the follicle develops up to the stage of theca internal but thereafter starts degrading. The LH pulse frequency is also low, and the threshold for the positive feedback of estradiol on LH surge is also very high [1]. So, there is no ovulation and no estrus. Gestational anestrus is common in all the animals. As there is a persistent corpus luteum present in the ovary throughout the gestation period, there is always an elevated level of progesterone. Progesterone has a negative effect on GnRH secretion and cyclicity stops. Though sometimes, cattle and buffalo can show estrus in the first few months of gestation. It is called gestational anestrus. The signs of estrus are indifferent from the nonpregnant animals in estrus, but the duration is shorter [2]. These animals also exhibit standing heat. The estrus should be carefully differentiated from true estrus to avoid undesirable effect on pregnant animals. At the end of gestation period, there is a decrease in progesterone level. Still the animals are unable to come into estrus cycle, known as postpartum anestrus. This anestrus provides some time for involution of the uterus so that animals can come into estrus subsequently. But, this duration should not be prolonged. Many times, due to lack of proper nutrition and several postpartum diseases, the animals do not show estrus. Proper care and management in the periparturient period can solve this issue. It is ideal to conceive the animal within 2 months of parturition to get one calf each year. When the animals are in lactation also, the estrus cycle can be disturbed especially in high yielders. A high level of prolactin hormone required for the milk synthesis can suppress the GnRH level. This is termed as lactational anestrus.

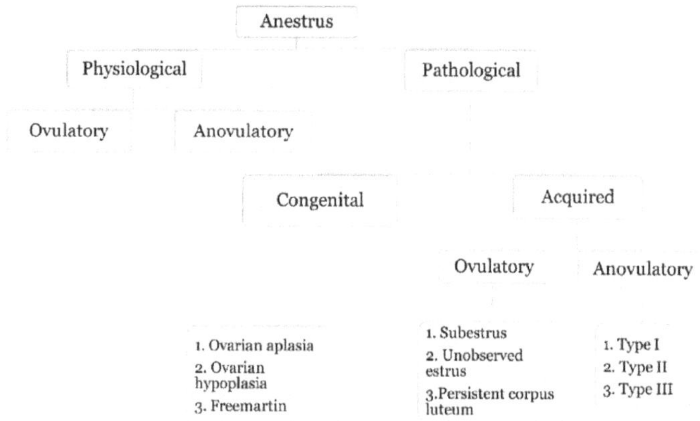

Figure 1. Classification of anestrus [1].

Pathological causes of anestrus can again be of two types, that is, congenital and hereditary causes of anestrus and acquired anestrus. Congenital and hereditary causes are observed in ovarian aplasia, ovarian hypoplasia, and freemartin.

Acquired anestrus can be ovulatory or anovulatory. Examples of ovulatory acquired anestrus are subestrus, unobserved estrus, and persistent corpus luteum. Acquired anovulatory anestrus has been classified into three type (I, II, and III) based on the stage of follicular growth [1]. In the case of type I, the follicles grow up to four millimeters and start regressing. In type II, the follicles grow further up to deviation and preovulatory stage but regress thereafter, and the next follicular wave starts. In type III, the follicle reaches up to the dominant stage but fails to ovulate and converts into persistent follicle.

4. INDUCTION OF ESTRUS

The problem of anestrus causes a huge economical loss to the farmers or producers. So, it needs to be solved immediately. Kumar et al. [1] have beautifully classified different ways of estrus induction. The estrus inducers can grossly be divided into two parts, that is, non-hormonal and hormonal. Non-hormonal treatments include plant-derived heat inducers, mineral supplementation, uterine and ovarian massage, and use of Lugol's iodine. The hormones that are used in estrus induction are estrogen, progesterone, GnRH, prostaglandin, insulin, and anti-prolactin-based treatment. All these treatment procedures are described below.

4.1 Non-hormonal treatment

4.1.1 Plant-deriv+ed heat inducers

Different plant extracts are being used for the treatment of anestrus traditionally. Several estrus-inducing herbal medicines are available in Indian market. The efficacy of estrus-inducing preparations like Prajana, Janova, Estrona, and Sajani is well established [3]. Other examples include Aloes, Heat-Up, Fertivet, Heat-raj, etc. These can be applied in delayed puberty, postpartum anestrus, and other problems. Though they can induce estrus in crossbred cows, the conception rate is remained unchanged. Aegle marmelos and Murraya koenigii are two medicinal plants used for the treatment of reproductive problems in livestock as well as laboratory animals [4–6]. Feeding the leaves of these plants individually or combined can help in starting the cascade of reproductive cycle. It is believed that they act like the gonadotropins. The other possible mechanism behind its efficacy is the antioxidant effect of the plant-derived substances enhancing the luteal function. The demand and usefulness of the plant-derived medicines are increasing day by day. As these are easily available, are economical, and have fewer side effects, these preparations can be successfully utilized especially in village level. Many times, the poor farmers cannot afford the cost of the hormonal estrus inducers which are not always available also. In this situation, herbal mixtures have emerged as a better option. A large comparative study is required to use these drugs as alternative to hormones.It is also recommended that these should be used along with vitamin and mineral supplementation. Kumar and Singh [7] have also reported about the use of the pigeon waste in estrus induction. They fed 100 gm dried pigeon waste for 3 days to anestrus cows and heifers and successfully induced estrus in 40% cows and 44% heifers. This may be due to the high iron, zinc, and other mineral content in the pigeon waste.

4.1.2 Mineral supplementation

Minerals have an important role in the reproduction of domestic animals, and their deficiency can cause several reproductive disorders. Deficiency of calcium is very common in postpartum cattle. Any alteration in Ca:P ration can affect the pituitary secretion and subsequently ovarian function [8]. This can cause delayed puberty, irregular estrus, etc. The optimum ratio of Ca:P should be within 1.5:1–2.5:1. Excess calcium is also harmful as it can disturb the absorption of other minerals. Phosphorus is a very important mineral for the normal reproduction. In the case of phosphorus deficiency, several disorders can be observed like delayed maturity, low conception rate, inactive ovary, etc. [8]. There are reports of other reproductive problems in areas with phosphorus deficiency. It includes silent estrus, delayed puberty, irregular estrus, and long inter-calving period [9]. Sodium and potassium are also necessary for maintaining normal reproductive physiology and energy metabolism, though excess consumption of potassium can cause a problem.

Other trace minerals like zinc, selenium, cobalt, iodine, chromium, etc. also have a prominent role in the reproduction of domestic animals. Animals can come into anestrus if proper nutrition is not provided. So, feeding management should be the first approach to prevent the problem of anestrus. Minerals should be supplemented in optimum quantity. The use of area-specific mineral mixture should be encouraged.

4.1.3 Uterine and ovarian massage

It is the most economical method for the treatment of anestrus. In this method, gentle massage of the uterus and ovary is done perrectally. There are reports which state about its utilization in estrus induction. There is no clear mechanism of action of this method. Possibly, it can be attributed to increased blood circulation on the surface of the ovary and stimulation of ovarian intrinsic factors [10, 11].

Application of this method needs experts who have a good idea about the anatomy of female reproductive system.

4.1.4 Lugol's iodine

Intrauterine application of Lugol's iodine can effectively induce estrus in cattle, buffalo, etc. [12, 13]. A dose of 20–30 ml is sufficient for treatment. It also shows a good conception rate with cost-effectiveness. It actually acts as uterine irritant and increases blood supply there. It can also stimulate the hypothalamus for the secretion of GnRH, and thus the reproductive cycle is regained [13].

4.2 Hormonal treatment

4.2.1 Estrogen

Estrogen is a very important hormone for the reproductive cycle of the animals. Administration of estrogen can help the animal to come into estrus [1], though it may be ovulatory or anovulatory. If a dominant follicle is present in the ovary, there will be ovulation. If no dominant follicle is present, it can be anovulatory. Estrogen promotes the ovulation through LH surge as estrogen shows a positive feedback effect toward the pituitary at this time. Use of estrogen is limited nowadays due to its side effects. Prolonged administration of estrogen can cause cystic ovary, peristalsis of the oviduct, etc. [1]. These can also lead to several infections like ovaritis, adhesion, etc.

4.2.2 Progesterone

Progesterone is secreted from the corpus luteum in a normal estrus cycle. With the decrease in the progesterone level, the follicles start growing. The same situation can be mimicked externally. Progesterone can be administered externally for a certain duration, and its withdrawal can cause induction of estrus. Several intravaginal progesterone-releasing devices are available. It includes CIDR (controlled internal drug release), PRID (progesterone-releasing intravaginal device), etc. Ear implant of progesterone is also available. These devices are generally used for 7–9 days and can be combined with other hormones like GnRH, prostaglandin F2α (PGF2α), etc. [1]. Other ways to use progesterone are oral progesterone compound and intramuscular injection.

4.2.3 GnRH

GnRH and its analogues can be successfully used to induce estrus in animals. It induces ovulation, if mature follicle is present by inducing the LH surge. GnRH can improve conception at the timed artificial insemination (Al) after estrous synchronization with prostaglandin F2α [14]. GnRH given after PGF may enhance fertility through its direct or indirect (via LH secretion) action on the ovulatory follicle, and it may act in a similar fashion at insemination after spontaneous estrus [15].

Gonadotropin-releasing hormone improved fertility at first postpartum inseminations in some studies [15], but not all investigations [16]. Increasing progesterone after insemination may be one way to improve fertility in cattle. It is possible that LH released by GnRH could enhance fertility through its effects on luteal function [17].

4.2.4 Prostaglandin

For persistent corpus luteum and subestrus, PGF2α is the treatment of choice. Successful management of silent estrus in cattle and buffaloes can be done by the natural or synthetic analogue of PGF2α as a single dose with a reasonable degree [18, 19]. PGF2α is only effective between days 6 and 16 of the cycle and in the presence of active corpus luteum. Administration of 25 mg of natural PGF2α intramuscular or 250–500 μg of synthetic ones is required to regress the CL in both cattle and buffaloes [1]. Pursley et al. [20] described Ovsynch protocol may be used to treat subestrus or unobserved estrus.

4.2.5 Insulin

Encouraging results have been found in the use of insulin for induction of estrus in animals either alone or in combination [21–23]. The recommended dose is 0.25 IU/kg body weight subcutaneously for 3–5 days. Promising results for management of anestrus in cattle have been observed with the use of GnRH or eCG pretreated with insulin [22, 23] and buffaloes [21, 24]. Insulin enhances the follicular growth in true anestrus buffalo which is a prerequisite for GnRH to be effective [24].

4.2.6 Anti–prolactin

Summer anestrus in buffaloes could be due to hyperprolactinemia, with this assumption bromocriptine, an anti-prolactin drug [25], has been used. Melatonin is also known to suppress prolactin secretion [26]; however, melatonin has been reported as stimulator of both GnRH and gonadotrophin secretions in buffaloes. As the plasma concentration of melatonin is low during summer, induction of estrus and ovulation by using melatonin implants have been reported by Ghuman et al. [27] in all treated summer anestrus buffalo heifers; however, the time taken to induce estrus and ovulation was highly variable (4–36 days).

5. SYNCHRONIZATION OF ESTRUS

The manipulation of the estrous cycle or induction of estrus brings a large percentage of a group of females into estrus at a short, predetermined time [28]. One of the advanced managemental processes through which the humane errors and managemental costs could be minimized is synchronization of estrus. It is predominantly useful in sheep, where timely heat detection is difficult due to exhibitions of less external heat symptoms and also in large herd of cattle. It helps in fixing the breeding time within a short predefined period and thereby scheduling the parturition time at the most favorable season in which newborns can be reared in suitable environment with ample food for augmenting their survivability. As timely breeding of the animals is possible with this technique, fertility in farm animals may be expected toward the upper side. By improving the production efficiency of animals, estrus synchronization provides more economic returns to the owner.

Synchronization can shorten the breeding period to less than 5 days, instead of females being bred over a 21-day period, depending on the treatment regimen.

Production of a uniform group of calves for the future replacement in the animal farm is another important benefit of this program. The current and future aspect of estrous synchronization is to focus on combining traditional methods of controlling cycle length with the follicular development manipulation. The combination of GnRH with the prostaglandin F2α [20]and progesterone [29]-based synchronization program has shown a novel direction in the estrus synchronization of cattle with the follicular development manipulation.

5.1 What is the basic approach for estrus synchronization?

To control the timing of the onset of estrus by controlling the length of the estrous cycle is the basic approach for the estrus synchronization. Various approaches for controlling cycle length are as follows:

1. Prostaglandin administration to regress the corpus luteum of the animal before the time of natural luteolysis

2. Progesterone or synthetic progestin administration to suppress ovarian activity temporarily
3. Creating estrous synchrony by using gonadotropin-releasing hormone or an analogue, which causes ovulation of a large follicle, helps in synchronizing estrous cycle in anestrous female.

5.2 Methods of estrus synchronization

5.2.1 Prostaglandin treatment

Luteolytic agent such as prostaglandin F2α, or an analogue, which causes the regression of the corpus luteum can be used to synchronize estrus [30, 31].

Administration of PGF2α is only effective from 8 to 17 days of the estrous cycle when functional corpus luteum is available in one of the ovaries. Fertility is high after prostaglandin synchronization. Synchronization of estrus and fertility with this product are good in cyclic females but not in non-cycling cows.

a. One-shot prostaglandin: In this method a single injection of prostaglandin is given to cyclic females, and then these females are bred as they express estrus.
b. Two-shot prostaglandin: In this method two injections of prostaglandins are given at an interval of 10–14 days [32] once the stage of estrous cycle in the cows is unknown and detection of estrus is not required before or between injections.

5.2.2 Progesterone treatment

High levels of progesterone in the female's system are maintained with the help of progestogens [33], even after the regression of the corpus luteum. After the progestin removal, synchrony of estrus occurs up to 2–5 days. Melengestrol acetate (MGA) (oral feeding), Syncro-Mate-B (SMB) (ear implant), and CIDR (intravaginal device) are the commercial products which fall into this category. The longer the progestin was administered to cattle, the higher the rate of estrous synchronization, but the fertility of the synchronized animals was lower. Kaltenbach et al. [34] and Wiltbank [35] reported that the estradiol was luteolytic when administered early in the bovine estrous cycle. Combining progestin treatment and estradiol administration at the initiation enabled the period of progestin to be shortened (9–14 days) without reducing the percentage of animals exhibiting a synchronized estrus. This treatment regimen was the basis for the commercial products Syncro-Mate-B, PRID, and CIDR. Administration of progestin at "sub-luteal" levels demonstrated that it inhibits estrus and ovulation and synchronizes estrus in cattle, but that a persistent, estrogen-secreting follicle develops when progestin treatment extends the estrous cycle [36].

5.2.2.1 Techniques of progesterone treatment

a. MGA feeding: MGA was added to feed such that females received 0.5 mg/head/day for 14 days and if MGA was administered, cyclic females begin to show estrus.

This estrus was subfertile, and it was recommended that females should be bred on the second estrus following MGA removal [37].

b. Syncro-Mate-B (ear implant) treatment late in the estrous cycle (>14 days) in cow gives lower conception rates. The ideal time for SMB treatment to begin is between the 8th and 12th day of the estrous cycle to maximize estrus response.
c. Application of CIDR.

CIDR insert for cattle is made by molding a thin layer of silicon and progesterone mixture (10% w/w) around a nylon spine under high temperature. It contains 1.38 g progesterone and is designed to maintain higher blood concentrations of progesterone to at least 2 ng/ml for up to 10 days. The CIDR is easily inserted into the vagina and has good retention capacity (2.5% loss rate is normal); a flexible nylon tail is attached to it for easy removal. The CIDR provides an exogenous source of the progesterone, and its removal on treatment day 7 results in a rapid fall in plasma progesterone levels, which results in estrus synchronization in those animals responding to treatment.

5.2.3 GnRH-based treatment

Estrus synchronization and fertility with a combination of GnRH and prosta-glandin F2α are good for cyclic females, and this combination may induce cyclicity in cows experiencing postpartum anestrus [20]. The new methods of estrus synchronization more precisely and control the time of ovulation more exactly in order to allow a single, timed insemination without the need for detection of behavioral estrus. Administration of GnRH during the estrous cycle in bovines causes regression or ovulation of the dominant follicle and initiates the emergence of a new wave of follicular growth [20]. Ovsynch, CO-Synch, Select-Synch, and Hybrid-Synch are the four systems for synchronization of estrus with GnRH-PG combinations.

At day 1 GnRH injection is used to program follicle growth in cyclic females and to induce ovulation in anestrous females, and PGF2α on day 8 induces regression of CL that is present to cause a decline in progesterone. Then on days 10–11, the second GnRH is given which induces ovulation of dominant follicles that have been preprogrammed by the first GnRH treatment. The major GnRH programs that do not involve use of the CIDR are described as follows:

a. GnRH-PGF system: This represents the simplest GnRH-based system. A common name for this system is "Select-Synch." In this system a single dose of GnRH and prostaglandin was injected on day 1 and day 8, respectively. Some cows (8%) exhibit estrus up to 48 hours before PGF (day 6). The early estrous are fertile and cows can be inseminated 12 hours after detection. The peak estrous response occurs 2–3 days after PGF with a range of 1–5 days. With this system, a minimum of 5 days of estrous detection after PGF and 2 days prior PGF is required to detect most heats.
b. GnRH-PGF + GnRH system: This system is a GnRH-PGF system in which second

GnRH injection is given to all or some cows between 48 and 72 hours after PGF (days 2–3), with timed AI on all or a portion of the herd.

In Ovsynch program, an injection of GnRH on day 1, an injection of prostaglandin on day 8, a second injection of GnRH on day 10, and then a timed insemination on day 11 are given [20]. The first GnRH injection alters follicular growth by inducing ovulation of the dominant follicle in the ovaries after the GnRH injection to form a new or additional CL [20]. Thus, estrus usually does not occur until a PGF2α injection regresses the natural CL and the secondary CL which is formed from the follicle induced to ovulate by the first GnRH injection. Based on transrectal ultrasonographic evidence, a new group of follicles appear in the ovaries, within 1–2 days after the first injection of GnRH [38]. From those follicles, a newly developed dominant follicle emerges, matures, and can ovulate after estrus is induced by PGF2α, or it can be induced to ovulate after a second GnRH injection. This GnRH release luteinizing hormone, the natural ovulation-inducing hormone of the estrous cycle. The stage of the estrous cycle when Ovsynch was initiated also affects synchronization and conception rate [38]. Ravi Kumar and Asokan [39] reported higher conception rate in subestrus buffaloes initiating the treatment with Ovsynch during the later stages of estrous cycle, but conception rate was nil in anestrus buffaloes though incidence of cyclicity was observed due to the treatment. Benefits of this program are as follows: there is tight synchronization of estrus, most females respond to the program, and it boosts estrus in non-cycling cows that are at least 30 days postpartum.

In CO-Synch program, an injection of GnRH on day 1, an injection of prostaglandin on day 8, and then a second injection of GnRH with breeding on day 10 are given. The benefits are as follows: there is tight synchronization of estrus, most females respond to the program, and it boosts estrus in non-cycling cows that are at least 30 days postpartum.

The Hybrid-Synch program is applied with an injection of GnRH on day 1, an injection of prostaglandin on day 8, and then estrous detection and breeding from day 8 to 11. Second injection of GnRH was given to the females which were not observed in estrus from day 8 to 11 and were bred on day 11. Hybrid-Synch program has a lower cost and less handling compared with Ovsynch and CO-Synch but more than Select-Synch. The program appears to have the highest conception rates among all GnRH-prostaglandin programs.

c. Progesterone in combination with GnRH-PG:

Oral administration of MGA to the cows for 14 days is performed, and 10 days after the withdrawal of MGA, GnRH injection was given. PGF2α is given after 7 days of GnRH injection. Patterson et al. [29] reported that 80% of the cows showed estrus within 48–96 hours after PGF2α injection.

5.2.4 CIDR to GnRH-based protocol

Failure to synchronize cyclic animals appropriately or to induce fertile ovulation potentially in anestrous females can have major effects on the success of a synchronization program. This CIDR to GnRH-based program has the potential to decrease losses in each of these areas. The most common use of this system comprises insertion of the CIDR on day 1 and its withdrawal on day 8. GnRH injection is given on the day of CIDR insertion and CIDR is kept in situ for 7 days. Injection of prostaglandin is given on the day of CIDR withdrawal, and then the second GnRH injection is given after 2 days of prostaglandin injection.

The primary advantage of inclusion of the CIDR in this program is that it guarantees that females will be exposed to progesterone during the period between day 1 and day 8. This progesterone exposure will result in normal (21 days) rather than short (10 days) cycles in earlier anestrous cows. Moreover, the withdrawal of a progestin has been demonstrated to induce onset of cycles in some anestrous females; the likelihood of an ovulation is enhanced. A second advantage to inclusion of the CIDR in this program is that the early heats (day 6 to day 9) that are inherent to these systems are prevented. The progesterone released by the CIDR will prevent estrus and ovulation between days 1 and 9.

5.2.5 Management Interference

Management has a significant role in animal reproductive. Effective nutritional management of the herd is crucial for the successful implementation of various synchronization programs in both cows and heifers. Management strategies such as timed insemination and calf removal have been documented as effective for estrus synchronization and can be utilized in various synchronization programs for enhanced outcomes. Typically, conception rates after timed insemination are inferior to those observed during visual assessment. Nonetheless, this diminished conception rate may be offset by the decreased control associated with timed insemination.

The suckling frequency of calves elicits a hormonal response that suppresses the return to estrus, as observed in beef cows. The temporary removal of calves, in conjunction with further synchronization methods, enhances estrus synchrony and conception rates in cattle. A 48-hour calf removal alone has been demonstrated to induce synchronization and cyclicity in certain cows. This approach is appropriate; nonetheless, it necessitates improved management and adequate facilities to avoid the reuniting of separated cows and calves.

REFERENCES

4. Kumar PR, Singh SK, Kharche SD, Govindaraju CS, Kumar B. Review article anestrus in cattle and Buffalo: Indian perspective. Advances in Animal and Veterinary Sciences. 2014;2(3):124-138

5. Thomas I, Dobson H. Oestrus during pregnancy in the cow. The Veterinary Record. 1989;124(15):387-390

6. Pugashetti B, Shivkumar MC, Chandrakal GK, Kulkarni VS. Effect of heat inducing preparations on postpartum anoestrus in Holstein Friesian x Deoni cows. Karnataka Journal of Agricultural Science. 2009;22(2):460-461

7. Das GK, Mehrotra S, Narayanan K, Kumawat BL, De Kumar U, Khan TA. Estrus induction response and fertility performance in delayed pubertal heifers treated with Aegle marmelos and Murraya koenigii. Journal of Animal Research. 2016;6(1):151-156

8. Mehrotra S, Umashankar J, Majumder AC, Agarwal SK. Effect of indigenous medicinal plants on onset of puberty in immature female rats. Journal of Animal Reproduction. 2003;24(2):131-133

9. Satheshkumar S, Punniamurthy N. Estrus induction by supplementation of Murraya koenigii in anestrus heifers. Indian Journal of Animal Reproduction. 2009;30(2):66-67

10. Kumar N, Singh M. Alternate Medicine in Animal Reproduction. 2017. Retrieved from: http://www.hillagric. ac.in/edu/covas/vpharma/winter school/lectures/17.pdf

11. Yasothai R. Importance of minerals on reproduction in dairy cattle. International Journal of Science, Enviroment and Technology. 2014;3(6):2081-2083

12. Choudhary S, Singh A. Role of nutrition in reproduction: A review. Intas Polivet. 2004;5(2):229-234

13. Monget P, Monniaux D. Growth factors and control of folliculogenesis. Journal of Reproduction and Fertility. 2019;49:321-333

14. Romaniuk J. Treatment of ovarian afunction in cows. Medycyna Weterynaryjna. 1973;29:296-298

15. Gupta R, Thakur MS, Sharma A. Estrus induction and fertility response in true anestrus buffaloes using Lugol's iodine. Veterinary World. 2011;4(2):77-78

16. Pandey P, Pandey A, Sinha AK, Singh B. Studies on the effect of Lugol's iodine on reproductive efficiency of dairy cattle. Annual Review and Research in Biology. 2011;1(2):33-36

17. Hansel W, Fortune J. The application of ovulation control. In: Crighton DB, Haynes NB, Foxcroft GR, Lamming GE, editors. Control of Ovulation. London: Butterworths; 1978. pp. 237-263

18. Nakao T, Narita S, Tanaka K, Hara H, Shirakawa J, Noshiro H, et al. Improvement of first-service pregnancy rate in cows with gonadotropinreleasing hormone analog. Theriogenology. 1983;20:111-119

19. Stevenson JS, Schmidt MK, Call EP. Gonadotropin-releasing hormone and conception of Holsteins. Journal of Dairy Science. 1984;67:140-145

20. Kunkel RN, Hagele WC, Mills AC. Effect of recipient pro-gesterone supplementation on morula and blastocysts survival. Journal of Animal Science. 1977;45(1):181

21. Nautiyal H, Shanker U, Agarwal SK. Synchronization of oestrus using double injection regimen of PGF2α in buffaloes. Indian Veterinary Medicine Journal. 1998;22:99-100

22. Singh M, Sood P, Vasistha NK, Singh C. Study on the use of prostaglandin F2α in treatment of suboestrus cows. The Indian Veterinary Journal. 2001;78:815-816

23. Pursley JR, Mee MO, Wiltbank MC. Synchronization of ovulation in dairy cows using PGF2α and GnRH. Theriogenology. 1995;44:915-923

24. Gupta V, Thakur MS, Agrawal RG, Quadri MA, Shukla SN. Effect of pretreatment with insulin on ovarian and fertility response in true anestrus buffaloes to gonadotrophin- releasing hormone. Buffalo Bulletin. 2010;29(3):172-179

25. Shukla SN, Agarwal SK, Shanker U, Varshney VP, Majumdar AC. Ovarian function and restoration of fertility using insulin in acyclic dairy cattle. The Indian Journal of Animal Sciences. 2005a;75:1135-1139

26. Shukla SN, Agarwal SK, Shanker U, Varshney VP, Majumdar AC. Modulation of ovarian response in anoestrous cattle treated with insulin alone and in combination with GnRH. Indian Journal of Animal Reproduction. 2005b;26(2):159-164

27. Ramoun AA, Serur BH, Fattouh E- SM, Darweish SA, Abou El-Ghait HA. Enhancing follicular growth as a prerequisite for GnRH treatment of true anestrum in buffalo. Animal Reproduction Science. 2012;132:29-35

28. Verma HK, Sidhu SS, Panqwanker GR, Dhablania DC. Treatment of summer anoestrus in buffaloes with Bromocriptine. Indian Journal of Animal Reproduction. 1992;13:190-192

29. Wuliji T, Litherland A, Goetsch AL, Sahlu T, Ruchala R, Dawson LJ, et al. Evaluation of melatonin and bromocriptine administration in Spanish goats: Effects on the out of season breeding performance in spring, kidding rate and fleece weight of does. Small Ruminant Research. 2003;49:31-40

30. Ghuman SP, Singh J, Honparkhe M, Dadarwal D, Dhaliwal GS, Jain AK. Induction of ovulation of ovulatory size non–ovulatory follicles and initiation of ovarian cyclicity in summer anoestrous buffalo heifers (Bubalus bubalis) using melatonin implants. Reproduction of Domestic Animals. 2010;45(4):600-607

31. Odde KJ. A review of synchronization of estrus in postpartum cattle. Journal of Animal Science. 1990;68:817-830

32. Patterson DJ, Kojima MF, Smith JE. A review of methods to synchronize estrus in beef cattle. Journal of Animal Science. 2003;56:7-10

33. King GJ, Robertson HA. A two injection schedule with prostaglandin F2α for the regulation of the ovulatory cycle of cattle. Theriogenology. 1974;1:123-128

34. Roche JF. Control of estrous in dairy cows with a synthetic analogue of prostaglandin F2α. Veterinary Research Communications. 1977;1:121-129

35. Cooper MJ. Control of oestrous cycles of heifers with a synthetic prostaglandin analogue. Veterinary Record. 1974;95:200-203

36. Nellore JE, Cole HH. The hormonal control of estrus and ovulation in beef heifer. Journal of Animal Science. 1956;15:650-661

37. Kaltenbach CC, Niswender GD, Zimmerman DR, Wiltbank JN. Alteration of ovarian activity in cycling, pregnant and hysterectomized heifers with exogenous estrogens. Journal of Animal Science. 1964;23:995-1001

38. Wiltbank JN. Modification of ovarian activity in the bovines following injection of oestrogen and gonadotrophin. Journal of Reproduction and Fertility. Supplement. 1966;1:1-8

39. Cupp A, Garcia-Winder M, Zumudio A, Mariscal V, Wehrman M, Kojima N, et al. Two concentrations of progesterone (P4) in circulation have a differential effect on pattern of ovarian follicular development in the cow. Biology of Reproduction. 1992;45(1):106

40. Imwalle DB, Fernandez D l, Schillo KK. Melengestrol acetate blocks the preovulatory surge of luteinizing hormone, the expression of behavioral estrus, and ovulation in beef heifers. Journal of Animal Science. 2002;80:1280-1284

41. Vasconcelos JLM, Schafer JE, Stegner MR. A review of methods to synchronize. Theriogenology. 1999;52:1067-1078

42. Ravikumar K, Asokan SA. Veterinary aspects of milk production. The Indian Veterinary Journal. 2008;85:388-392

8 Chapter

BOVINE MASTITIS: PART I

1. INTRODUCTION: AN OVERVIEW

Bovine mastitis is a significant bacterial illness affecting dairy cattle globally. Mastitis incurs significant economic losses for dairy producers and the milk processing sector due to diminished milk production, changes in milk composition, milk wastage, heightened replacement expenses, additional labor, treatment costs, and veterinary services. [1]. Annual economic losses due to bovine mastitis are estimated to be $2 billion in the United States [2], $400 million in Canada (Canadian Bovine Mastitis and Milk Quality Research Network-CBMQRN), and $130 million in Australia [3]. Many factors including host, pathogen, and environmental factors influence the development of mastitis; however, inflammation of the mammary gland is usually a consequence of adhesion, invasion, and colonization of the mammary gland by one or more contagious (Staphylococcus aureus, Streptocococcus agalactiae, Corynebacterium bovis, Mycoplasmsa bovis, etc.) or environmental (coliform bacteria, environmental Streptococcus spp. and some coagulase negative Staphylococcus spp., many other minor pathogens) mastitis pathogens.

2. ETIOLOGY OF MASTITIS

Over 135 various microorganisms have been identified from bovine mastitis. The most common bovine mastitis pathogens are classified as contagious and environmental mastitis pathogens [4]. This classification depends upon their distribution in their natural habitat and mode of transmission from their natural habitat to the mammary glands of dairy cows [5]. It is important to mention that all pathogens lists as environmental or contagious may not be strictly environmental or strictly contagious; some of them may transmit both ways. Environmental mastitis pathogens exist in the cow's environment, and they can cause infection at any time. Environmental mastitis pathogens are difficult to control because they are in the environment of dairy cows and can transmit to the mammary glands at any time, whereas contagious mastitis pathogens exist in the infected udder or on the teat skin and transmit from infected to non-infected udder during milking by milker's hand or milking machine liners. Environmental mastitis pathogens include a wide range of organisms, including coliform bacteria (Escherichia coli, Klebsiella spp., Enterobacter spp., and Citrobacter spp), environmental Streptococcus spp. (Streptococcus uberis, Streptococcus dysgalactiae, Streptococcus equi, Streptococcus zooepidemicus, Streptococcus equinus, Streptococcus canis, Streptococcus parauberis, and others), Trueperella pyogenes, which was previously called Arcanobacterium pyogenes or Corynebacterium pyogenes and environmental coagulase-negative Staphylococcus species (CNS) (S. chromogenes, S. simulans, S. epidermidis, S. xylosus, S. haemolyticus, S. warneri, S. sciuri, S. lugdunensis, S. caprae, S. saccharolyticus, and others) [4, 6–9] and others such as Pseudomonas, Proteus, Serratia, Aerococcus, Listeria, Yeast and Prototheca that are increasingly found as mastitis-causing pathogens on some farms [10, 11].

Contagious mastitis pathogens primarily exist in the infected mammary glands or on the cow's teat skin and transmit from infected to non-infected mammary glands during milking by milker's hand or milking machine liners. Mycoplasma spp. may spread from cow to cow through aerosol transmission and invade the udder subsequent to bacteremia. The most frequent contagious mastitis pathogens are coagulase-positive Staphylococcus aureus, Streptococcus agalactiae, Mycoplasma bovis, and Corynebacterium bovis [11, 12]. The prevalence of mastitis caused by these different mastitis pathogens varies depending on herd management practices, geographical location, and other environmental conditions [13]. These different causative agents of mastitis have a multitude of virulence factors that make treatment and prevention of mastitis difficult.

2.1 Environmental mastitis pathogens

It is important to mention that all environmental mastitis pathogens may not be strictly environmental, and some of them may transmit both ways (contagious and environmental). However, the vast majority of these organisms are in the environment of dairy cows, and they transmit from these environmental sources to the udder of a cow at any time of the lactation cycle.

2.1.1 Streptococcus uberis mastitis

Streptococcus uberis is one of the environmental mastitis pathogens that accounts for a significant proportion of subclinical and clinical mastitis in lactating and nonlactating cows and heifers [14]. This organism is commonly found in the bedding material, which facilitates infection of mammary glands at any time [15]. Some report also indicated the possibility of contagious transmission of Streptococcus uberis [16].

S. uberis has various mechanisms of virulence that increases the chances of this organism establishing infection. These include a capsule, which evades phagocytosis, adherence to, and invasion into mammary epithelial cells [17, 18].

S. uberis adheres to epithelial cells using different mechanisms, including the formation of pedestals [19] and bridge formation through Streptococcus uberis adhesion molecule (SUAM) and lactoferrin [20–22]. This attachment is specific and mediated through a bridge formation between Streptococcus uberis adhesion molecule (SUAM) [23, 24] on S. uberis surface and lactoferrin, which is in the mammary secretion and has a receptor on the mammary epithelial surface [20, 22]. This interaction creates a molecular bridge that enhances S. uberis adherence to and internalization into mammary epithelial cells most likely via caveolae-dependent endocytosis and potentially allows S. uberis to evade host defense mechanisms [22, 24]. These factors increase the pathogenicity of S. uberis to cause mastitis. The sua gene is conserved among strains of S. uberis isolated from geographically diverse areas [9, 13], and a sua deletion mutant of S. uberis is defective in adherence to and internalization into mammary epithelial cells [14].

2.1.2 Coagulase-negative Staphylococcus species (CNS)

More recently, coagulase-negative Staphylococcus species (CNS) such as S. chromogenes, S. simulans, S. xylosus, S. haemolyticus, S. hyicus, and S. epidermidis are increasingly isolated from bovine milk [7, 25–27] with S. chromogenes being the most increasingly diagnosed species as a cause of subclinical mastitis. Staphylococcus chromogenes [28] and other CNS [4, 8] have been shown to cause subclinical infections in dairy cows that reduce the prevalence of contagious mastitis pathogens.

Staphylococcus chromogenes is most commonly isolated from mammary secretions rather than from the environment itself [8, 29]. S. chromogenes consistently isolated from the cow's udder and teat skin [30], and some studies showed that it causes long-lasting, persistent subclinical infections [26]. The CNS causes high somatic cell counts in milk on some dairy farms [29, 31]. Woodward et al. [32] evaluated the normal teat skin flora and found that 25% of the isolates exhibited the ability to prevent the growth of some mastitis pathogens. An in vitro study conducted on S. chromogenes showed that this organism could inhibit the growth of major mastitiscausing pathogens such as Staph. aureus, Strep. dysgalactiae, and Strep. uberis [28].

In a study conducted on conventional and organic Canadian dairy farms, CNS were found in 20% of the clinical samples [33]. Recently, mastitis caused by CNS increasingly became more problematic in dairy herds [30, 34–36]. However, mastitis caused by CNS is less severe compared to mastitis caused by Staphylococcus aureus [26].

2.1.3 Coliform mastitis

Coliform bacteria such as Escherichia, Klebsiella, and Enterobacter are a common cause of mastitis in dairy cows [37]. The most common species, isolated in more than 80% of cases of coliform mastitis, is Escherichia coli [38, 39]. E. coli usually infects the mammary glands during the dry period and progresses to inflammation and clinical mastitis during the early lactation with local and sometimes severe systemic clinical manifestations. Some reports indicated that the severity of E. coli mastitis is mainly determined by cow factors rather than by virulence factors of E. coli [40]. However, recent molecular and genetic studies showed that the pathogenicity of E. coli is entirely dependent on the FecA protein that enables E. coli to actively uptake iron from ferric-citrate in the mammary gland [41]. The severity of the clinical mastitis and peak E. coli counts in mammary secretions are positively correlated. Intramammary infection with E. coli induced expression and release of pro-inflammatory cytokines [42, 43]. Recently, it has been shown with mouse mastitis models that IL-17A and Th17 cells are instrumental in the defense against E. coli intramammary infection [44, 45]. However, the role of IL-17 in bovine E. coli mastitis is not well defined. The result of recent vaccine efficacy study against E. coli mastitis suggested that cell-mediated immune response has more protective effect than humoral response [46]. However, the cytokine signaling pathways that lead to efficient bacterial clearance are not clearly defined.

2.2 Contagious mastitis pathogens

2.2.1 Coagulase-positive Staphylococcus aureus

Coagulase-positive Staphylococcus aureus is one of the most common contagious mastitis pathogens in dairy cows, with an estimated incidence rate of 43–74% [47, 48]. Staphylococcus aureus is grouped under the family Staphylococcaceae and genus Staphylococcus. It is a gram-positive, catalase and coagulase-positive, non-spore forming, oxidase negative, non-motile, cluster forming, and facultative anaerobe [49]. The coagulase test is not an absolute test for the confirmation of the diagnosis of S. aureus from the cases of bovine mastitis, but more than 95% of all coagulase-positive staphylococci from bovine mastitis belong to S. aureus [50]. Other coagulase-positive species include S. aureus subsp. anaerobius causes lesion in sheep; S. pseudintermedius causes pyoderma, pustular dermatitis, pyometra, otitis externa, and other infections in dogs and cats; S. schleiferi subsp. coagulans causes otitis externa (inflammation of the external ear canal) in dogs; S. hyicus is coagulase variable (some strains are positive and some others are negative), species that causes mastitis in dairy cows, exudative epidermitis (greasy pig disease) in pigs; and S. delphini causes purulent cutaneous lesions in dolphins.

S. aureus can infect many host species, including humans. In humans, S. aureus causes a wide variety of illnesses ranging from mild skin infection to a life-threatening systemic infection. It has been reported that certain strains of S. aureus with specific tissue tropism can be adapted to infect specific tissue such as the mammary gland [51]. Furthermore, a study by McMillan [52] showed distinct lineages of S. aureus in bovine, ovine, and caprine species. S. aureus strains can be host specific, meaning that they are found more commonly in a specific species [51]. Some studies showed that S. aureus that causes mastitis belong to certain dominant clones, which are frequently responsible for clinical and subclinical mastitis in a herd at certain geographic areas, indicating that the control measures may need to be directed against specific clones in a given area [53–55]. However, because S. aureus is such a big problem in human health, cross-infection has been an important research topic. Several studies have reported cases of cross-infection in several different species [56–58]. In the dairy industry, there have been reports of human origin methicillin-resistant S. aureus infecting bovine mammary glands [59, 60]. These studies add to the unease that strains can gain new mutations or virulence factors and adapt to cross the interspecies boundary relatively rapidly [61].

Although the incidence of S. aureus mastitis can be reduced with hygienic milking practices and a good management system, it is still a major problem for dairy farms, with a prevalence of 66% among farms tested in the United States [62]. The prevalence of S. aureus mastitis varies from farm to farm because of variation in hygienic milking practices and overall farm management differences on the application of control measures for contagious mastitis pathogens. Good hygiene in the milking parlor can significantly reduce the occurrence of new S. aureus mastitis in the herd, but it does not remove existing cases within a herd [63]. Neave et al. concluded that it is nearly impractical to keep all udder quarters of dairy cows free of all pathogens at all times. Since this early observation by Neave et al. [63], many studies have confirmed that management practices can reduce new cases of intramammary infection (IMI) [9, 64] but cannot eliminate existing infections. In the United States, the prevalence of clinical and subclinical S. aureus mastitis ranged from 10 to 45% [65] and 15 to 75%, respectively.

2.2.1.1 Virulence factors of S. aureus

Staphylococcus aureus has many virulence factors that can be grouped broadly into two major classes. These include (1) secretory factors which are surface localized structural components that serve as virulence factors and (2) secretory virulence factors which are produced by bacteria cells and secreted out of cells and act on different targets in the host body. Both non-secretory and secretory virulence factors together help this pathogen to evade the host's defenses and colonize mammary glands.

2.3 Non-secretory factors

Some of surface localized structural components that serve as virulence factors include membrane-bound proteins, which include collagen-binding protein, fibrinogen-binding protein, elastin-binding protein, penicillin-binding protein, and lipoteichoic acid. Similarly, cell wall-bound factors such as peptidoglycan, lipoteichoic acid, teichoic acid, protein A, β-Lactamase, and proteases serve as non-secretory virulence factors. Other cell surface-associated virulence factors include exopolysaccharides, which comprises capsule, slime, and biofilm. Overall, S. aureus has over 24 surface proteins and 13 secreted proteins that are involved in immune evasion [66] and about 15–26 proteins for biofilm formation [67, 68].

Surface proteins, such as staphylococcal protein A (SpA), clumping factors A and B (ClfA and ClfB) [69–71], fibrinogen-binding proteins [72], iron-regulated surface determinants (IsdA, IsdB, and IsdH) [69, 73], fibronectin-binding proteins A and B [74], biofilm associated protein (BAP) and exopolysaccharides (capsule, slime, and biofilms) [75–79], play roles in S. aureus adhesion to and invasion into host cells [80]. The BAP expression enhances biofilm production and the BAP gene is only found in S. aureus strain from bovine origin [81–83]. Evaluation of BAP gene of S. aureus from bovine and human isolates using polymerase chain reaction restriction fragment length polymorphism (PCR-RFLP) showed that bovine and human isolates are not closely related [84]. Thus, some host-specific evolutionary factors may have been developed between both strain types.

Biofilms are considered an important virulence factor in the pathogenesis of bovine S. aureus mastitis [77, 78]. Slime, an extracellular polysaccharide layer, acts as a barrier against phagocytosis and antimicrobials. It also helps with adhesion to a surface [85]. If a biofilm forms in a mammary gland, it will protect those bacteria from antimicrobials and the host's immune system [77, 78]. In addition, once the biofilm matures and the immune attack has subsided, the biofilm can break open and allow reinfection of the mammary gland [86]. There are many contributors to biofilm production, such as polysaccharide intercellular adhesin (PIA) also known as poly-N-acetyl-β (1-6)-glucosamine (PNAG), MSCRAMMS, teichoic acids, and extracellular DNA (eDNA) [75, 76] that are known to help these bacteria cells to hold onto a surface [87]. Various proteins encoded by intercellular adhesion loci such as icaA, icaB, icaC, and icaD are involved in PIA production which in turn result in biofilm formation [75, 76]. Vasudevan et al. [88] evaluated the correlation of slime production and presence of the intercellular adhesion (ica) genes with biofilm production. These authors [88] found that all tested isolates were positive for icaA and icaD genes, and most tested isolates produce slime, but not all slime positives produced biofilms in vitro. Similarly, a study in Poland found that all isolates were positive for icaA and icaD [80] genes. While adhesion is promoted with biofilm production, the bap gene prevents the invasion of host cells [83]. Despite the presence of the ica gene strongly support biofilm production, the presence of the ica gene is not mandatory for biofilm production since S. aureus lacking ica gene can still produce biofilm through other microbial surface components recognizing adhesive matrix molecules (MSCRAM) and secreted proteins [89, 90].

2.4 Secretory factors

Some of the known secretory virulence factors are toxins which include staphylococcal enterotoxins, non-enteric exfoliative toxins, toxic shock syndrome toxin 1, leucocidin, and hemolysins (alpha, beta, delta, and gamma) [91, 92]. Similarly, enzymes such as coagulase, staphylokinase, DNAase, phosphatase, lipase, phospho- lipase, and hyaluronidase serve as virulence factors of S. aureus [93].

2.4.1 Hemolysins

S. aureus isolates from bovine mastitis produce alpha (α), beta (β), gamma (γ), and delta (δ) hemolysins that cause hemolysis of red blood cells of the host [94] and all are antigenically distinct. α-hemolysin is a pore-forming toxin that binds to a disintegrin and metalloproteinase domain-containing protein-10 (ADAM10) receptor resulting in pore formation and cellular necrosis [95, 96]. It is also known to increase the inflammatory response and decrease macrophage function [97]. α-hemolysin damages the plasma membrane of the epithelial cell resulting in leakages of low-molecular-weight molecules from the cytosol and death of the cell [98]. It is produced by 20–50% of strains from bovine IMI [99]. A study reported that the α-hemolysin might be required for a cell to cell interaction during biofilm formation [100]. β-hemolysin hydrolyzes the sphingomyelin present in the plasma membrane resulting in increased permeability with progressive loss of cell surface charge [101]. It is produced by 75–100% of S. aureus strains from bovine IMI [99]. α-hemolysin expression requires specific growth conditions in vitro because its growth is inhibited by agar [102]. α-hemolysin producing strains cause complete hemolysis of sheep red blood cells, whereas β-hemolysin producing strains cause partial hemolysis within 24 h of incubation at 37°C [103]. Partial hemolysis caused by β-hemolysin becomes completely lysed after further storage at 4–15°C, which is also expressed as hot-cold lysis [104]. β-hemolysin producing strains are the most frequent isolates from animals [105]. δ-hemolysin causes complete hemolysis of red blood cells of wide range of species including human, rabbit, sheep, horse, rat, guinea pig, and some fish erythrocytes. δ-hemolysin migrates more slowly through agar than the α-hemolysin so the effect takes longer time to express. Double (α- and β-) hemolysin producing strains caused complete hemolysis in the middle with partial hemolysis on the peripheral area around each colony [105]. γ-hemolysin is produced by almost every strain of S. aureus, but γ-hemolysin is not identifiable on blood agar plates, due to the inhibitory effect of agar on toxin activity [106].

2.4.2 Enterotoxins Enterotoxins

These toxins are heat stable and can resist pasteurization. S. aureus produces staphylococcal enterotoxins A, B, C, D, E, G, H, I, and J–Q as well as toxic shock syndrome toxin 1 (tsst-1) [105, 107, 108]. Enterotoxins can get into the food chain through the consumption of contaminated food and cause food poisoning [109]. Staphylococcal enterotoxins tend to contaminate dairy products and cause foodborne illness [110, 111]. Staphylococcal enterotoxins G to Q (SEG–SEQ) are prevalent among S. aureus isolates from cases of bovine mastitis and are also implicated in the pathogenesis of mastitis. Some of these toxins are known to function as superantigens that cause increased immunological reactivity in the host [110]. Some studies showed that about 20% of S. aureus isolates from IMI produce toxic shock syndrome toxin-1 [109, 112]. Toxic shock syndrome toxin causes toxic shock syndrome and can be fatal [113]. Besides the superantigenic effect of enterotoxins, their role in the pathogenesis of mastitis is unknown. It may be specific to each strain or area based on selective pressures in the habitat [114]. Enterotoxin prevalence seems to vary between geographical regions. The strains producing enterotoxin C have been isolated relatively frequently from cases of bovine mastitis [108, 115, 116].

Enterotoxins are believed to have a role in the development of mastitis since S. aureus isolates from cases of mastitis had a high prevalence of enterotoxins than isolates from milk of cows without mastitis [117, 118]; however, staphylococcal entero- toxins expressions are controlled by several regulatory elements [119] that respond to a variety of different micro-environmental stimuli and the exact mechanisms by which enterotoxins contribute to the development of mastitis are not clearly known and yet to be determined.

In addition to specific virulence factors, Staphylococcus aureus also possesses different mechanisms or traits such as biofilm formation, adhesion to and invasion into mammary epithelial cells, and formation of small colony variant (SCV) that enable this pathogen to resist host defense mechanisms. The ability of S. aureus to invade mammary epithelial cells during mastitis plays a significant role in the pathogenesis of S. aureus. Internalized bacteria can hide from the host's immune system inside the host cell and continue to multiply inside the host cell [120]. There may be many mechanisms that S. aureus uses to invade into host cells, and each mechanism can be strain dependent. S. aureus strains have a fibronectin-binding protein that can link to the fibronectin on the mammary epithelial cell surface. Fibronectin binding protein is thought to be a common way for the bacteria cells to invade bovine mammary epithelial cells. Fibronectin-binding protein-deficient strains cannot invade host cells [121]. The presence of a capsule prevents adherence to epithelial cells [122, 123].

Adhesion is the first step in the formation of biofilm or the invasion of host cells, which protects the bacteria from the host immune system and facilitates chronic infection [124]. Adhesion is dependent on surface proteins called adhesins, which help the bacterium to recognize and attach to host cells. Staphylococci are coated with a wide variety of surface proteins that help them to adhere to host cells and extracellular matrix components. Microbial surface components recognizing adhesive matrix molecules (MSCRAMMs) of the host are the most common surface proteins that are involved in adhesion [124]. The ability to bind to host tissue or the host's cell surface is a pivotal part of the bacteria's pathogenicity because adhesion is typically the first step in the invasion and biofilm formation [125, 126].

Adhesion to and invasion into epithelial cells [124], intracellular survival in macrophages [127], and epithelial cells allow them to avoid detection by the host immune system and resist treatment with antibiotics [120]. Due to its poor response to treatments, S. aureus infections often become chronic with a low cure rate [128]. Treatment of Staphylococcus aureus mastitis with cloxacillin cured only 25% of the clinical cases and 40% of subclinical cases in the study by Tyler and Baggot [129]. Staphylococcus aureus also has a known ability to form biofilms [77, 78, 86] and acquire antimicrobial-resistance genes via horizontal resistance gene transfer, which enables this bacterium to develop antimicrobial resistance [130, 131].

The mode of transmission from infected mammary glands or colonized udder skin to healthy mammary glands is through contact during milking procedures with milker's hand, towel, and milking machine [58]. S. aureus usually causes subclinical or chronic infections and is difficult to clear with antibiotic treatment [132].

2.4.3 Streptococcus agalactiae

The most important virulence factor of S. agalactiae is the capsular polysaccharide [133], which protects this bacterium from being engulfed by macrophages and subsequently phagocytosed [133]. Another virulence factor of S. agalactiae is the Rib protein, which confers resistance to proteases. Emaneini et al. [133] found that the Rib encoding gene (rib) was detected in 89% of the isolates from bovine origin. Streptococcus agalactiae causes persistent infections that are usually difficult to clear without antibiotic treatment [134]. Though Streptococcus agalactiae is highly contagious, it has good response to treatment with antibiotics, which makes it possible to eliminate from herds with current mastitis control measures [129]. Since the adoption of hygienic milking practices, the incidence of mastitis caused by S. agalactiae has dramatically decreased and is now rarely observed in dairy herds [135].

2.4.4 Mycoplasma mastitis

Mastitis caused by Mycoplasma spp. is a growing concern in the United States. It is believed that this organism has been underreported due to the difficulty of isolation by culture method [136]. The incidence of Mycoplasma mastitis varies across the globe, with a 3.2% prevalence rate in the United States that may increase to 14.4% in larger herd size of greater than 500 cows [47, 48, 62, 137]. A risk factor for Mycoplasma mastitis increase with herd size, and most of the Mycoplasma mastitis cases are subclinical infections with outbreaks linked to asymptomatic carriers [138]. Pathogenesis of most Mycoplasma spp. infection is characterized by adherence to and internalization into host cells resulting in colonization of the host with immune modulation without causing severe disease [138]. Mycoplasma species lack a cell wall, thus not sensitive to beta-lactam antibiotics, but showed sensitivity to non-beta-lactam antibiotics [139].

3. ROUTES OF ENTRY OF MASTITIS PATHOGENS TO THE UDDER

In general, it is believed that mastitis pathogens gain entrance to the udder through teat opening into the teat canal and from the teat canal into the intramammary area during the reverse flow of milk due to vacuum pressure fluctuation of the milking machine [9]. However, the detailed mechanism of mastitis pathogen colonization of the mammary gland may vary among species of bacteria and the virulence factors associated with particular strain in each species. An example of this is in some cases; it has been shown that E. coli can penetrate the teat canal without the reverse flow of milk [9]. Some of the major mastitis pathogens, such as E. coli [140], Staphylococcus aureus, and Streptococcus uberis [20–22] can adhere to and subsequently invade into the mammary epithelial cells. This adherence and subsequent invasion into mammary epithelial cells allow them to persist in the intracellular area as well as to escape the host immune defenses attack and action of antimicrobial drugs [120, 140–144]. Dogan et al. [145] compared E. coli strains known to cause chronic infections with strains known to cause acute infections and found that chronic strains were more invasive to the epithelial cells, leading to the difficulty in clearance and persistent infection compared to acute strains. S. aureus enters the mammary gland through the teat opening and subsequently multiply in the mammary gland where they may form biofilms, attach to, and internalize into the mammary epithelial cells causing inflammation of mammary glands characterized by swelling, degeneration of epithelial cells, and epithelial erosions and ulcers [146, 147].

4. CLINICAL MANIFESTATION OF MASTITIS

Depending on clinical signs, mastitis can also be divided into clinical and subclinical mastitis. Clinical mastitis is characterized by visible inflammatory changes (abnormalities) in the mammary gland tissue such as redness, swelling, pain, increased heart, and abnormal changes in milk color (watery, bloody, and blood tinged) and consistency (clots or flakes) [9]. Clinical mastitis can be acute, peracute, subacute, or chronic. Acute mastitis is a very rapid inflammatory response characterized by systemic clinical signs which include fever, anorexia, shock, as well as local inflammatory changes in the mammary gland and milk. Peracute mastitis is manifested by a rapid onset of severe inflammation, pain, and systemic symptoms that resulted in a severely sick cow within a short period of time. Subacute mastitis is the most frequently seen form of clinical mastitis characterized by few local signs of mild inflammation in the udder and visible changes in milk such as small clots.

Chronic mastitis is a long-term recurring, persistent case of mastitis that may show few symptoms of mastitis between repeated occasional flare-ups of the disease where signs are visible and can continue over periods of several months. Chronic mastitis often leads to irreversible damage to the udder from the repeated occurrences of the inflammation, and often these cows are culled.

Subclinical mastitis is the inflammation of the mammary gland that does not create visible changes in the milk or the udder. Subclinical mastitis is an infection of mammary gland characterized by non-visible inflammatory changes such as a high somatic cell count coupled with shedding of causative bacteria through milk [9]. During this inflammatory process, the milk samples showed a rapid increase of somatic cells, characterized by increased number of neutrophils in the secretion [146, 148]. Despite increased recruitment of somatic cells into infected mammary glands, evidenced by an increased number of neutrophils, infection usually does not clear but became subclinical. Intramammary infections during early lactation may become acute clinical mastitis characterized by gangrene development due congestion and thrombosis (blockage) of blood supply to the tissue but most new infection during late lactation or dry period become acute or chronic mastitis [149, 150].

The increase in somatic cell count during subclinical infections leads to a decrease in useful components in the milk, such as lactose and casein [151]. Lactose is the sugar found in milk, and casein is one of the major proteins in milk and decreases in these two components affect the quality and quantity of milk yield [9]. During mastitis, there is an increase in lipase and plasmin, which have a detrimental effect on the quantity and quality of milk due to the breakdown of milk fat and casein [9]. Subclinical infections can reduce milk production by 10–12% when just one-quarter is infected [152]. These subclinical infections cause some of the greatest unseen economic [20] losses because of their detrimental impact on production and milk quality without showing visible signs of infection [152].

5. RISK FACTORS FOR MASTITIS

There are host-, pathogen-, and environmental-related risk factors that predispose dairy cows to mastitis. The host risk factors include age (parity), stage of lactation, somatic cell count, breed, the anatomy of the mammary glands/ morphology of udder and teat (diameter of teat canal and conformation of the udder), and immune competence (immunity) [153] (Figure 1). The environmental risk factors include the proper functioning status of milking machine, udder trauma, sanitation, climate, nutrition, management, season, and housing condition [154]

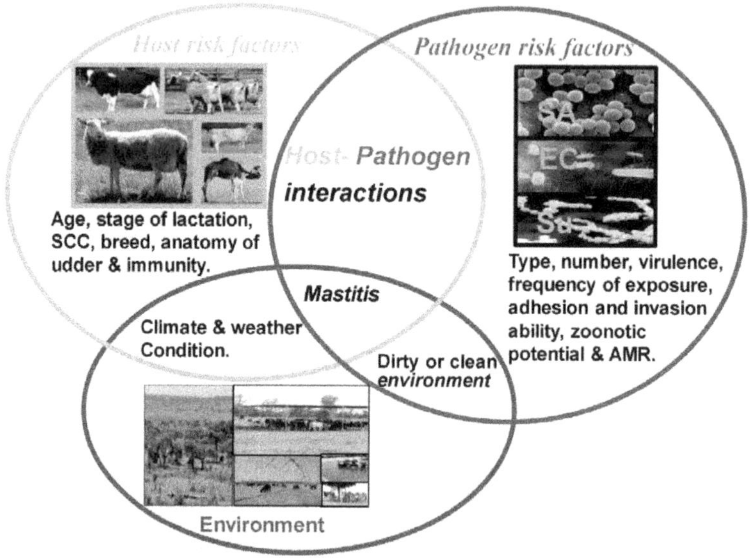

Figure 1. Risk factors for mastitis. SA, Staphylococcus aureus; EC, Escherichia coli; SU, Streptococcus uberis; SCC, somatic cell count; AMR, antimicrobial resistance.

(Figure 1). The pathogen risk factors include type (bacteria, fungi, yeast, and algae), number (large number and small number), virulence (highly, moderate, or less virulent), frequency of exposure (dirty farm floor, dirty milking machine, and dirty teat drying towels frequently expose to pathogen; clean floor, clean milking machine, and clean teat drying towels less exposure to pathogens), ability to resist flushing out of the glands by milk (ability to adhere or attach to and invade or internalize into mammary epithelial cells), zoonotic (transmit from cow to human or vice versa) potential, and resistance to antimicrobials [4] (Figure 1). The warm, humid, and moist climate favors the growth of bacteria and increases the chances of intramammary infection (IMI) and mastitis development [154]. The incidence of mastitis varies from farm to farm due to the combined effects of these different factors that increase the risk of disease development.

Dairy cows are highly susceptible to IMI during the early dry period due to increased colonization of teat skin with bacteria. Bacterial colonization of teat increases during the early dry period because of an absence of hygienic milking practices including pre-milking washing and drying of teats [155], as well as pre- and post-milking teat dipping in antiseptic solutions [156, 157] that are known to reduce teat end colonization and infection. An udder infected during the early dry period usually manifests clinical mastitis during the transition period because of increased production of parturition inducing immunosuppressive hormones [158, 159], negative energy balance [160], and physical stress during calving [161].

6. ROLE OF MASTITIS ON PUBLIC HEALTH

Mastitis is increasingly becoming a public health concern due to the ability of the causative bacterial pathogens and/or their products, such as enterotoxins, toenter the food supply and cause foodborne diseases [109, 162], especially through the consumption of raw milk [29] and undercooked meat of culled dairy cows due to chronic mastitis that are usually sold to the slaughter (abattoir) for meat consumption. The Center for Disease Control (CDC) estimated that roughly 48 million people in the United States a year become sick from foodborne diseases [163]. Foodborne pathogens have been detected in bulk tank milk in multiple studies [164–167]. These authors found that the number of foodborne pathogens detected in bulk tank milk vary with location, management practices, hygiene, and number of animals on the farm [165]. Similarly, a study on bulk tank milk from east Tennessee and southwest Virginia by Rohrbach et al. [168] showed that 32.5% of the samples analyzed contained one or more foodborne pathogens. Even dairy producers who used proper hygienic milking practices, pre- and post-milking teat disinfectant and antibiotic dry cow therapy, had foodborne pathogens in their bulk tank milk [164]. The isolation of these foodborne pathogens from bulk tank milk samples across the United States demonstrate the threat that mastitis pathogens and zoonotic mastitis causing pathogens create on public health if raw milk is consumed or if these pathogens make it through processing.

7. CONCISE SUMMARY

Bovine mastitis is the predominant multifactorial illness affecting dairy cattle globally. Mastitis incurs significant economic losses for dairy producers and the milk processing sector due to diminished milk production, changes in milk composition, rejected milk, elevated replacement costs, additional labor, treatment expenses, and veterinary services. Numerous factors, including pathogens, hosts, and environmental conditions, might affect the onset of mastitis. Mastitis, the inflammation of the mammary gland, typically results from the adhesion, invasion, and colonization of the gland by one or more pathogens, including Staphylococcus aureus, Streptococcus uberis, and Escherichia coli.

REFERENCES

1. Petrovski K, Trajcev M, Buneski G. A review of the factors affecting the costs of bovine mastitis. Journal of the South African Veterinary Association. 2006;77:52-60
2. NMC. The Cost of Mastitis: Dairy Insight Research 2005/2006: Final report. 2005
3. Ismail ZB. Mastitis vaccines in dairy cows: Recent developments and recommendations of application. Veterinary world. 2017;10:1057

4. Bradley AJ. Bovine mastitis: An evolving disease. The Veterinary Journal. 2002;164:116-128
5. Calvinho LF, Oliver SP. Invasion and persistence of streptococcus dysgalactiae within bovine mammary epithelial cells. Journal of Dairy Science. 1998;81:678-686
6. Becker K, Heilmann C, Peters G. Coagulase-negative staphylococci. Clinical Microbiology Reviews. 2014;27:870-926
7. De Vliegher S, Fox LK, Piepers S, McDougall S, Barkema HW. Invited review: Mastitis in dairy heifers: Nature of the disease, potential impact, prevention, and control. Journal of Dairy Science. 2012;95:1025-1040
8. Piessens V, Van Coillie E, Verbist B, Supre K, Braem G, Van Nuffel A, et al. Distribution of coagulase-negative staphylococcus species from milk and environment of dairy cows differs between herds. Journal of Dairy Science. 2011;94:2933-2944
9. Blowey RW. Mastitis Control in Dairy Herds. 2nd ed. Cambridge, Mass, MA: CABI; 2010
10. Cameron M, Saab M, Heider L, McClure JT, Rodriguez-Lecompte JC, Sanchez J. Antimicrobial susceptibility patterns of environmental streptococci recovered from bovine milk samples in the maritime provinces of Canada. Front Vet Sci. 2016;3:79
11. Bobbo T, Ruegg PL, Stocco G, Fiore E, Gianesella M, Morgante M, et al. Associations between pathogen- specific cases of subclinical mastitis and milk yield, quality, protein composition, and cheese-making traits in dairy cows. Journal of Dairy Science. 2017;100:4868-4883
12. Barkema HW, Green MJ, Bradley AJ, Zadoks RN. Invited review: The role of contagious disease in udder health. Journal of Dairy Science. 2009;92:4717-4729
13. Oliver S, Mitchell B. Prevalence of mastitis pathogens in herds participating in a mastitis control program1. Journal of Dairy Science. 1984;67:2436-2440
14. Smith KL, Todhunter D, Schoenberger P. Environmental mastitis: Cause, prevalence, prevention1, 2. Journal of Dairy Science. 1985;68:1531-1553
15. Bramley AJ. Sources of streptococcus uberis in the dairy herd: I. Isolation from bovine faces and from straw bedding of cattle. Journal of Dairy Research. 1982;49:369-373
16. Zadoks RN, Gillespie BE, Barkema HW, Sampimon OC, Oliver SP, Schukken YH. Clinical, epidemiological and molecular characteristics of Streptococcus uberis infections in dairy herds. Epidemiology and Infection. 2003;130:335-349

17. Almeida R, Oliver S. Antiphagocytic effect of the capsule of Streptococcus uberis. Zoonoses and Public Health. 1993;40:707-714

18. Oliver S, Almeida R, Calvinho L. Virulence factors of Streptococcus uberis isolated from cows with mastitis. Zoonoses and Public Health. 1998;45:461-471

19. Matthews K, Almeida R, Oliver S. Bovine mammary epithelial cell invasion by Streptococcus uberis. Infection and Immunity. 1994;62:5641-5646

20. Almeida RA, Kerro Dego O, Headrick SI, Lewis MJ, Oliver SP. Role of Streptococcus uberis adhesion molecule in the pathogenesis of Streptococcus uberis mastitis. Veterinary Microbiology. 2015;179:332-335

21. Almeida RA, Fang W, Oliver SP. Adherence and internalization of Streptococcus uberis to bovine mammary epithelial cells are mediated by host cell proteoglycans. FEMS Microbiology Letters. 1999;177:313-317

22. Patel D, Almeida RA, Dunlap JR, Oliver SP. Bovine lactoferrin serves as a molecular bridge for internalization of Streptococcus uberis into bovine mammary epithelial cells. Veterinary Microbiology. 2009;137:297-301

23. Fang W, Oliver SP. Identification of lactoferrin-binding proteins in bovine mastitis-causing Streptococcus uberis. FEMS Microbiology Letters. 1999;176:91-96

24. Almeida RA, Luther DA, Park HM, Oliver SP. Identification, isolation, and partial characterization of a novel Streptococcus uberis adhesion molecule (SUAM). Veterinary Microbiology. 2006;115:183-191

25. Vanderhaeghen W, Piepers S, Leroy F, Van Coillie E, Haesebrouck F, De Vliegher S. Invited review: Effect, persistence, and virulence of coagulase-negative Staphylococcus species associated with ruminant udder health. Journal of Dairy Science. 2014;97:5275-5293

26. Taponen S, Pyorala S. Coagulase- negative staphylococci as cause of bovine mastitis- not so different from Staphylococcus aureus? Veterinary Microbiology. 2009;134:29-36

27. Nyman AK, Fasth C, Waller KP. Intramammary infections with different non-aureus staphylococci in dairy cows. Journal of Dairy Science. 2018;101:1403-1418

28. De Vliegher S, Opsomer G, Vanrolleghem A, Devriese L, Sampimon O, Sol J, et al. In vitro growth inhibition of major mastitis pathogens by Staphylococcus chromogenes originating from teat apices of dairy heifers. Veterinary Microbiology. 2004;101:215-221

29. Gillespie BE, Headrick SI, Boonyayatra S, Oliver SP. Prevalence and persistence of coagulase-negative Staphylococcus species in three dairy research herds. Veterinary Microbiology. 2009;134:65-72

30. Taponen S, Bjorkroth J, Pyorala S. Coagulase-negative staphylococci isolated from bovine extramammary sites and intramammary infections in a single dairy herd. The Journal of Dairy Research. 2008;75:422-429

31. Fry PR, Middleton JR, Dufour S, Perry J, Scholl D, Dohoo I. Association of coagulase-negative staphylococcal species, mammary quarter milk somatic cell count, and persistence of intramammary infection in dairy cattle. Journal of Dairy Science. 2014;97:4876-4885

32. Woodward W, Besser T, Ward A, Corbeil L. In vitro growth inhibition of mastitis pathogens by bovine teat skin normal flora. Canadian Journal of Veterinary Research. 1987;51:27

33. Levison L, Miller-Cushon E, Tucker A, Bergeron R, Leslie K, Barkema H, et al. Incidence rate of pathogen-specific clinical mastitis on conventional and organic Canadian dairy farms. Journal of Dairy Science. 2016;99:1341-1350

34. Pyorala S, Taponen S. Coagulase- negative staphylococci-emerging mastitis pathogens. Veterinary Microbiology. 2009;134:3-8

35. Taponen S, Koort J, Bjorkroth J, Saloniemi H, Pyorala S. Bovine intramammary infections caused by coagulase-negative staphylococci may persist throughout lactation according to amplified fragment length polymorphism-based analysis. Journal of Dairy Science. 2007;90:3301-3307

36. Taponen S, Liski E, Heikkila AM, Pyorala S. Factors associated with intramammary infection in dairy cows caused by coagulase-negative staphylococci, Staphylococcus aureus, Streptococcus uberis, Streptococcus dysgalactiae, Corynebacterium bovis, or Escherichia coli. Journal of Dairy Science. 2017;100:493-503

37. Hogan J, Larry SK. Coliform mastitis. Veterinary Research. 2003;34:507-519

38. Botrel MA, Haenni M, Morignat E, Sulpice P, Madec JY, Calavas D. Distribution and antimicrobial resistance of clinical and subclinical mastitis pathogens in dairy cows in Rhone-Alpes, France. Foodborne Pathogens and Disease. 2010;7:479-487

39. Bradley AJ, Leach KA, Breen JE, Green LE, Green MJ. Survey of the incidence and aetiology of mastitis on dairy farms in England and Wales. The Veterinary Record. 2007;160:253-257

40. Burvenich C, Van Merris V, Mehrzad J, Diez-Fraile A, Duchateau L. Severity of E. coli mastitis is mainly determined by cow factors. Veterinary Research. 2003;34:521-564

41. Blum SE, Goldstone RJ, Connolly JPR, Reperant-Ferter M, Germon P, Inglis NF, et al. Postgenomics characterization of an essential genetic determinant of mammary pathogenic Escherichia coli. MBio. 2018;9(2):e00423-18

42. Petzl W, Zerbe H, Gunther J, Seyfert HM, Hussen J, Schuberth HJ. Pathogen-specific responses in the bovine udder. Models and immunoprophylactic concepts. Research in Veterinary Science. 2018;116:55-61

43. Petzl W, Zerbe H, Gunther J, Yang W, Seyfert HM, Nurnberg G, et al. Escherichia coli, but not Staphylococcus aureus triggers an early increased expression of factors contributing to the innate immune defense in the udder of the cow. Veterinary Research. 2008;39:18

44. Zhao Y, Zhou M, Gao Y, Liu H, Yang W, Yue J, et al. Shifted T helper cell polarization in a murine Staphylococcus aureus mastitis model. PLoS One. 2015;10:e0134797

45. Porcherie A, Gilbert FB, Germon P, Cunha P, Trotereau A, Rossignol C, et al. IL-17A is an important effector of the immune response of the mammary gland to Escherichia coli infection. Journal of Immunology. 2016;196:803-812

46. Herry V, Gitton C, Tabouret G, Reperant M, Forge L, Tasca C, et al. Local immunization impacts the response of dairy cows to Escherichia coli mastitis. Scientific Reports. 2017;7:3441

47. USDA APHIS U. Antibiotic Use on U.S. Dairy Operations, 2002 and 2007 (infosheet, 5p, October, 2008) [Online]. 2008a. Available from: https://www.aphis.usda.gov/animal_health/nahms/ dairy/downloads/dairy07/Dairy07_is_AntibioticUse_1.pdf [Accessed: 23 March 2020]

48. USDA APHIS U. United States Department of Agriculture, Animal Plant Health Inspection Service National Animal Health Monitoring System. Highlights of Dairy 2007 Part III: Reference of dairy cattle health and management practices in the United States, 2007 (info sheet 4p, October, 2008) [Online]. 2008b. Available from: https://www.aphis.usda.gov/animal_health/nahms/dairy/downloads/ dairy07/Dairy07_ir_Food_safety.pdf [Accessed: 23 March 2020]

49. Takahashi T, Satoh I, Kikuchi N. Phylogenetic relationships of 38 taxa of the genus Staphylococcus based on 16S rRNA gene sequence analysis. International Journal of Systematic Bacteriology. 1999;49(Pt 2):725-728

50. Fox LK, Hancock DD. Effect of segregation on prevention of intramammary infections by Staphylococcus aureus. Journal of Dairy Science. 1989;72:540-544

51. van Leeuwen WB, Melles DC, Alaidan A, Al-Ahdal M, Boelens HA, Snijders SV, et al. Host-and tissue-specific pathogenic traits of Staphylococcus aureus. Journal of Bacteriology. 2005;187:4584-4591

52. McMillan K, Moore SC, McAuley CM, Fegan N, Fox EM. Characterization of Staphylococcus aureus isolates from raw milk sources in Victoria, Australia. BMC Microbiology. 2016;16:169

53. Graber HU, Naskova J, Studer E, Kaufmann T, Kirchhofer M, Brechbuhl M, et al. Mastitis-related subtypes of bovine Staphylococcus aureus are characterized by different clinical properties. Journal of Dairy Science.2009;92:1442-1451

54. Capurro A, Aspan A, Artursson K, Waller KP. Genotypic variation among Staphylococcus aureus isolates from cases of clinical mastitis in Swedish dairy cows. Veterinary Journal. 2010;185:188-192

55. Anderson KL, Lyman RL. Long- term persistence of specific genetic types of mastitis-causing Staphylococcus aureus on three dairies. Journal of Dairy Science. 2006;89:4551-4556

56. Simoons-Smit A, Savelkoul P, Stoof J, Starink T, Vandenbroucke- Grauls C. Transmission of Staphylococcus aureus between humans and domestic animals in a household. European Journal of Clinical Microbiology and Infectious Diseases. 2000;19:150-152

57. Rodgers JD, McCullagh JJ, McNamee PT, Smyth JA, Ball HJ. Comparison of Staphylococcus aureus recovered from personnel in a poultry hatchery and in broiler parent farms with those isolated from skeletal disease in broilers. Veterinary Microbiology. 1999;69:189-198

58. Zadoks R, Van Leeuwen W, Kreft D, Fox L, Barkema H, Schukken Y, et al. Comparison of Staphylococcus aureus isolates from bovine and human skin, milking equipment, and bovine milk by phage typing, pulsed-field gel electrophoresis, and binary typing. Journal of Clinical Microbiology. 2002;40:3894-3902

59. Monecke S, Kuhnert P, Hotzel H, Slickers P, Ehricht R. Microarray based study on virulence-associated genes and resistance determinants of Staphylococcus aureus isolates from cattle. Veterinary Microbiology. 2007;125:128-140

60. Türkyılmaz S, Tekbıyık S, Oryasin E, Bozdogan B. Molecular epidemiology and antimicrobial resistance mechanisms of methicillin- resistant Staphylococcus aureus isolated from bovine milk. Zoonoses and Public Health. 2010;57:197-203

61. Pantosti A, Sanchini A, Monaco M. Mechanisms of antibiotic resistance in Staphylococcus aureus. Future Microbiology. 2007;2:323-334

62. USDA APHIS U. Part III: Health Management and Biosecurity in US Feedlots, 1999. US Department of Agriculture [Online]. 2000. Available from: https://www.aphis.usda.gov/animal_health/nahms/dairy/downloads/ dairy07/Dairy07_ir_Food_safety.pdf [Accessed: 23 December 2020]

63. Neave F, Dodd F, Kingwill R, Westgarth D. Control of mastitis in the dairy herd by hygiene and management. Journal of Dairy Science. 1969;52:696-707

64. Hillerton J, Berry E. Treating mastitis in the cow a tradition or an archaism. Journal of Applied Microbiology. 2005;98:1250-1255

65. Sischo W, Heider LE, Miller G, Moore D. Prevalence of contagious pathogens of bovine mastitis and use of mastitis control practices. Journal of the American Veterinary Medical Association. 1993;202:595-600

66. McCarthy AJ, Lindsay JA. Genetic variation in Staphylococcus aureus surface and immune evasion genes is lineage associated: Implications for vaccine design and host-pathogen interactions. BMC Microbiology. 2010;10:173

67. Brady RA, Leid JG, Camper AK, Costerton JW, Shirtliff ME. Identification of Staphylococcus aureus proteins recognized by the antibody- mediated immune response to a biofilm infection. Infection and Immunity. 2006;74:3415-3426

68. den Reijer PM, Sandker M, Snijders SV, Tavakol M, Hendrickx AP, van Wamel WJ. Combining in vitro protein detection and in vivo antibody detection identifies potential vaccine targets against Staphylococcus aureus during osteomyelitis. Medical Microbiology and Immunology. 2017;206:11-22

69. Clarke SR, Foster SJ. Surface adhesins of Staphylococcus aureus. Advances in Microbial Physiology. 2006;51:187-224

70. Hauck CR, Ohlsen K. Sticky connections: Extracellular matrix protein recognition and integrin- mediated cellular invasion by Staphylococcus aureus. Current Opinion in Microbiology. 2006;9:5-11

71. Speziale P, Pietrocola G, Rindi S, Provenzano M, Provenza G, Di Poto A, et al. Structural and functional role of Staphylococcus aureus surface components recognizing adhesive matrix molecules of the host. Future Microbiology. 2009;4:1337-1352

72. Burke FM, McCormack N, Rindi S, Speziale P, Foster TJ. Fibronectin-binding protein B variation in Staphylococcus aureus. BMC Microbiology. 2010;10:160

73. Zecconi A, Scali F. Staphylococcus aureus virulence factors in evasion from innate immune defenses in human and animal diseases. Immunology Letters. 2013;150:12-22

74. Camussone CM, Calvinho LF. Virulence factors of Staphylococcus aureus associated with intramammary infections in cows: Relevance and role as immunogens. Revista Argentina de Microbiología. 2013;45:119-130

75. Gotz F. Staphylococcus and biofilms. Molecular Microbiology. 2002;43:1367-1378

76. Otto M. Staphylococcal biofilms. Current Topics in Microbiology and Immunology. 2008;322:207-228

77. Donlan RM, Costerton JW. Biofilms: Survival mechanisms of clinically relevant microorganisms. Clinical Microbiology Reviews. 2002;15:167-193
78. Stewart PS, Costerton JW. Antibiotic resistance of bacteria in biofilms. Lancet. 2001;358:135-138
79. Foster TJ, Geoghegan JA, Ganesh VK, Hook M. Adhesion, invasion and evasion: The many functions of the surface proteins of Staphylococcus aureus. Nature Reviews. Microbiology. 2014;12:49-62
80. Szweda P, Schielmann M, Milewski S, Frankowska A, Jakubczak A. Biofilm production and presence of Ica and bap genes in Staphylococcus aureus strains isolated from cows with mastitis in the eastern Poland. Polish Journal of Microbiology. 2012;61:65-69
81. Cucarella C, Solano C, Valle J, Amorena B, Lasa I, Penades JR. Bap, a Staphylococcus aureus surface protein involved in biofilm formation. Journal of Bacteriology. 2001;183:2888-2896
82. Lasa I, Penadés JR. Bap: A family of surface proteins involved in biofilm formation. Research in Microbiology. 2006;157:99-107
83. Valle J, Latasa C, Gil C, Toledo- Arana A, Solano C, Penadés JR, et al. Bap, a biofilm matrix protein of Staphylococcus aureus prevents cellular internalization through binding to GP96 host receptor. PLoS Pathogens. 2012;8:e1002843
84. Cucarella C, Tormo MÁ, Ubeda C, Trotonda MP, Monzón M, Peris C, et al. Role of biofilm-associated protein bap in the pathogenesis of bovine Staphylococcus aureus. Infection and Immunity. 2004;72:2177-2185
85. Milanov D, Lazić S, Vidić B, Petrović J, Bugarski D, Šeguljev Z. Slime production and biofilm forming ability by Staphylococcus aureus bovine mastitis isolates. Acta Veterinaria. 2010;60:217-226
86. Melchior MB, Vaarkamp H, Fink-Gremmels J. Biofilms: A role in recurrent mastitis infections? Veterinary Journal. 2006;171:398-407
87. Dhanawade NB, Kalorey DR, Srinivasan R, Barbuddhe SB, Kurkure NV. Detection of intercellular adhesion genes and biofilm production in Staphylococcus aureus isolated from bovine subclinical mastitis. Veterinary Research Communications. 2010;34:81-89
88. Vasudevan P, Nair MKM, Annamalai T, Venkitanarayanan KS. Phenotypic and genotypic characterization of bovine mastitis isolates of Staphylococcus aureus for biofilm formation. Veterinary Microbiology. 2003;92:179-185
89. O'Gara JP. Ica and beyond: Biofilm mechanisms and regulation in Staphylococcus epidermidis and Staphylococcus aureus. FEMS Microbiology Letters. 2007;270:179-188

90. Otto M. Staphylococcal infections: Mechanisms of biofilm maturation and detachment as critical determinants of pathogenicity. Annual Review of Medicine. 2013;64:175-188

91. Aydin A, Sudagidan M, Muratoglu K. Prevalence of staphylococcal enterotoxins, toxin genes and genetic-relatedness of foodborne Staphylococcus aureus strains isolated in the Marmara region of Turkey. International Journal of Food Microbiology. 2011;148:99-106

92. Rogolsky M. Nonenteric toxins of Staphylococcus aureus. Microbiological Reviews. 1979;43:320-360

93. Wadstrom T. Biological properties of extracellular proteins from Staphylococcus. Annals of the New York Academy of Sciences. 1974;236:343-361

94. Bramley AJ, Patel AH, O'Reilly M, Foster R, Foster TJ. Roles of alpha- toxin and beta-toxin in virulence of Staphylococcus aureus for the mouse mammary gland. Infection and Immunity. 1989;57:2489-2494

95. Berube BJ, Bubeck WJ. Staphylococcus aureus alpha-toxin: Nearly a century of intrigue. Toxins (Basel). 2013;5:1140-1166

96. Otto M. Staphylococcus aureus toxins. Current Opinion in Microbiology. 2014;17:32-37

97. Songer JG, Post KW. Veterinary Microbiology-E-Book: Bacterial and Fungal Agents of Animal Disease. St. Louis, Missouri: Elsevier Health Sciences; 2004

98. Kerro Dego O, Nederbragt H. Factors involved in the early pathogenesis of bovine Staphylococcus aureus mastitis with emphasis on bacterial adhesion and invasion. A review. The veterinary quarterly. 2002;24:181-198

99. Sutra L, Poutrel B. Virulence factors involved in the pathogenesis of bovine intramammary infections due toStaphylococcus aureus. Journal of Medical Microbiology. 1994;40:79-89

100. Caiazza NC, O'toole G. Alpha- toxin is required for biofilm formation by Staphylococcus aureus. Journal of Bacteriology. 2003;185:3214-3217

101. Low DKR, Freer JH. Biological effects of highly purified B-lysin (sphingomyelinase) from S. aureus. FEMS letters. 1977;2:133-138

102. O'Callaghan RJ, Callegan MC, Moreau JM, Green LC, Foster TJ, Hartford OM, et al. Specific roles of alpha- toxin and beta-toxin during Staphylococcus aureus corneal infection. Infection and Immunity. 1997;65:1571-1578

103. Essmann F, Bantel H, Totzke G, Engels IH, Sinha B, SchulzeOsthoff K, et al. Staphylococcus aureus alpha-toxin-induced cell death: Predominant

necrosis despite apoptotic caspase activation. Cell Death and Differentiation. 2003;10:1260-1272

104. Smyth CJ, Mollby R, Wadstrom T. Phenomenon of hot- cold hemolysis: Chelator-induced lysis of sphingomyelinase-treated erythrocytes. Infection and Immunity. 1975;12:1104-1111

105. Dinges MM, Orwin PM, Schlievert PM. Exotoxins of Staphylococcus aureus. Clinical Microbiology Reviews. 2000;13:16-34

106. Prevost G, Couppie P, Prevost P, Gayet S, Petiau P, Cribier B, et al. Epidemiological data on Staphylococcus aureus strains producing synergohymenotropic toxins. Journal of Medical Microbiology. 1995;42:237-245

107. Srinivasan V, Sawant AA, Gillespie BE, Headrick SJ, Ceasaris L, Oliver SP. Prevalence of enterotoxin and toxic shock syndrome toxin genes in Staphylococcus aureus isolated from milk of cows with mastitis. Foodborne Pathogens and Disease. 2006;3:274-283

108. Matsunaga T, Kamata S-I, Kakiichi N, Uchida K. Characteristics of Staphylococcus aureus isolated from peracute, acute and chronic bovine mastitis. Journal of Veterinary Medical Science. 1993;55:297-300

109. Hennekinne J-A, De Buyser M-L, Dragacci S. Staphylococcus aureus and its food poisoning toxins: Characterization and outbreak investigation. FEMS Microbiology Reviews. July 2012; 36(4):815-836

110. Bergdoll MS, Chu FS, Borja CR, Huang I-Y, Weiss KF. The staphylococcal enterotoxins. Japanese Journal of Microbiology. 1967;11:358-368

111. Kong C, H-m N, Nathan S. Targeting Staphylococcus aureus toxins: A potential form of anti-virulence therapy. Toxins. 2016;8:72

112. Kenny K, Reiser RF, Bastida- Corcuera FD, Norcross NL. Production of enterotoxins and toxic shock syndrome toxin by bovine mammary isolates of Staphylococcus aureus.Journal of Clinical Microbiology. 1993;31:706-707

113. Todd J, Fishaut M, Kapral F, Welch T. Toxic-shock syndrome associated with phage-group-I staphylococci. The Lancet. 1978;312:1116-1118

114. Moon J, Lee A, Kang H, Lee E, Joo Y, Park YH, et al. Antibiogram and coagulase diversity in staphylococcal enterotoxin-producing Staphylococcus aureus from bovine mastitis. Journal of Dairy Science. 2007;90:1716-1724

115. Stephan R, Annemüller C, Hassan A, Lämmler C. Characterization of enterotoxigenic Staphylococcus aureus strains isolated from bovine mastitis in north-East Switzerland. Veterinary Microbiology. 2001;78:373-382

116. Cenci-Goga B, Karama M, Rossitto P, Morgante R, Cullor J. Enterotoxin production by Staphylococcus aureus isolated from mastitic cows. Journal of Food Protection. 2003;66:1693-1696

117. Piccinini R, Borromeo V, Zecconi A. Relationship between S. aureus gene pattern and dairy herd mastitis prevalence. Veterinary Microbiology. 2010;145:100-105

118. Piechota M, Kot B, Zdunek E, Mitrus J, Wicha J, Wolska MK, et al. Distribution of classical enterotoxin genes in staphylococci from milk of cows with- and without mastitis and the cowshed environment. Polish Journal of Veterinary Sciences. 2014;17:407-411

119. Fisher EL, Otto M, Cheung GYC. Basis of virulence in enterotoxin- mediated staphylococcal food poisoning. Frontiers in Microbiology. 2018;9:436

120. Almeida RA, Matthews KR, Cifrian E, Guidry AJ, Oliver SP. Staphylococcus aureus invasion of bovine mammary epithelial cells. Journal of Dairy Science. 1996;79:1021-1026

121. Lammers A, Nuijten PJ, Smith HE. The fibronectin binding proteins of Staphylococcus aureus are required for adhesion to and invasion of bovine mammary gland cells. FEMS Microbiology Letters. 1999;180:103-109

122. Cifrian E, Guidry A, O'Brien C, Marquardt W. Effect of alpha-toxin and capsular exopolysaccharide on the adherence of Staphylococcus aureus to cultured teat, ductal and secretory mammary epithelial cells. Research in Veterinary Science. 1995;58:20-25

123. Hensen S, Pavičić M, Lohuis J, Poutrel B. Use of bovine primary mammary epithelial cells for the comparison of adherence and invasion ability of Staphylococcus aureus strains. Journal of Dairy Science. 2000;83:418-429

124. Josse J, Laurent F, Diot A. Staphylococcal adhesion and host cell invasion: Fibronectin-binding and other mechanisms. Frontiers in Microbiology. 2017;8:2433

125. Loffler B, Tuchscherr L, Niemann S, Peters G. Staphylococcus aureus persistence in non-professional phagocytes. International Journal of Medical Microbiology. 2014;304:170-176

126. Moormeier DE, Bayles KW. Staphylococcus aureus biofilm: A complex developmental organism. Molecular Microbiology. 2017;104:365-376

127. Fowler T, Wann ER, Joh D, Johansson S, Foster TJ, Hook M. Cellular invasion by Staphylococcus aureus involves a fibronectin bridge between the bacterial fibronectin-binding MSCRAMMs and host cell beta-1 integrins. European Journal of Cell Biology. 2000;79:672-679

128. Abdi RD, Gillespie BE, Vaughn J, Merrill C, Headrick SI, Ensermu DB, et al. Antimicrobial resistance of] Staphylococcus aureus isolates from dairy cows and genetic diversity of resistant isolates. Foodborne Pathogens and Disease. 2018;15:449-458

129. Tyler JW, Wilson RC, Dowling P. Treatment of subclinical mastitis. The Veterinary Clinics of North America. Food Animal Practice. 1992;8:17-28

130. Brüssow H, Canchaya C, Hardt W-D. Phages and the evolution of bacterial pathogens: From genomic rearrangements to lysogenic conversion. Microbiology and Molecular Biology Reviews. 2004;68:560-602

131. Owens W, Ray C, Watts J, Yancey R. Comparison of success of antibiotic therapy during lactation and results of antimicrobial susceptibility tests for bovine mastitis. Journal of Dairy Science. 1997;80:313-317

132. Carter E, Kerr D. Optimization of DNA-based vaccination in cows using green fluorescent protein and protein a as a prelude to immunization against staphylococcal mastitis. Journal of Dairy Science. 2003;86:1177-1186

133. Emaneini M, Jabalameli F, Abani S, Dabiri H, Beigverdi R. Comparison of virulence factors and capsular types of Streptococcus agalactiae isolated from human and bovine infections. Microbial Pathogenesis. 2016;91:1-4

134. Farnsworth R. Indications of Contagious and Environmental Mastitis Pathogens in a Dairy Herd. USA: Annual Meeting of National Mastitis Council; 1987

135. Hillerton JE, Berry EA. The management and treatment of environmental streptococcal mastitis. Veterinary Clinics of North America: Food Animal Practice. 2003;19:157-169

136. Nicholas R, Ayling R, McAuliffe L. Mycoplasma mastitis. Veterinary Record. 2007;160:382-382

137. USDA APHIS U. United States Department of Agriculture, Animal Plant Health Inspection Service National Animal Health Monitoring System. Injection Practices on U.S. Dairy Operations, 2007 (Veterinary Services Info Sheet 4 p, February 2009) [Online]. 2009. Available from https://www.aphis.usda.gov/animal_health/nahms/ dairy/downloads/dairy07/Dairy07_ is_InjectionPrac_1.pdf [Accessed: 23 March 2020]

138. Fox LK. Mycoplasma mastitis: Causes, transmission, and control. Veterinary Clinics: Food Animal Practice. 2012;28:225-237

139. Jasper DE. Bovine mycoplasmal mastitis. Advances in Veterinary Science and Comparative Medicine. 1981;25:121-157

140. Dogan B, Klaessig S, Rishniw M, Almeida R, Oliver S, Simpson K, et al. Adherent and invasive Escherichia coli are associated with persistent bovine mastitis. Veterinary Microbiology. 2006;116:270-282

141. Almeida RA, Dogan B, Klaessing S, Schukken YH, Oliver SP. Intracellular fate of strains of Escherichia coli isolated from dairy cows with acute or chronic mastitis. Veterinary Research Communications. 2011;35:89-101

142. Bayles KW, Wesson CA, Liou LE, Fox LK, Bohach GA, Trumble W. Intracellular Staphylococcus aureus escapes the endosome and induces apoptosis in epithelial cells. Infection and Immunity. 1998;66:336-342

143. Craven N, Anderson JC. Phagocytosis of Staphylococcus aureus by bovine mammary gland macrophages and intracellular protection from antibiotic action in vitro and in vivo. The Journal of Dairy Research. 1984;51:513-523

144. Zhao S, Gao Y, Xia X, Che Y, Wang Y, Liu H, et al. TGF-β1 promotes Staphylococcus aureus adhesion to and invasion into bovine mammary fibroblasts via the ERK pathway. Microbial Pathogenesis. 2017;106:25-29

145. Perez-Casal J, Prysliak T, Kerro Dego O, Potter AA. Immune responses to a Staphylococcus aureus GapC/B chimera and its potential use as a component of a vaccine for S. aureus mastitis. Veterinary Immunology and Immunopathology. 2006;109:85-97

146. Gudding R, McDonald J, Cheville N. Pathogenesis of Staphylococcus aureus mastitis: Bacteriologic, histologic, and ultrastructural pathologic findings. American Journal of Veterinary Research. 1984;45:2525-2531

147. Zecconi A, Cesaris L, Liandris E, Dapra V, Piccinini R. Role of several Staphylococcus aureus virulence factors on the inflammatory response in bovine mammary gland. Microbial Pathogenesis. 2006;40:177-183

148. Harmon R. Physiology of mastitis and factors affecting somatic cell counts1. Journal of Dairy Science. 1994;77:2103-2112

149. Keefe G. Update on control of Staphylococcus aureus and Streptococcus agalactiae for management of mastitis. The Veterinary Clinics of North America. Food Animal Practice. 2012;28:203-216

150. Zecconi A. Staphylococcus aureus mastitis: What we need to know to con. Israel Journal of Veterinary Medicine. 2010;65:93-99

151. Malek dos Reis CB, Barreiro JR, Mestieri L, MADF P, dos Santos MV. Effect of somatic cell count and mastitis pathogens on milk composition in Gyr cows. BMC Veterinary Research. 2013;9:67

152. Akers RM, Nickerson SC. Mastitis and its impact on structure and function in the ruminant mammary gland. Journal of Mammary Gland Biology and Neoplasia. 2011;16:275-289

153. Sordillo LM, Streicher KL. Mammary gland immunity and mastitis susceptibility. Journal of Mammary Gland Biology and Neoplasia. 2002;7:135-146

154. Hogan J, Smith K. 1987. A practical look at environmental mastitis. The compendium on continuing education for the practicing veterinarian (USA). Gibson H, Sinclair LA, Brizuela CM, Worton HL, Protheroe RG. Effectiveness of selected premilking teat-cleaning regimes in reducing teat microbial load on commercial dairy farms. Letters in Applied Microbiology. 2008;46:295-300

155. Gleeson D, O'Brien B, Flynn J, O'Callaghan E, Galli F. Effect of pre- milking teat preparation procedures on the microbial count on teats prior to cluster application. Irish Veterinary Journal. 2009;62:461-467

156. Dufour S, Frechette A, Barkema HW, Mussell A, Scholl DT. Invited review: Effect of udder health management practices on herd somatic cell count. Journal of Dairy Science. 2011;94:563-579

157. Mordak R, Stewart PA. Periparturient stress and immune suppression as a potential cause of retained placenta in highly productive dairy cows: Examples of prevention. Acta Veterinaria Scandinavica. 2015;57:84

158. Drackley JK. ADSA foundation scholar award. Biology of dairy cows during the transition period: The final frontier? Journal of Dairy Science. 1999;82:2259-2273

159. Esposito G, Irons PC, Webb EC, Chapwanya A. Interactions between negative energy balance, metabolic diseases, uterine health and immune response in transition dairy cows. Animal Reproduction Science. 2014;144:60-71

160. Bach A. Associations between several aspects of heifer development and dairy cow survivability to second lactation. Journal of Dairy Science. 2011;94:1052-1057

161. Oliver SP, Jayarao BM, Almeida RA. Foodborne pathogens, mastitis, milk quality, and dairy food safety. In: Proceedings of National Mastitis Council (NMC), 44th meeting, January 16-19. Orlando, FL; 2005. pp. 3-27

162. Scallan E, Hoekstra RM, Angulo FJ, Tauxe RV, Widdowson M-A, Roy SL, et al. Foodborne illness acquired in the United States—Major pathogens. Emerging Infectious Diseases. 2011;17:7-15

163. Jayarao BM, Henning DR. Prevalence of foodborne pathogens in bulk tank milk1. Journal of Dairy Science. 2001;84:2157-2162

164. Gillespie BE, Oliver SP. Simultaneous detection of mastitis pathogens, Staphylococcus aureus, Streptococcus uberis, and Streptococcus agalactiae by multiplex real-time polymerase chain reaction. Journal of Dairy Science. 2005;88:3510-3518

165. Steele ML, Mcnab WB, Poppe C, Griffiths MW, Chen S, Degrandis SA, et al. Survey of Ontario bulk tank raw Milk for food-borne pathogens. Journal of Food Protection. 1997;60:1341-1346

166. Van Kessel J, Karns J, Gorski L, McCluskey B, Perdue M. Prevalence of Salmonellae, Listeria monocytogenes, and fecal coliforms in bulk tank milk on US dairies. Journal of Dairy Science. 2004;87:2822-2830

167. Rohrbach BW, Draughon FA, Davidson PM, Oliver SP. Prevalence of Listeria monocytogenes, Campylobacter jejuni, Yersinia enterocolitica, and Salmonella in bulk tank milk: Risk factors and risk of human exposure. Journal of Food Protection. 1992;55:93-97

9 Chapter MASTITIS: CONTROL AND PREVENTION PART II

1. INTRODUCTION: AN OVERVIEW

Although the current ten-point mastitis control strategies, particularly effective against contagious mastitis pathogens, yield substantial benefits when completely implemented, their adoption is inconsistent among farmers, resulting in mastitis remaining the most prevalent and expensive disease affecting dairy cattle globally.

Despite extensive research over several decades aimed at creating effective vaccines for significant bacterial mastitis pathogens, including Staphylococcus aureus, Streptococcus uberis, and E. coli in dairy cows, the intramammary immune mechanisms remain inadequately understood, thereby sustaining dependence on antibiotic treatments for mastitis management in dairy cows. Reliance on antibiotics is unsustainable due to their limited effectiveness and the heightened possibility of developing antimicrobial-resistant bacteria, which present significant public health dangers. Most immunization efforts aimed at preventing mastitis have concentrated on augmenting humoral immunity. The investigation into the development of vaccinations that elicit a protective cellular immune response in the mammary gland has been insufficient. The capacity to stimulate cellular immunity, particularly through neutrophil activation and recruitment to the mammary gland, is a crucial strategy in mastitis management; however, the extent and duration of heightened cellular influx into the mammary gland can result in elevated somatic cell counts and diminished milk quality. The sustainable control measure involves the development of effective vaccines that can elicit robust and balanced cellular and humoral immunity, hence preventing production losses and diminishing the clinical severity of mastitis without provoking a prolonged inflammatory response.

2. HYGIENIC CONTROL MEASURES

Current mastitis control programs devised in the 1960s based on teat disinfection, antibiotic therapy, and culling of chronically infected cows have led to considerable progress in controlling contagious mastitis pathogens such as Streptococcus agalactiae and Staphylococcus aureus. However, these procedures are much less effective against environmental pathogens, particularly Streptococcus uberis and

E. coli which accounts for a significant proportion of subclinical and clinical mastitis in lactating and nonlactating cows and heifers [1–4]. The National Mastitis Council developed a 5-point mastitis control program in 1969 to control the incidence rate of mastitis. This 5-point mastitis control program includes (1) dipping teats in an antiseptic solution before and after milking, (2) proper cleaning and maintenance of milking equipment, (3) early detection and treatment of infected animals, (4) dry cow therapy with long acting antibiotics to reduce duration of existing infection and to prevent new intramammary infection, and (5) finally culling chronically infected animals [5, 6]. Later, it was updated to a 10-point plan, which includes more steps such as establishing udder health goals, maintain clean, dry, and comfortable environment, proper milking procedures, proper maintenance and use of milking equipment, good record keeping, management of clinical mastitis during lactation, effective dry cow management including blanket dry cow therapy, maintenance of good biosecurity for contagious pathogens and marketing chronically infected cows, regular monitoring of udder health status, and periodic review of mastitis control program [7]. Though these hygienic milking practices and control measures decrease bacterial spreading, transmission, and subsequent infection, it does not fully prevent infections from establishing. Dairy farmers utilize antimicrobials as a prophylactic treatment for the prevention of mastitis or as therapeutics to treat cases of mastitis [8].

3. USE OF ANTIMICROBIALS FOR TREATMENT AND PREVENTION OF MASTITIS

Antibiotics are used extensively in food-producing animals to combat disease and to improve animal productivity. On dairy farms, antibiotics are used for treatment and prevention of diseases affecting dairy cows, particularly mastitis, and are often administered routinely to entire herds to prevent mastitis during the dry or non-lactating period. Use of antibiotics in food-producing animals has resulted in healthier, more productive animals; lower disease incidence and prevalence rates, reduced morbidity and mortality; and production of abundant quantities of nutritious, high-quality, and low-cost food for human consumption. In spite of these benefits, there is considerable concern from public health, food safety, and regulatory perspectives about use of antibiotics in food-producing animals [9]. There has been a growing concern with the extensive use of antimicrobials in production animals, especially non-therapeutic usage such as dry cow therapy in the case of dairy production, because of potential emergence and spread of antimicrobial resistant bacteria. There has been an increased incidence of antimicrobial resistant bacteria both in human and animal medical services.

In almost all dairy farms in the US and many other countries, intramammary infusion of long-acting antimicrobials to dairy cows at dry-off is a routine practice to prevent bacterial IMI during the dry period. Over 90% of dairy farms in the US infuse all udder quarters of all cows with antimicrobial (blanket dry cow therapy) regardless of their health status [8, 10, 11]. Antibiotics are also heavily used in dairy farms for the treatment of cases of mastitis and other diseases of dairy cows such as metritis, endometritis, retained placenta, lameness, and pneumonia. Similarly, antibiotics are also used for the treatment of neonatal calf diarrhea and pneumonia in dairy calves. This practice exposes a large number of animals to antimicrobials and increases the use of antimicrobials in dairy farms. Antimicrobials for the treatment of mastitis are given through intramammary infusion as well as administered parenterally to dairy herd for the treatment of clinical (acute or peracute) mastitis and other periparturient diseases of dairy cows such as metritis, endometritis, retained placenta, and others like lameness and pneumonia. Antimicrobial treatment for neonatal diarrhea and pneumonia are also given through parenteral routes. Some farms also feed waste milk (discarded milk during antibiotic treatment, milk after parturition before allowed into the bulk tank) to heifer calves, which puts their gastrointestinal tract (GIT) microbiota under antibiotics pressure. Antibiotics infused into the mammary glands can be excreted to the environment through leakage of milk from the antibiotic-treated udder or absorbed into the body and enter the blood circulation and biotransformed (pharmacokinetics) in the liver or kidney and excreted from the body through urine or feces into the environments. Therefore, both parenteral and intramammary administration of antibiotics has a significant impact on other commensals or opportunistic bacteria in the gastrointestinal tract of dairy cows. This practice exposes large numbers of healthy cows to antimicrobials and also increases the use of antimicrobials in dairy farms, which in turn creates intense pressure on microbes in animals' body and farm environments.

Intramammary infection may progress to clinical or subclinical mastitis [12]. Clinically infected udder is usually treated with antimicrobial, whereas subclinically infected udder may not be diagnosed immediately and treated but remained infected and shedding bacteria through milk throughout lactation. The proportion of cure following treatment of mastitis varies and the variation in cure rate is multi-factorial including cow factors (age or parity number, stage of lactation, and duration of infection, etc.), management factors (detection and diagnosis of infection and time from detection to treatment, availability of balanced nutrition, sanitation, etc.), factors related to antimicrobial use patterns (type, dose, route, frequency, and duration), and pathogen factors (type, species, number, pathogenicity or virulence, resistance to antimicrobial, etc.) [13, 14].

The most common antibiotics used to treat mastitis include cephalosporins (53.2%), followed by lincosamide (19.4%) and non-cephalosporin β-lactam antibiotics (19.1%) [8]. The problem with the use of non-selective blanket antimicrobials administration to dairy cows as a prophylactic control of mastitis is that they put selective pressure on both mastitis-causing bacteria as well as commensal bacteria in the animals' body [15, 16]. The ultimate result may not be different but the exposure level to antibiotics and its biotransformed products are different for the bacteria in the gut, in the mammary glands, and dairy farm environments during use of antimicrobials for prevention and treatment of mastitis and other diseases of dairy cattle. This selective pressure can result in antimicrobial resistant bacteria that become difficult to clear and persistent on farms and spread among animals [17]. The antimicrobial resistant bacteria or their genes may spread from these sources to human or animals or to other bacteria. McAllister et al. [18] found that CNS could potentially transfer penicillin, cephalosporins, and fluoroquinolones resistant genes to S. aureus. The transfer of these antibiotic resistance genes could lead to the development of antimicrobial resistant bacteria including methicillinresistant S. aureus (MRSA) [18]. Treatment of Staphylococcus aureus mastitis with antibiotics is of limited success which may dictate the culling of the animal [14, 19]. Until recently, MRSA was a common antimicrobial resistant strain mainly found in human hospitals; however, recent findings indicated that it has also been increasingly isolated from cattle herds [20]. The major problem with MRSA is that it is mostly resistant to multiple commonly used antimicrobials (multidrug resistant) and difficult to control and eliminate [21]. On an average, the cure rate of lactating cow therapy against S. aureus mastitis is about 30% or less [22]. Currently, there is no effective vaccine against bovine S. aureus mastitis [23], and since treatment is of limited efficacy, control of S. aureus mastitis focuses on prevention of contamination and spread, rather than treatment [14, 19].

Antimicrobial resistance is a growing problem in Staphylococcus aureus mastitis. Antimicrobial resistance helps bacteria to stay alive after treatment with antibiotics and some of the mechanisms of resistance are the presence of antimicrobial resistance genes that can spread by horizontal transfer from bacteria to bacteria by mobile genetic elements such as plasmids, phages, and pathogenicity islands [24]. This resistance can also occur through random mutations when the bacteria are under stress [25]. In the cases of mastitis, the prevalence of antimicrobial resistant bacteria seems to be increasing at least for some antimicrobials. Studies reported over 50% of isolates that cause mastitis were resistant to either beta lactam drugs or penicillin [26]. In human medicine, methicillin resistant S. aureus (MRSA) is a huge problem because MRSA strains are resistant to most of antibiotics making them very difficult or impossible to treat. There have also been reports of cases of bovine mastitis caused by MRSA [27–30]. Some report that these infections are due to the human strain, but others have found MRSA strains of bovine origin [21, 31]. These authors suggested that MRSA strains isolated from bovine probably gain resistance from human MRSA strain through transfer of resistance genes [32].

Waller et al. [33] evaluated the antimicrobial susceptibility of CNS and found a difference across the species on β-lactamase production. Similarly, Sawant et al. [34] found that 18% and 46 of the S. chromogenes and S. epidermidis isolates produce β-lactamase, respectively. Sampimon et al. [35] also found a 70% resistance to penicillin in S. epidermidis, but more importantly found that 30% of the CNS were resistant to more than one antimicrobial.

From antimicrobial resistance perspective, environmental mastitis pathogens are very important for two reasons: (1) some members of environmental mastitis pathogens are either normal microflora or opportunistic pathogens in the gastrointestinal tract of dairy cows and frequently exposed to antimicrobials directly through oral or indirectly through parenteral routes; (2) despite strain variation, some of them are highly pathogenic for human (for example, E. coli 0157:H7 is normal microflora in the rectum of cattle). Of significant concern is the potential for human infection by antimicrobial-resistant environmental mastitis pathogens such as extended-spectrum beta-lactam resistant E. coli directly through contact with carrier animal or indirectly through the food chain. Some of the Gramnegative environmental mastitis pathogens, such as E. coli, Klebsiella pneumoniae, Acinetobacter baumannii, Pseudomonas aeruginosa, and Enterobacter spp. are the greatest threat to human health due to the emergence of strains that are resistant to all or most available antimicrobials [36, 37].

In general, the antimicrobial resistance of mastitis pathogens varies with dairy farms and bacterial species within and among dairy farms [11, 38–42]. However, the antimicrobial-resistance status of human pathogenic environmental mastitis pathogens, especially the resistance status of Gram-negative environmental mastitis pathogens in the family of Enterobacteriaceae, is yet to be determined. Monitoring antimicrobial resistance patterns of bacterial isolates from cases of mastitis is important for treatment decisions and proper design of mitigation measures. It also helps to determine emergence, persistence, and potential risk of the spread of antimicrobial-resistant bacteria and resistome to human, animal, and environment [17, 43]. The prudent use of antimicrobials in dairy farms reduces emergence, persistence, and spread of antimicrobial-resistant bacteria and resistome from dairy farms to human, animal, and environment.

4. VACCINES

Several vaccine studies were conducted over the years as controlled experimental and field trials. Some of the most common mastitis pathogens that have been targeted for vaccine development are S. aureus, S. agalactiae, S. uberis, and E. coli [44]. Most of these experimental and some commercial vaccines are bacterins which are inactivated whole organism, and some vaccines contained subunits of the organism such as surface proteins [45], toxins, or polysaccharides.

All coliform mastitis vaccine formulations use Gram-negative core antigens to produce non-specific immunity directed against endotoxin (LPS) [44]. The principle of these bacterins is based upon their ability to stimulate production of antibodies directed against common core antigens that Gram-negative bacteria share. These vaccines do not prevent new intramammary infection but significantly reduced the clinical severity of the infection [46–48]. Experimental challenge studies have demonstrated that J5 vaccines are able to reduce bacterial counts in milk and resulted in fewer and less severe clinical symptoms [47]. Vaccinated cows may become infected with Gram-negative mastitis pathogens at the same rate as control animals but have a lower rate of development of clinical mastitis [48], reduced duration of infection [46], less loss of milk production, culling, and death losses [49, 50]. The Eviracor®J5 E. coli vaccine (Zoetis, Kalamazoo, MI), [51, 52], as well as the UBAC® S. uberis vaccine (Hipra, Amir, Spain), [53] are similar to vaccination with nonspecific killed whole bacterial cells (bacterin vaccines), achieving only partial reduction in clinical severity of mastitis.

Despite several mastitis vaccine trials conducted against S. aureus mastitis [54–65], all field trials have either been unsuccessful or had limited success. There are two commercial vaccines for Staphylococcus aureus mastitis on the market, Lysigin® (Boehringer Ingelheim Vetmedica, Inc., St. Joseph, MO) in the United States and Startvac® (Hipra S.A, Girona, Spain) in Europe and Canada [66]. None of these vaccines confer protection in field trials as well as under controlled experimental studies [54, 58, 62, 67]. Several field trials and controlled experimental studies have been conducted testing the efficacy of Lysigin® and Startvac® and results from those studies have shown some interesting results, namely a reduced incidence, severity, and duration of mastitis in vaccinated cows compared to non-vaccinated control cows [54, 62, 68]. Contrary to these observations, other studies failed to find an effect on improving udder health or showed no difference between vaccinated and non-vaccinated control cows [66, 69]. None of these bacterin-based vaccines prevents new S. aureus IMI [54, 58, 62, 67]. Differences found in these studies are mainly due to methodological differences (vaccination schedule, route of vaccination, challenge model, herd size, time of lactation, etc.) in testing the efficacy of these vaccines. It is critically important to have a good infection model that mimics natural infection and a model that has 100% efficacy in causing infection. Without a good challenge model, the results from vaccine efficacy will be inaccurate.

5. CONCISE SUMMARY

Contemporary mastitis management initiatives rely on teat disinfection, antibiotic treatment, and the culling of chronically sick cows. No singular vaccine is effective against any mastitis pathogen. The physiological characteristics of mammary glands, wherein induced systemic immune responses must traverse from the body into the glands, combined with the dilution of effector immune responses by the substantial volume of milk and the capacity of mastitis-causing bacteria to evolve immune evasion strategies and resistance to antimicrobials, complicate the management of mastitis significantly. Nonetheless, the development of enhanced and efficacious vaccinations that surmount these limitations through rapidly increasing genetic, genomic, and immunological technologies is a sustainable intervention strategy.

The administration of antibiotics in food-producing animals contributes to heightened antimicrobial resistance in dairy cattle and agricultural settings. Antimicrobial resistance among dairy pathogens, especially bacterial strains responsible for mastitis in dairy cattle, is not escalating at an alarming rate. Antimicrobial resistance in Gram-negative bacteria, particularly those that mostly cause human diseases, is exceedingly high in dairy cow and dairy farm conditions. The transmission of antimicrobial-resistant mastitis pathogens and/or foodborne pathogens to humans may occur via direct contact with animals or indirectly through the food chain, particularly if contaminated unpasteurized milk or dairy products derived from tainted raw milk are ingested. This underscores the critical rationale for avoiding the consumption of raw milk. Similarly, antibiotic-resistant bacteria contaminating meat from culled dairy cows can readily transfer to humans through the consumption of undercooked meat.

We advocate for the judicious application of antibiotics in dairy farms. Strategies for the judicious use of antibiotics in treatment include identifying the pathogen responsible for the infection, evaluating its susceptibility or resistance patterns to select the most suitable antibiotic, and ensuring a sufficiently prolonged treatment duration to maintain effective antibiotic concentrations for pathogen eradication. Alternatives to antibiotics for sustaining animal health and productivity include preventative measures such as vaccination, enhanced nutrition, environmental sanitation, application of teat sealants, and selection for genetic traits associated with disease resistance. Additionally, advancements in rapid pathogen detection and characterization systems will undoubtedly be crucial in strategies designed to enhance dairy productivity while ensuring the safety of dairy products for human consumption.

REFERENCES

1. Hogan JS, Smith KL, Hoblet KH, Schoenberger PS, Todhunter DA, Hueston WD, et al. Field survey of clinical mastitis in low somatic cell count herds. Journal of Dairy Science. 1989;72:1547-1556

2. Oliver SP. Frequency of isolation of environmental mastitis-causing pathogens and incidence of new intramammary infection during the nonlactating period. American Journal of Veterinary Research. 1988;49:1789-1793

3. Oliver SP, Gillespie BE, Headrick SI, Lewis MJ, Dowlen HH. Prevalence, risk factors and strategies for controlling mastitis in heifers during the periparturient period. International Journal of Applied Research in Veterinary Medicine. 2005;3:150-162

4. Todhunter DA, Smith KL, Hogan JS. Environmental streptococcal intramammary infections of the bovine mammary gland. Journal of Dairy Science. 1995;78:2366-2374

5. Neave F, Dodd F, Kingwill R, Westgarth D. Control of mastitis in the dairy herd by hygiene and management. Journal of Dairy Science. 1969;52:696-707

6. Blowey RW. Mastitis Control in Dairy Herds. 2nd ed. Cambridge, MA: CABI, Cambridge, Mass; 2010

7. Middleton JR, Saeman A, Fox LK, Lombard J, Hogan JS, Smith KL. The National Mastitis Council: A global organization for mastitis control and milk quality, 50 years and beyond. Journal of Mammary Gland Biology and Neoplasia. 2014;19:241-251

8. USDA APHIS. Antibiotic use on U.S. dairy operations, 2002 and 2007 (infosheet, 5p, October, 2008). 2008a. Available from: https://www.aphis.usda.gov/animal_health/nahms/dairy/downloads/dairy07/Dairy07_is_AntibioticUse_1.pdf [Accessed: 23 March 2020]

9. Oliver SP, Murinda SE, Jayarao BM. Impact of antibiotic use in adult dairy cows on antimicrobial resistance of veterinary and human pathogens: A comprehensive review. Foodborne Pathogens and Disease. 2011;8:337-355

10. USDA APHIS. United States Department of Agriculture, Animal Plant Health Inspection Service National Animal Health Monitoring System. Highlights of Dairy 2007 Part III: reference of dairy cattle health and management practices in the United States, 2007 (Info Sheet 4p, October, 2008). 2008b. Available from: https:// www.aphis.usda.gov/animal_health/ nahms/dairy/downloads/ dairy07/ Dairy07_ir_Food_safety.pdf [Accessed: 23 March 2020]

11. Mathew AG, Cissell R, Liamthong S. Antibiotic resistance in bacteria associated with food animals: A United States perspective of livestock production. Foodborne Pathogens and Disease. 2007;4:115-133

12. Seegers H, Fourichon C, Beaudeau F. Production effects related to mastitis and mastitis economics in dairy cattle herds. Veterinary Research. 2003;34:475-491

13. Bradley AJ, Green MJ. Factors affecting cure when treating bovine clinical mastitis with cephalosporin-based intramammary preparations. Journal of Dairy Science. 2009;92:1941-1953

14. Barkema HW, Schukken YH, Zadoks RN. Invited review: The role of cow, pathogen, and treatment regimen in the therapeutic success of bovine Staphylococcus aureus mastitis. Journal of Dairy Science. 2006;89:1877-1895
15. Barber DA, Miller GY, McNamara PE. Models of antimicrobial resistance and foodborne illness: Examining assumptions and practical applications. Journal of Food Protection. 2003;66:700-709
16. Barbosa TM, Levy SB. The impact of antibiotic use on resistance development and persistence. Drug Resistance Updates. 2000;3:303-311
17. Normanno G, La Salandra G, Dambrosio A, Quaglia N, Corrente M, Parisi A, et al. Occurrence, characterization and antimicrobial resistance of enterotoxigenic Staphylococcus aureus isolated from meat and dairy products. International Journal of Food Microbiology. 2007;115:290-296
18. McAllister T, Yanke L, Inglis G, Olson M. Is antibiotic use in dairy cattle causing antibiotic resistance. Advanced Dairy Science and Technology. 2001;13:229-247
19. McDougall S, Parker KI, Heuer C, Compton CW. A review of the prevention and control of heifer mastitis via non-antibiotic strategies. Veterinary Microbiology. 2009;134:177-185
20. Haran KP, Godden SM, Boxrud D, Jawahir S, Bender JB, Sreevatsan S. Prevalence and characterization of Staphylococcus aureus, including methicillin-resistant Staphylococcus aureus, isolated from bulk tank milk from Minnesota dairy farms. Journal of Clinical Microbiology. 2012;50:688
21. Holmes MA, Zadoks RN. Methicillin resistant S. aureus in human and bovine mastitis. Journal of Mammary Gland Biology and Neoplasia. 2011;16:373-382
22. Mellenberger R, Keirk J. Mastitis Control Program for Staphylococcus aureus Infected Dairy Cows. Davis, California: Vetmed. Ucdavis. edu; 2001
23. Pereira UP, Oliveira DG, Mesquita LR, Costa GM, Pereira LJ. Efficacy of Staphylococcus aureus vaccines for bovine mastitis: A systematic review. Veterinary Microbiology. 2011;148:117-124
24. Brussow H, Canchaya C, Hardt WD. Phages and the evolution of bacterial pathogens: From genomic rearrangements to lysogenic conversion. Microbiology and Molecular Biology Reviews. 2004;68:560-602
25. Pantosti A, Sanchini A, Monaco M. Mechanisms of antibiotic resistance in Staphylococcus aureus. Future Microbiology. 2007;2:323-334
26. De Oliveira A, Watts J, Salmon S, Aarestrup FM. Antimicrobial susceptibility of Staphylococcus aureus isolated from bovine mastitis in Europe and the United States. Journal of Dairy Science. 2000;83:855-862

27. Jamali H, Radmehr B, Ismail S. Short communication: Prevalence and antibiotic resistance of Staphylococcus aureus isolated from bovine clinical mastitis. Journal of Dairy Science. 2014;97:2226-2230

28. Luini M, Cremonesi P, Magro G, Bianchini V, Minozzi G, Castiglioni B, et al. Methicillin-resistant Staphylococcus aureus (MRSA) is associated with low within-herd prevalence of intramammary infections in dairy cows: Genotyping of isolates. Veterinary Microbiology. 2015;178:270-274

29. Savic NR, Katic V, Velebit B. Characteristics of coagulase-positive staphylococci isolated from milk in cases of subclinical mastitis. Acta Veterinaria (Beograd). 2014;64:115-123

30. Silva NC, Guimaraes FF, Marcela de PM, Gomez-Sanz E, Gomez P, Araujo-Junior JP, et al. Characterization of methicillin-resistant coagulase-negative staphylococci in milk from cows with mastitis in Brazil. Antonie Van Leeuwenhoek. 2014;106:227-233

31. Gentilini E, Denamiel G, Llorente P, Godaly S, Rebuelto M, DeGregorio O. Antimicrobial susceptibility of Staphylococcus aureus isolated from bovine mastitis in Argentina. Journal of Dairy Science. 2000;83:1224-1227

32. Feßler A, Scott C, Kadlec K, Ehricht R, Monecke S, Schwarz S. Characterization of methicillin- resistant Staphylococcus aureus ST398 from cases of bovine mastitis. Journal of Antimicrobial Chemotherapy. 2010;65:619-625

33. Waller KP, Aspán A, Nyman A, Persson Y, Andersson UG. CNS species and antimicrobial resistance in clinical and subclinical bovine mastitis. Veterinary Microbiology. 2011;152:112-116

34. Sawant A, Gillespie B, Oliver S. Antimicrobial susceptibility of coagulase-negative Staphylococcus species isolated from bovine milk. Veterinary Microbiology. 2009;134:73-81

35. Sampimon OC. Coagulase-Negative Staphylococci Mastitis in Dutch Dairy Herds. Utrecht, The Netherlands: Utrecht University; 2009

36. Wyres KL, Holt KE. Klebsiella pneumoniae as a key trafficker of drug resistance genes from environmental to clinically important bacteria. Current Opinion in Microbiology. 2018;45:131-139

37. Wyres KL, Hawkey J, Hetland MAK, Fostervold A, Wick RR, Judd LM, et al. Emergence and rapid global dissemination of CTX-M-15-associated Klebsiella pneumoniae strain ST307. The Journal of Antimicrobial Chemotherapy. 2019;74:577-581

38. Abdi RD, Gillespie BE, Vaughn J, Merrill C, Headrick SI, Ensermu DB, et al. Antimicrobial resistance of Staphylococcus aureus isolates from dairy cows

and genetic diversity of resistant isolates. Foodborne Pathogens and Disease. 2018;15:449-458

39. Erskine RJ, Walker RD, Bolin CA, Bartlett PC, White DG. Trends in antibacterial susceptibility of mastitis pathogens during a seven-year period. Journal of Dairy Science. 2002;85:1111-1118
40. Kalmus P, Aasmae B, Karssin A, Orro T, Kask K. Udder pathogens and their resistance to antimicrobial agents in dairy cows in Estonia. Acta Veterinaria Scandinavica. 2011;53:4
41. Myllys V, Asplund K, Brofeldt E, Hirvela-Koski V, Honkanen-Buzalski T, Junttila J, et al. Bovine mastitis in Finland in 1988 and 1995 changes in prevalence and antimicrobial resistance. Acta Veterinaria Scandinavica. 1998;39:119-126
42. Saini V, McClure JT, Leger D, Keefe GP, Scholl DT, Morck DW, et al. Antimicrobial resistance profiles of common mastitis pathogens on Canadian dairy farms. Journal of Dairy Science. 2012;95:4319-4332
43. Durso LM, Cook KL. Impacts of antibiotic use in agriculture: What are the benefits and risks? Current Opinion in Microbiology. 2014;19:37-44
44. Ismail ZB. Mastitis vaccines in dairy cows: Recent developments and recommendations of application. Veterinary World. 2017;10:1057
45. Merrill C, Ensermu DB, Abdi RD, Gillespie BE, Vaughn J, Headrick SI, et al. Immunological responses and evaluation of the protection in dairy cows vaccinated with staphylococcal surface proteins. Veterinary Immunology and Immunopathology. 2019;214:109890
46. Hogan JS, Smith KL, Todhunter DA, Schoenberger PS. Field trial to determine efficacy of an Escherichia coli J5 mastitis vaccine. Journal of Dairy Science. 1992;75:78-84
47. Hogan JS, Weiss WP, Smith KL, Todhunter DA, Schoenberger PS, Sordillo LM. Effects of an Escherichia coli J5 vaccine on mild clinical coliform mastitis. Journal of Dairy Science. 1995;78:285-290
48. Hogan JS, Weiss WP, Todhunter DA, Smith KL, Schoenberger PS. Efficacy of an Escherichia coli J5 mastitis vaccine in an experimental challenge trial. Journal of Dairy Science. 1992;75:415-422
49. Allore HG, Erb HN. Partial budget of the discounted annual benefit of mastitis control strategies. Journal of Dairy Science. 1998;81:2280-2292
50. DeGraves FJ, Fetrow J. Partial budget analysis of vaccinating dairy cattle against coliform mastitis with an Escherichia coli J5 vaccine. Journal of the American Veterinary Medical Association. 1991;199:451-455

51. Wilson DJ, Grohn YT, Bennett GJ, González RN, Schukken YH, Spatz J. Comparison of J5 vaccinates and controls for incidence, etiologic agent, clinical severity, and survival in the herd following naturally occurring cases of clinical mastitis. Journal of Dairy Science. 2007;90:4282-4288
52. Wilson DJ, Mallard BA, Burton JL, Schukken YH, Grohn YT. Association of Escherichia coli J5-specific serum antibody responses with clinical mastitis outcome for J5 vaccinate and control dairy cattle. Clinical and Vaccine Immunology. 2009;16:209-217
53. Collado R, Montbrau C, Sitja M, Prenafeta A. Study of the efficacy of a Streptococcus uberis mastitis vaccine against an experimental intramammary infection with a heterologous strain in dairy cows. Journal of Dairy Science. 2018;101:10290-10302
54. Bradley AJ, Breen J, Payne B, White V, Green MJ. An investigation of the efficacy of a polyvalent mastitis vaccine using different vaccination regimens under field conditions in the United Kingdom. Journal of Dairy Science. 2015;98:1706-1720
55. Lee JW, O'Brien CN, Guidry AJ, Paape MJ, Shafer-Weaver KA, Zhao X. Effect of a trivalent vaccine against Staphylococcus aureus mastitis lymphocyte subpopulations, antibody production, and neutrophil phagocytosis. Canadian Journal of Veterinary Research. 2005;69:11-18
56. Leitner G, Lubashevsky E, Glickman A, Winkler M, Saran A, Trainin Z. Development of a Staphylococcus aureus vaccine against mastitis in dairy cows. I. Challenge trials. Veterinary Immunology and Immunopathology. 2003;93:31-38
57. Luby CD, Middleton JR. Efficacy of vaccination and antibiotic therapy against Staphylococcus aureus mastitis in dairy cattle. The Veterinary Record. 2005;157:89-90
58. Middleton JR, Ma J, Rinehart CL, Taylor VN, Luby CD, Steevens BJ. Efficacy of different Lysigin formulations in the prevention of Staphylococcus aureus intramammary infection in dairy heifers. The Journal of Dairy Research. 2006;73:10-19
59. O'Brien CN, Guidry AJ, Douglass LW, Westhoff DC. Immunization with Staphylococcus aureus lysate incorporated into microspheres. Journal of Dairy Science. 2001;84:1791-1799
60. O'Brien CN, Guidry AJ, Fattom A, Shepherd S, Douglass LW, Westhoff DC. Production of antibodies to Staphylococcus aureus serotypes 5, 8, and 336 using poly(DL-lactide-co-glycolide) microspheres. Journal of Dairy Science. 2000;83:1758-1766

61. Rivas AL, Tadevosyan R, Quimby FW, Lein DH. Blood and milk cellular immune responses of mastitic non-periparturient cows inoculated with Staphylococcus aureus. Canadian Journal of Veterinary Research. 2002;66:125-131

62. Schukken YH, Bronzo V, Locatelli C, Pollera C, Rota N, Casula A, et al. Efficacy of vaccination on Staphylococcus aureus and coagulase- negative staphylococci intramammary infection dynamics in 2 dairy herds. Journal of Dairy Science. 2014;97:5250-5264

63. Shkreta L, Talbot BG, Diarra MS, Lacasse P. Immune responses to a DNA/ protein vaccination strategy against Staphylococcus aureus induced mastitis in dairy cows. Vaccine. 2004;23:114-126

64. Shkreta L, Talbot BG, Lacasse P. Optimization of DNA vaccination immune responses in dairy cows: Effect of injection site and the targeting efficacy of antigen-bCTLA-4 complex. Vaccine. 2003;21:2372-2382

65. Smith GW, Lyman RL, Anderson KL. Efficacy of vaccination and antimicrobial treatment to eliminate chronic intramammary Staphylococcus aureus infections in dairy cattle. Journal of the American Veterinary Medical Association. 2006;228:422-425

66. Freick M, Frank Y, Steinert K, Hamedy A, Passarge O, Sobiraj A. Mastitis vaccination using a commercial polyvalent vaccine or a herd-specific Staphylococcus aureus vaccine. Tierärztliche Praxis Ausgabe G: Großtiere/ Nutztiere. 2016;44:219-229

67. Middleton JR, Luby CD, Adams DS. Efficacy of vaccination against staphylococcal mastitis: A review and new data. Veterinary Microbiology. 2009;134:192-198

68. Piepers S, Prenafeta A, Verbeke J, De Visscher A, March R, De Vliegher S. Immune response after an experimental intramammary challenge with killed Staphylococcus aureus in cows and heifers vaccinated and not vaccinated with Startvac, a polyvalent mastitis vaccine. Journal of Dairy Science. 2017;100:769-782

69. Landin H, Mork MJ, Larsson M, Waller KP. Vaccination against Staphylococcus aureus mastitis in two Swedish dairy herds. Acta Veterinaria Scandinavica. 2015;57:81

10
Chapter

CURRENT STATUS OF ANTIMICROBIAL RESISTANCE AND PROSPECTS FOR NOVEL VACCINES AGAINST PRINCIPAL BACTERIAL PATHOGENS OF BOVINE MASTITIS

1. INTRODUCTION: AN OVERVIEW

1.1 Antibiotic use in dairy farms and antimicrobial resistance

Economic losses due to bovine mastitis is estimated to be $2 billion in the United States alone [1]. Most studies showed that there is no widespread, emerging resistance among mastitis pathogens [2–4] in dairy farms. Some studies showed that the antimicrobial resistance of mastitis pathogens varies with dairy farms and bacterial species within and among dairy farms [4–9]. However, antimicrobial resistance patterns of human pathogenic bacteria and their resistome in dairy farms might be of significant concern.

On average, starting from calving (giving birth) dairy cow is milked (in lactation) for about 300 days and then dried off (stop milking) for about 60 days before they calve again. Under the ideal dairy farming condition, a dairy cow should become pregnant within 60 days of calving, and the lactation cycle continues (Figure 1).

The goal of a dry period is to give them a break from milking so that milk-producing cells regenerate, multiply, and ready for the next cycle of lactation. The incidence of intramammary infection (IMI) by bacteria is high during the early dry period and transition periods [10]. In general, for a dairy cow, a transition period, also known as the periparturient period, is a time range from three weeks before parturition (non-milking time) until three weeks after calving (milking time). It is a transition time from non-milking to milking.

Dairy cows are susceptible to mastitis during early non-lactating (dry period) and transition periods [11, 12], especially new infection with environmental pathogens (Streptococcus spp. and coliform) are highest during the first two weeks after drying off and last two weeks before calving [13] compared to contagious mastitis pathogens such as S. aureus [14]. The incidence of intramammary infection is high during the early dry period because of an absence of hygienic milking practices such as pre-milking teat washing and drying [15], preand post-milking teat dipping in antiseptic solutions [16, 17], that are known to reduce teat end colonization by bacteria and infection. An udder infected during the early dry period usually manifests clinical mastitis during the transition period [18] because of increased production of parturition inducing immunosuppressive hormones [19], negative energy balance [12], and physical stress during calving [20].

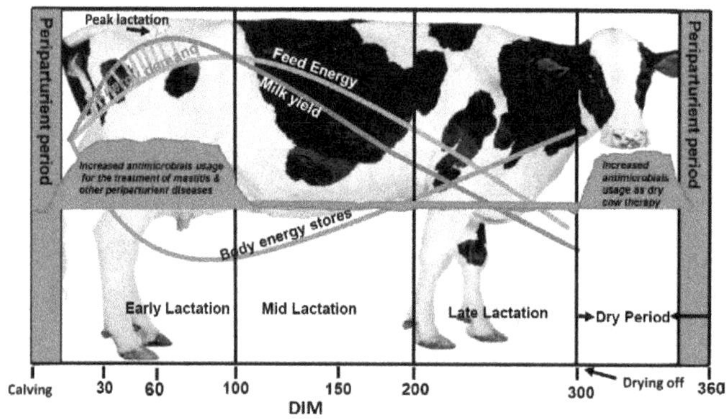

Figure 1. Antimicrobials usage patterns during the lactation cycle. DIM: Days in milk, yellow star: Peak lactation at 60 DIM, green bars: Energy demand that requires the mobilization of body energy reserve at the expense of losing bodyweight, red bumps showed increased usage of antimicrobials.

Cows are naturally protected against intramammary infections during the dry period by physical barriers such as the closure of teat opening by smooth muscle (teat sphincter) and the formation of a keratin plug, fibrous structural proteins (scleroproteins) [21, 22], in the teat canal produced by teat canal epithelium [23]. Keratin contains a high concentration of fatty acids, such as lauric, myristic, and palmitoleic acids, which are associated with reduced susceptibility to infection and stearic, linoleic, and oleic acids that are associated with increased susceptibility to infection. Keratin also contains antibacterial proteins that can damage the cell wall of some bacteria by disrupting the osmoregulatory mechanism [23]. However, the time of teat canal closure varies among cows. Some studies showed that 50% of teat canals were classified as closed by seven days after drying off, 45% closed over the following 50–60 days after drying off, and 5% had not closed by 90 days after dry off [24]. Teats that do not form a plug-like keratin seal are believed to be most susceptible to infection. Infusion of long-acting antimicrobials into the udder at drying-off (dry cow therapy) has been the major management tool for the prevention of IMI during the dry period, as well as to clear IMI established during the previous lactation [24].

In the United States and many other countries at the end of lactation (at drying off), all cows regardless of their health status, are given an intramammary infusion of long-acting antimicrobials (blanket dry cow therapy) to prevent IMI by bacteria during the dry period [3, 25]. Because of increased concern on the use of blanket dry cow therapy for its role in driving antimicrobial resistance, selective dry cow therapy (intramammary infusion of antimicrobials into only quarters that have tendency or risk of infection) has been under investigation [26, 27]. Some recent studies showed that the use of bacteriological culture-based selective dry cow therapy at drying-off did not negatively affect cow health and performance during early lactation [26, 27]. In general, dairy farms are one of the largest users of antimicrobials including medically important antimicrobials [28]. Some of the antimicrobials used in dairy farms include beta-lactams (penicillins, Ampicillin, oxacillin, penicillin novobiocin), extended-spectrum beta-lactams (third-generation cephalosporins, e.g., ceftiofur), aminoglycosides (streptomycin), macrolides (erythromycin), lincosamide (pirlimycin), tetracycline, sulfonamides, and fluoroquinolones [28–30]. Antimicrobials are also heavily used in dairy farms for the treatment of cases of mastitis [3, 25, 31] and other diseases of dairy cows such as metritis, retained placenta, lameness, diarrhea, pneumonia, [32–36] and neonatal calf diarrhea [37]. Over 90% of dairy farms in the US infuse all udder quarters of all cows with antimicrobial regardless of their health status [7, 25, 38]. According to dairy study in 2007 that was conducted in 17 major dairy states in the United States, 85.4% of farms use antibiotics for mastitis, 58.6% for lameness, 55.8% for diseases of the respiratory system, 52.9% for diseases of reproductive system, 25% for diarrhea or gastrointestinal infections and 6.9% for all other health problems [3, 25]. Cephalosporins were the most widely used antibiotics for the treatment of mastitis, followed by lincosamides and non-cephalosporin beta-lactam antibiotics [3, 25]. The two most commonly used antibiotics for dry cow therapy are Penicillin G/dihydrostreptomycin and cephalosporins [3, 25]. Antimicrobials were administered for the prevention and treatment of mastitis and other diseases of dairy cattle mainly through intramammary infusion and intramuscular route (USDA APHIS, 2009a). Antimicrobials infused into the mammary glands can be excreted to the environment through leakage of milk from the antimicrobial-treated udder or absorbed into the body and enter the blood circulation and biotransformed in the liver or kidney and excreted from the body through urine or feces into the environments [39–42]. Similarly, antimicrobials administered through parenteral routes for the treatment of acute or peracute mastitis or other diseases of dairy cows will enter the blood circulation and biotransformed in the liver or kidney and excreted from the body through urine or feces into the environments [39–42]. Therefore, both parenteral and intramammary administration of antibiotics has a significant impact on other commensals or opportunistic bacteria in the gastrointestinal tract of dairy cows and farm environments.

In addition to the use of antimicrobials for the prevention and treatment of mastitis and other diseases of dairy cattle, some farms also feed raw waste milk or pasteurized waste milk from antibiotic-treated cows to dairy calves. Feeding of raw waste milk or pasteurized waste milk from antibiotic-treated cows to calves increases pressure on gut microbes such as E. coli to became antimicrobial-resistant [43–45]. Aust et al. [43] showed that the proportion of antimicrobial-resistant E. coli, especially cephalosporin-resistant E. coli isolates, was significantly higher in calves fed waste milk or pasteurized waste milk from antimicrobial treated cows than calves fed bulk tank milk from non-antibiotic treated cows. However, pasteurized waste milk from cows not treated with antimicrobials is acceptable to be feed to young calves [43] but it is not known if pasteurization prevents the transfer of antimicrobial-resistant genes to microbes in the calve's gut. Some studies also showed that feeding pasteurized waste milk from antimicrobial treated cows to calves increased the presence of phenotypic resistance to ampicillin, cephalothin, ceftiofur, and florfenicol in fecal E. coli compared with milk replacer-fed calves [45]. However, the presence of resistance to sulfonamides, tetracyclines, and aminoglycosides was common in dairy calves regardless of the source of milk, suggesting other driving factors for resistance development [45]. It has been suggested that antimicrobial residues present in waste milk have a non-specific effect at a lower taxonomical level [44]. Collectively, these non-prudent antimicrobials usage practices in dairy farms expose a large number of animals in dairy farms to antimicrobials and also increases the use of antimicrobials in dairy farms, which in turn creates intense pressure on microbes in animals' body especially commensal and opportunistic microbes in the gastrointestinal tract and farm environments.

Some of these commensal bacteria in the animal body are serious human pathogens (e.g., E. coli 0157:H7). Staphylococcus aureus is one of the pathogens with a known ability to develop antimicrobial resistance and established S. aureus infections are persistent and difficult to clear. The failure to control these infections leads to the presence of reservoirs in the dairy herd, which ultimately leads to the spread of the infection and the culling of the chronically infected cows [46, 47].

Monitoring antimicrobial resistance patterns of bacterial isolates from cases of mastitis is important for treatment decisions and proper design of mitigation measures. It also helps to determine emergence, persistence, and potential risk of the spread of antimicrobial-resistant bacteria and resistome to human, animal, and environment [48, 49]. The prudent use of antimicrobials in dairy farms reduce emergence, persistence, and spread of antimicrobial-resistant bacteria and resistome from dairy farms to human, animal, and environment.

1.2 Transmission of antimicrobial-resistant bacteria from dairy farms to human

Most studies showed that there is no widespread, emerging resistance among mastitis pathogens [2–4] in dairy farms. However, dairy farms may serve as a source of antimicrobial-resistant human pathogenic bacteria. Extensive use of thirdgeneration cephalosporins (3GCs) in dairy cattle for the prevention and treatment of mastitis [3, 25, 28] and other diseases of dairy cattle [31, 32] can result in the carriage of extended-spectrum beta-lactamase producing Enterobacteriaceae (ESBL Ent) [50, 51]. Third and fourth-generation cephalosporins are commonly used for the treatment of invasive Gram-negative bacterial infections in humans [52–54].

In 2017, there were an estimated 197,400 cases of ESBL Ent among hospitalized patients and 9100 estimated deaths in the US alone [55]. Among Enterobacteriaceae, Escherichia coli (E. coli) is the most common bacteria that reside in the gut as normal microflora or opportunist pathogen of animals and humans. However, certain pathogenic strains can cause diseases such as mastitis in cattle, neonatal calf diarrhea in calves and hemorrhagic enteritis, and more life-threatening conditions such as hemolytic uremic syndrome and urinary tract infections in humans. New strains of multi-drug resistant foodborne pathogens that produce extended-spectrum beta-lactamases that inactivate nearly all beta-lactam antibiotics have been reported [30]. Ceftiofur is the most common 3GC used in dairy cattle operations [56]. The 3GCs are also critically important antibiotics for the treatment of serious infections caused by Enterobacteriaceae such as Escherichia coli (E. coli) and Salmonella spp. in humans [57, 58]. The use of structurally and chemically similar antibiotics in dairy cattle production and human medicine may lead to co-resistance or cross-resistance [52–54]. Some of the species of Gram-negative environmental mastitis pathogens, such as E. coli, Klebsiella pneumoniae, Acinetobacter spp., Pseudomonas spp., Enterobacter spp. are the greatest threat to human health due to the emergence of strains that are resistant to all or most available antimicrobials [59, 60].

The resistance of Enterobacteriaceae to 3GC is mainly mediated by the production of extended-spectrum beta-lactamase enzymes (ESBLs) that breakdown 3GC [61]. E. coli is one of the most frequently isolated Enterobacteriaceae carrying ESBL genes (blaCTX-M, blaSHV, blaTEM, and blaOXA) families [62–64]. These ESBL genes are usually carried on mobile plasmids along with other resistance genes such as tetracycline, quinolones, and aminoglycosides. E. coli resides in the gastrointestinal tract of cattle as normal or opportunistic microflora, but some strains (for e.g.,

0157:H7) cause serious infection in humans [58], indicating that cattle could serve as a reservoir of ESBLs producing E. coli (ESBLs E. coli) for human.

In the US, the occurrence of ESBLs E. coli in the dairy cattle was reported a decade ago from Ohio [52] and few previous studies reported the occurrence and an increase in the trend of ESBLs E. coli in the dairy cattle production system [52, 53, 65–67]. However, recent studies increasingly showed the rise of ESBLs E. coli in the cattle [51, 52, 65, 67]. Similarly, reports from the Center for Disease Control (CDC) showed a continuous increase in the number of community-associated human infections caused by ESBLs-producing Enterobacteriaceae [55]. This CDC report showed a 9% average annual increase in the number of hospitalized patients from ESBLs pathogens in six consecutive years (from 2012 to 2017). As a result, the human health sector tends to blame dairy farms that routinely use the 3GC for the rise of ESBLs pathogens such as E. coli [55, 68]. However, despite the general believe of possibility of transmission of antimicrobial-resistant bacteria from dairy farms to humans directly through contact or indirectly through food chain, there was no clear evidence-based data that showed the spread of antimicrobial-resistant bacteria from the dairy production system to humans. The opinion of the scientific community on the factors that drive the emergence and spread of antimicrobial-resistant bacteria also varies [69]. Transmission of an antimicrobial-resistant pathogen to humans could occur if contaminated unpasteurized milk and/or undercooked meat from culled dairy cows due to chronic mastitis is consumed [70]. So it is crucial to pasteurize milk or cook meat properly to reduce the risk of infection by antimicrobial-resistant bacteria [71]. It is not known, if pasteurization or proper cooking prevents the transfer of resistant genes from milk or meat to commensal or opportunistic bacteria in the human gastrointestinal tract (GIT), or the GIT of calves fed pasteurized waste milk. Mechanisms of antibiotic resistance gene transfer from resistant to susceptible bacteria are not well known, and killing resistant pathogens alone may not be good enough to prevent the transfer of the resistance gene. Non-prudent use of antimicrobials in dairy farms increases selection pressure, which could result in the emergence, persistence, and horizontal transfer of antimicrobial-resistant determinants from resistant to non-resistant bacteria. Bacteria exchange resistance genes through mobile genetic elements such as plasmids, bacteriophages, pathogenicity islands, and these genes may ultimately enter bacteria pathogenic to humans or commensal or opportunistic bacterial pathogens. The prudent use of antimicrobials in dairy farms requires identification of the pathogen causing mastitis, determining the susceptibility/resistance of the pathogen, and proper dose, duration, and frequency of treatment to ensure effective concentrations of the antibiotic to eliminate the pathogen.

2. PROSPECTS FOR EFFECTIVE VACCINES AGAINST MAJOR BACTERIAL MASTITIS PATHOGENS

Despite decades of research to develop effective vaccines against major bacterial bovine mastitis pathogens such as Staphylococcus aureus, Streptococcus uberis, and E. coli, the effective intramammary immune mechanism is still poorly understood, perpetuating reliance on antibiotic therapies to control mastitis in dairy cows. Dependence on antimicrobials is not sustainable because of their limited efficacy [46, 47] and increased risk of emergence of antimicrobial-resistant bacteria that pose serious public health threats [4, 72–74]. Neither of the two currently available commercial Bacterin vaccines against S. aureus (Table 1), Lysigin® (Boehringer Ingelheim Vetmedica, Inc., St. Joseph, MO) in the USA and Startvac® (Hipra, Girona, Spain) in Europe and other countries, confer protection from new intramammary infection under field trials as well as under controlled experimental challenge studies [75–81].

There are four commercial vaccines against E. coli mastitis which include 1) the Eviracor®J5 (Zoetis, Kalamazoo, MI), [82, 83], 2) Mastiguard®, 3) J-VAC® (Merial-Boehringer Ingelheim vet medical, Inc., Duluth, GA) and 4) ENDOVAC- Bovi® (IMMVAC) (Endovac Animal Health, Columbia, MO) (Table 1). The Endovac-bovi® is a cross-protective vaccine made of genetically engineered R/17 mutant strain of Salmonella typhimurium and the core somatic antigen mutant J-5 strain of E. coli combined with an immune-potentiating adjuvant (IMMUNEPlus®). Endovac-bovi significantly reduces diseases caused by Gram-negative bacteria producing various endotoxins and protects against E. coli mastitis and other endotoxin-mediated diseases caused by E. coli, Salmonella, Pasteurella multocida, and Mannheimia hemolytica. The UBAC® (Hipra, Amir, Spain) [84] is a recently developed vaccine against S. uberis mastitis with label claim of partial reduction in clinical severity of S. uberis mastitis.

Table 1. Commercialized and experimental vaccines against major bovine mastitis pathogens.

Mastitis Pathogen	Vaccine	Vaccine component	Protective effect	Reference
	Commercial			
S. aureus	Lysigin®	Bacterin: Somaticantigen containingphage types I, II, III,IV with differentstrains of S. aureus	Reduced SCC, clinical mastitis, and chronicIMI	[85–87]
	"	"	Field-based studies concluded no such effect	[80, 81,88–90]

	Startvac®	Bacterin: E. coli J5and S. aureus CP type8 with SAAC	Decreased duration of IMI, transmissibility of S. aureus, coliforms, and CNS	[77]
	"	"	Use of the vaccine was not associated with adecrease in mastitis	[75]
	Bestvac® Vs Startvac	herd-specific autologous vaccine compared with Startvac®	Both vaccines decreased herd prevalence of S. aureusmastitis but no other differences in terms of improvement of udder health	[78]
	Experimental			
	Whole-cell lysate	Bacterin encapsulated in biodegradable microspheres	Induced antibodies that were more opsonicfor neutrophils and inhibited adhesion to mammary epithelium.	[91]
	Whole-cell lysate from two strains	Bacterin from twostrains (α and α + βhemolytic) plussupernatants fromnon-hemolytic strain	Vaccinated cows had70% protection from infection compared to less than 10% protection in control cows	[92]
	MASTIVAC I	Whole-cell lysate	Improved udder health in addition to specific protection against S.aureus infection	[93]
	Live pathogenic S.aureus through IM route	Live pathogenic S. aureus	Induce activationof immune cells inmammary gland and blood	[94]
	Fibronect in binding protein and clumping factor A	DNA primed and protein boosted	Induced cellular and humoral immune responses that provide partial protection against S. aureus	[95]
	Protein A of S. aureus with the green fluorescent protein	DNA	Induced humoral and cellular immune responses	[96]
	Plasmid encoding bacterial antigen β-gal	DNA	Induced humoral and cellular immune responses	[97]
	Polyvalent S. aureus Bacterin	Bacterin	Eliminated some cases of chronic intramammary S. aureus infections	[88]
	Lysigin® with three-isolates based experimental Bacterin	Bacterin	Lysigin reduced the clinical severity and duration of clinical disease. None of the experimental Bacterins has significant effects	[80]
	Polyvalent S. aureus Bacterin	Bacterin + antibiotic therapy	S. aureus intramammary infection cure rate increased	[89]

	Whole-cell lysate	Whole-cell trivalent vaccine containing CP types 5, 8 and 336 with FIA or Alum adjuvants	Elicited antibody responses specific to the 3 capsular polysaccharides	[98]
	CP conjugated to a protein and incorporated in polymicrospheres and emulsified in FIA	CP types 5, 8 and 336	Cows in both groups produced increased concentrations of I gG1, IgG2 antibodies, hyperimmune sera from immunized cows increased phagocytosis, decreased bacterial adherence to epithelial cells	[99]
	Polysaccharidero-tein conjugates in FIA	Polysaccharide-protein conjugate		
	SASP or SCSP	Surface proteins	Induced partial protection	[100]
	Vaccination with Efb and LukM		Induced increased titers in serum and milk	[101]
	Inactivated Bacterin	Bacterin	Partial protection	[102]
S. uberis	Commercial			
	UBAC®	Extract from biofilm-forming strains of S. uberis	Reduce clinical signs, bacterial count, temperature, daily milk yield losses and increased the number of quarters with isolation and somatic cell count <200,000 cells/mL of milk	[84]
	Experimental			
	Killed S. uberis cells	Bacterin	Reduced numbers of homologous S. uberis in milk	[103]
	Killed bacterial cells	Bacterin of S. uberis and S. agalactiae	Parenteral vaccination has no effect on streptococcal mastitis	[104, 105]
	Live S. uberis/ cutaneous route	Live S. uberis	Some protective effect only on the homologous strain	[106]
	GapC or chimeric CAMP factor	Protein	Reduction in inflammation	[107]
	PauA	protein	Partial protection	[108]
Coliform	Commercial			
	E. coli J5 Mastiguard® J Vac® Endovac-bovi® (IMMVAC)	Bacterin	Reduce bacterial counts in milk, duration of IMIand resulted in fewer clinical symptoms	[82, 83, 109–111]

SAAC: slime associated antigenic complex, SASP: Staphylococcus aureus surface proteins, SCSP: Staphylococcus chromogenes surface proteins, CP: Capsular polysaccharide, GapC: Glyceraldehyde-3-phosphate dehydrogenase C, pauA: plasminogen activator protein, FIA: Freund's incomplete adjuvant, Efb: fibrinogen-binding protein, LukM: leukocidin subunit M.

2.1 Intramammary immune mechanisms

Intramammary immunity can be induced locally in the mammary gland or systemically in the body and cross from the body into the mammary glands. Mammary gland pathogen that enters through teat opening interact with host innate defense system primarily with macrophages in the mammary gland. Macrophages recognize invading pathogens through its pattern recognition receptors (PRR) which binds to pathogen associated molecular patterns (PAMPs) and engulf and break down the foreign pathogen into small peptides and load on to MHC-II molecules move to the supramammary lymph nodes and display on its surface to the T cells. Naïve T cells bind with peptide on MHC-II molecule through its T- cell receptor and become activated and start secreting cytokines, which further stimulate B-cells to produce antibodies. Antibody produced by B-cells released into the blood circulation and depending on type of antibody may be released to the site of infection (e.g., IgG) and opsonize the infecting pathogen and subject them to destruction by opsono- phagocytic mechanisms. Antibodies may also remain on mucosal surfaces (e.g., IgA) and bind to invading pathogens and prevent them from binding to host cells or tissue and thereby prevent colonization and infection.

Intramammary infection (IMI) leads to increased somatic cell count in the milk or mammary secretion. Somatic cells are mainly white blood cells such as granulocytes (neutrophils, eosinophils, and basophils), monocytes or macrophages, and lymphocytes, which are recruited to the mammary glands in response to mammary gland infection to fight off infection. A small proportion of mammary epithelial cells that produce milk are also shed through milk and are included in the somatic cell count. So, somatic cells are white blood cells and mammary epithelial cells.

Milk somatic cell count (SCC) increases when there is mammary gland infection (IMI) because of an inflammatory response to clear infection. In general, SCC is also an indicator of milk quality [112–116] because if there are few mammary pathogenic bacteria in the gland, the inflammatory response is less, and somatic cells recruitment into the gland is also low and vice versa. Bulk tank milk (BTM) is milk collected from all lactating dairy cows in a farm into a tank or multiple tanks. So BTSCC is somatic cell counts obtained from milk sample collected from a tank.

Intramammary infection may progress to clinical or subclinical mastitis [117]. Clinically infected udder usually treated with antimicrobial, whereas subclinically infected udder may not be diagnosed immediately and treated but remained infected and shedding bacteria through milk throughout lactation. The proportion of cure following treatment of mastitis varies and the variation in cure rate is multifactorial including cow factors (age or parity number, stage of lactation, and duration of infection, etc.), management factors (detection and diagnosis of infection and time from detection to treatment, availability of balanced nutrition, sanitation, etc.), factors related to antimicrobial use patterns (type, dose, route, frequency, and duration), and pathogen factors (type, species, number, pathogenicity or virulence, resistance to antimicrobial, etc.) [46, 118].

The dilution of effector humoral immune responses by large volume of milk coupled with the ability of mastitis causing bacteria to develop resistance to antimicrobials makes the control of mastitis very difficult. Therefore, the development of an alternative preventive tool such as a vaccine, which can overcome these limitations, has been a crucial focus of current research to decrease not only the incidence of mastitis but also the use of antimicrobials in dairy cattle farms.

Most vaccination strategies against mastitis have focused on the enhancement of humoral immunity. Development of vaccines that induce an effective cellular immune response in the mammary gland has not been well investigated. The ability to induce cellular immunity, especially neutrophil activation and recruitment into the mammary gland, is one of the key strategies in the control of mastitis, but the magnitude and duration of increased cellular recruitment into the mammary gland leads to a high number of somatic cells and poor-quality milk. So, effective balanced humoral and cellular immunity that clear intramammary infection in a short period of time is required. Several vaccine studies were conducted over the years under controlled experimental and field trials. The major bacterial bovine mastitis pathogens that have been targeted for vaccine development are S. aureus, S. uberis, and E. coli [119]. Most of these experimental and some commercial vaccines are Bacterins which are inactivated whole organism, and some vaccines contained subunits of the organism such as surface proteins [100], toxins, or polysaccharides.

2.2 Vaccine trials against Staphylococcus aureus mastitis

Staphylococcus aureus is one of the most common contagious mastitis pathogens, with an estimated incidence rate ranging from 43–74% [25, 38, 56, 120, 121].

Staphylococcus chromogenes is another increasingly reported coagulase-negative Staphylococcus species with an estimated quarter incidence rate of 42.7% characterized by high somatic cell counts [122–128]. In a study on conventional and organic Canadian dairy farms, coagulase-negative Staphylococcus species were found in 20% of the clinical samples [129]. Recently, mastitis caused by coagulase-negative Staphylococcus species increasingly became more problematic in dairy herds [125, 127, 130, 131].

Several staphylococcal vaccine efficacy trials showed that vaccination with Bacterin vaccines induced increased antibody titers in the serum and milk that are associated with partial protection [75–77, 80, 132–134] or no protection at all [78, 79, 81]. However, effective intramammary immune mechanisms against staphylococcal mastitis is still poorly understood. None of the commercially available Bacterin vaccines protects new intramammary infection [75, 77, 80, 81]. Dependence on antibiotics for the prevention and treatment of mastitis is not sustainable because of limited success [46, 47] and the emergence of antimicrobial- resistant bacteria that are major threat to human and animal health [72–74].

Despite several mastitis vaccine trials conducted against S. aureus mastitis [75, 77, 80, 88, 89, 91, 93–95, 97–99, 133] all field trials have either been unsuccessful or had limited success. There are two commercial vaccines for Staphylococcus aureus mastitis on the market, Lysigin® (Boehringer Ingelheim Vetmedica, Inc., St. Joseph, MO) in the United States and Startvac® (Hipra S.A, Girona, Spain) in Europe and Canada [78]. None of these vaccines confer protection under field trials as well as under controlled experimental studies [75, 77, 80, 81]. Several field trials and controlled experimental studies have been conducted testing the efficacy of Lysigin® and Startvac®, and results from those studies have shown some interesting results, namely a reduced incidence, severity, and duration of mastitis in vaccinated cows compared to non-vaccinated control cows [75–77]. Contrary to these observations, other studies failed to find an effect on improving udder health or showed no difference between vaccinated and non-vaccinated control cows [78, 79]. None of these Bacterin-based vaccines prevents new S. aureus IMI [75, 77, 80, 81]. Differences found in these studies are mainly due to methodological differences (vaccination schedule, route of vaccination, challenge model, herd size, time of lactation, etc.) in testing the efficacy of these vaccines. It is critically important to have a good infection model that mimics natural infection and a model that has 100% efficacy in causing infection. Without a good challenge model, the results from vaccine efficacy will be inaccurate.

The Startvac® (Hipra, Girona, Spain) is the commercially available vaccine in Europe and is a polyvalent vaccine that contains E. coli J5 and S. aureus strain SP140 [119]. In a field trial, Freick et al. [78] compared the efficacy of Startvac® with Bestvac® (IDT, Dessau-Rosslau, Germany) another herd-specific autologous commercial vaccine in a dairy herd with a high prevalence of S. aureus and found that the herd prevalence of S. aureus mastitis was lower in the Startvac® and Bestvac® vaccinated cows compared to the control cows. However, there were no other differences in terms of improvement of udder health. These authors [78] concluded that vaccination with Startvac® and Bestvac® did not improve udder health. In another field efficacy study on Startvac® in the UK, Bradley et al. [75] found that Startvac® vaccinated cows had clinical mastitis with reduced severity and higher milk production compared to non-vaccinated control cows [75].

Similarly, Schukken et al. [77] evaluated effect of Startvac® on the development of new IMI and the duration of infections caused by S. aureus and CNS. These authors [77] found that vaccinated cows had decreased incidence rate and a shorter duration of S. aureus and CNS mastitis. Piepers et al. [76], also tested the efficacy of Startvac®

through vaccination and subsequent challenge with a heterologous killed S. aureus strain and found that the inflammatory response in the vaccinated cows was less severe compared to the control cows. These authors [76] suggested that Startvac® elicited a strong Th2 immune response against S. aureus in vaccinated cows and was more effective at clearing bacteria compared to the control cows. Contrary to these observations, Landin et al. [135], evaluated the effects of Startvac® on milk production, udder health, and survival on two Swedish dairy herds with S. aureus mastitis problems and found no significant differences between the Startvac® vaccinated and non-vaccinated control cows on the health parameters they evaluated.

An experimental S. aureus vaccine made up of a combination of plasmids encoding fibronectin-binding motifs of fibronectin-binding protein (FnBP) and clumping factor A (ClfA), and plasmid encoding bovine granulocyte macrophage colony stimulatory factor, was used as a vaccine with a subsequent challenge with bacteria to test its protective effects [95]. These authors (Shkreta et al. 2004) found that their experimental vaccine-induced immune responses in the heifers that were partially protective upon experimental challenge [95]. Another controlled experimental vaccine efficacy study was conducted on the slime associated antigenic complex (SAAC) which is an extracellular component of Staphylococcus aureus, as vaccine antigen in which one group of cows were vaccinated with a vaccine containing a low amount of SAAC and another group with a high amount of SAAC and the unvaccinated group served as a control [136]. Upon intramammary infusion (challenge) with S. aureus, no difference in the occurrence of mastitis among all three groups despite the fact that the vaccine with high SAAC content induced higher production of antibodies compared to the vaccine with a low amount of SAAC [136]. Similarly, Pellegrino et al. [137], vaccinated dairy cows with an avirulent mutant strain of S. aureus and subsequently challenged with S. aureus 20 days after the second vaccination which resulted in no significant differences in the number of somatic cell count (SCC) or number of bacteria shedding through milk despite increased IgG antibody titer in the vaccinated cows compared to the control cows.

Some of the constraints affecting the successful development of effective mastitis vaccines are strain variation, the presence of exopolysaccharide (capsule, slime, biofilm) layer in most pathogenic strains of bacteria (Staph. aureus, Strep. uberis) which does not allow recognition of antibody-coated bacteria by phagocytic cells, dilution of immune effectors by milk [138, 139], the interaction between milk components and immune effectors [140] that reduce their effectiveness, and the ability of most mastitis-causing bacteria to attach and internalize into mammary epithelial cells. Furthermore, evaluation of mastitis vaccines is complicated by the absence of uniform challenge study models, and lack of uniform route(s) of vaccination, time of vaccination, adjuvants, and challenge dose. There is an increasing need for development of better vaccines that overcome these problems. Most mastitis vaccines are killed whole bacterial cells (Bacterin) vaccines [75, 77, 80, 88, 89, 91–95, 97–99] that are difficult to improve because of difficulty to specifically identify an immunogenic component that induced partial or some protective effect. In this regard, some of the current efforts to use a mixture of purified surface proteins as vaccine antigens [100] to induce immunity than killed whole bacterial cells (Bacterin) is encouraging. A better understanding of natural and acquired immunological defenses of the mammary gland coupled with detailed knowledge of the pathogenesis of each mammary pathogen should lead to the development of improved methods of reducing the incidence of mastitis in dairy cows.

2.3 Vaccine trials against Streptococcus uberis

S. uberis is ubiquitous in the cow's environment accounting for a significant number of mastitis cases. It is found on-farm in water, soil, plant material, bedding, flies, hay, and feces [141]. As such, S. uberis is remarkably adaptable, affecting lactating and dry cows, heifers, and multiparous cows, causing clinical or subclinical mastitis, and even being responsible for persistent colonization without an elevation in the somatic cell count [142, 143]. It has been described as an environmental pathogen [108, 144–146] with potential as a contagious pathogen [142, 143, 147]. S. uberis has ability to persist within the mammary gland which lead to chronic mastitis that is difficult to treat [148]. Coliform bacteria are a major cause of clinical mastitis [149, 150]. A vaccine that prevents S. uberis mastitis is not available, control measures are limited to the implementation of good management practices. Recently vaccine efficacy trial with extract of biofilm-forming strains of S. uberis (UBAC®) (Hipra, Amir, Spain), was reported to reduce clinical severity [84]. It is not clear what kind of adative immunity is induced by UBAC® S. uberis vaccine [84] and it only conferred partial reduction in clinical severity of mastitis. Multiple intramammary vaccinations of dairy cows with killed S. uberis cells resulted in the complete protection from experimental infection with the homologous strain [103]. Similarly, subcutaneous vaccination of dairy cows with live S. uberis followed by intramammary booster vaccination with S. uberis cell surface extract protected against challenge with the homologous strain but was less effective against a heterologous strain [106]. Vaccination with S. uberis glyceraldehyde phosphate dehydrogenase C (GapC) protein induced immune responses that confer a significant reduction in inflammation post-challenge [107, 151]. The pauA is a plasminogen activator and also binds active protease plasmin [152]. It has been postulated that acquisition of plasmin may promote invasion [153]. Vaccination of dairy cows with PauA induced increased antibody titers that conferred reduction in clinical severity [154]. However, mutation of pauA did not alter ability to grow in milk or to infect lactating bovine mammary glands. It appears that the ability to activate plasminogen through PauA does not play a major role in pathogenesis of S. uberis to either grow in milk or infect bovine mammary gland [155].

S. uberis expresses several surface associated proteins such as S. uberis adhesion molecule (SUAM) and extracellular matrix binding proteins, which allow it to adhere to and internalize into mammary epithelial cells, successfully inducing IMI [156–158]. The S. uberis adhesion molecule (SUAM) plays a central role in the adherence of S. uberis to mammary epithelial cells [159–162]. Vaccination of dairy cows with SUAM induced strong immune resposes in vaccinated cows [163].

The immune serum from SUAM vaccinated cows prevented S. uberis adhesion and invasion into mammary epithelial cells in vitro [163]. In vivo infusion of mammary quarters of dairy cows with S. uberis pre-incubated with immuneserum from SUAM vaccinated cows reduced clinical severity [164]. The SUAM gene deletion mutant strain is less pathogenic to mammary epithelial cells [165] and to dairy cows [159]. Controlled experimental efficacy studies using SUAM as vaccine antigen to control S. uberis mastitis showed that SUAM is immunogenic but the induced immunity was not protective. Following experimental IMI challenge with S. uberis, clinical signs emerged at about 48 h, along with increased levels of inflammatory cytokines including TNF-α, IL-1β, IL-6, and IL-8 in milk at 60 h post-infection [166]. Adaptive immune response cytokines such as IFN-γ promotes a cell-mediated immune response by enhancing functions such as macrophage bacterial killing, antigen presentation, cytotoxic T cell activation, and increased IgG2 levels. The IL-4 expression is associated with the antibody- mediated response, which is generally linked to parasite resistance, allergic reactions, and increased levels of IgG1 [167, 168]. This partial protection by the SUSP vaccine can be improved with dose optimization, appropriate adjuvant, route of injection, and timing of vaccination.

In conclusion, it is clear that Bacterin vaccines have some protective effect against homologous strains, and single surface protein is not effective. Therefore; use of multiple surface proteins may induce better immunity that prevents clinical disease and production losses.

2.4 Vaccine trials against E. coli mastitis

Coliform bacteria are a major cause of clinical mastitis [149, 150]. Coliforms include the genera Escherichia, Klebsiella, and Enterobacter [169]. Eighty to ninety percent of coliform intramammary infection (IMI) develop clinical mastitis, and 10% will be severe and could lead to death [150]. E. coli usually infects the mammary glands during the dry period and progresses to inflammation and clinical mastitis during the early lactation with local and sometimes severe systemic clinical manifestations.

Iron is an essential nutrient for the growth of coliforms [170]. However, free iron is limited in the bovine milk because most iron is bound to citrate and to a lesser extent to lactoferrin, transferrin, xanthine oxidase, and some caseins [171] and maintained at concentrations below levels required to support coliform growth [172]. To overcome this limited iron source, coliforms express multiple iron transport systems [173], which include synthesis of siderophores (e.g., enterobactin, aerobactin, ferrichrome) that bind iron with high affinity [174], the expression of iron-regulated outer membrane proteins (IROMP) that binds to ferric siderophore complexes to transport into bacterial cell and enzymes to utlize the chelated iron [173]. The siderophores are too large (600 to 1200 Da) to pass through the porin channels of the bacterial outer membrane [175, 176]. Therefore, the siderophores require specific IROMP to enable their passage across the bacterial outer membrane into the periplasm [177, 178]. The enterobactin is a siderophore with the highest affinity for iron, and it is produced by most pathogenic E. coli and Klebsiella spp. [179–181]. The aerobactin is another siderophore that was detected in only 12% of E. coli isolated from mastitis cases [182]. Enterobactin is the primary siderophore of Escherichia coli and many other Gram-negative bacteria [183]. Coliform bacteria also developed the ability to take up iron directly from naturally occurring organic iron-binding acids, including citrate [173, 184]. The citrate iron uptake system requires ferric dicitrate for induction [184]. More than 0.1 mM citrate is required for the induction of this system under iron-restricted conditions [184]. The ferric citrate transport system is the major iron acquisition system utilized by E. coli [173] to grow in the mammary gland. The mammary gland is an iron-restricted environment, and bovine milk contains approximately 7 mM citrate [185] which is ideal for induction of ferric citrate transport sytem.

Ferric enterobactin receptor, FepA, is an 81 kDa iron regulated outer membrane protein (IROMP), that binds to ferric enterobactin complex to transoport iron into the bacterial cell [186, 187]. Vaccination of dairy cows with FepA elicited an increased immunological response in serum and milk [188]. Bovine IgG directed against FepA inhibited the growth of coliform bacteria by interfering with the binding of the ferric enterobactin complex [189]. Ferric citrate receptor, FecA, is an 80.5-kDa IROMP that is responsible for the binding of ferric dicitrate [190] and transport into the bacterial cell. The FecA, is conserved among coliforms isolated from cases of naturally occurring mastitis [191]. The iron-regulated outer membrane proteins, FepA and FecA are ideal vaccine candidates because they are surface exposed, antigenic, and conserved among isolates from IMI.

Immunization of dairy cows with FepA induced significantly higher serum and whey anti-FepA IgG titers than in E. coli J5 vaccinates [188]. Results of in vitro growth inhibition studies demonstrated that antibody specific for blocking ferric enterobactin-binding site (anti-FepA) inhibited the growth of E. coli in vitro [192].

Cows immunized with FecA did have increased antibody titers in serum and mammary secretions compared with E. coli J5 immunization and unimmunized control cows [193, 194]. Antibody purified from colostrum inhibited the growth of E. coli when cultured in synthetic media modified to induce FecA expression [193]. Despite their antigenicity, the use of either FepA or FecA alone were not sufficient to prevent mastitis. The FecA and FepA are antigenically distinct [191].

Intramammary infection with E. coli induced expression and release of pro-inflammatory cytokines such as TNF-alpha, IL-8, IL-6, and IL-1 [195, 196]. Recently it has been shown with mouse mastitis models that IL-17A and Th17 cells are instrumental in the defense against E. coli IMI [197, 198]. However, the role of IL-17 in bovine E. coli mastitis is not well defined. Results of a recent vaccine efficacy study against E. coli mastitis suggested that cell-mediated immune response has more protective effect than humoral response [199]. The cytokine signaling pathways that lead to efficient bacterial clearance is not clearly defined.

The four coliform vaccines which include 1) J-5 Bacterin® (Zoetis, Kalamazoo, MI) [82, 83], 2) Mastiguard®, 3) J Vac® (Merial-Boehringer Ingelheim vet medical, Inc., Duluth, GA) and 4) Endovac-bovi® (IMMVAC) (Endovac Animal Health, Columbia, MO). Of the four coliform vaccines, J-5 Bacterin® and Mastiguard® are believed to have the same component, which is J5 Bacterin. The J Vac® is a different bacterin-toxoid. The Endovac-Bovi® contains mutant Salmonella typhimurium bacterin toxoid. All coliform mastitis vaccine formulations use gram-negative core antigens to produce non-specific immunity directed against endotoxin (LPS) [119]. The efficacy of these vaccines has been demonstrated in both experimental challenge trials and field trials in commercial dairy herds [109–111]. The principle of these bacterins is based upon their ability to stimulate the production of antibodies directed against common core antigens that gram-negative bacteria share. These vaccines are considered efficacious even though the rate of intramammary infection is not significantly reduced in vaccinated animals because they significantly reduce the clinical effects of the infection. Experimental challenge studies have demonstrated that J5 vaccines are able to reduce bacterial counts in milk and result in fewer clinical symptoms [109]. Vaccinated cows may become infected with gram- negative mastitis pathogens at the same rate as control animals but have a lower-rate of development of clinical mastitis [111], reduced the duration of IMI [110], reduced production, culling, and death losses [200, 201].

There is a growing necessity for the creation of efficacious vaccines targeting significant bacterial pathogens of bovine mastitis. A comprehensive grasp of the innate and adaptive immunological defenses of the mammary gland, alongside an in-depth knowledge of the pathogenesis of each breast pathogen, could facilitate the advancement of enhanced strategies to diminish the prevalence of mastitis in dairy cows. (Table 1).

REFERENCES

1. DeGraves FJ, Fetrow J. 1993. Economics of mastitis and mastitis control. The Veterinary Clinics of North America Food Animal Practice 9:421-434.
2. Erskine RJ, Cullor J, Schaellibaum M. Bovine mastitis pathogens and trends in resistance to antibacterial drugs, p. In (ed), Oliver SP, Murinda SE, Jayarao BM. 2011. Impact of antibiotic use in adult dairy cows on antimicrobial resistance of veterinary and human pathogens: a comprehensive review. Foodborne Pathog Dis 8:337-55.
3. Abdi RD, Gillespie BE, Vaughn J, Merrill C, Headrick SI, Ensermu DB, D'Souza DH, Agga GE, Almeida RA, Oliver SP, Kerro Dego O. 2018. A ntimicrobial Resistance of Staphylococcus aureus Isolates from Dairy Cows and Genetic Diversity of Resistant Isolates. Foodborne Pathog Dis 15:449-458.
4. Erskine RJ, Walker RD, Bolin CA, Bartlett PC, White DG. 2002. Trends in antibacterial susceptibility of mastitis pathogens during a seven-year period. J Dairy Sci 85:1111-8.
5. Kalmus P, Aasmae B, Karssin A, Orro T, Kask K. 2011. Udder pathogens and their resistance to antimicrobial agents in dairy cows in Estonia. Acta Vet Scand 53:4.
6. Mathew AG, Cissell R, Liamthong S. 2007. Antibiotic resistance in bacteria associated with food animals: a United States perspective of livestock production. Foodborne Pathog Dis 4:115-33.
7. Myllys V, Asplund K, Brofeldt E, Hirvela-Koski V, Honkanen-Buzalski T, Junttila J, Kulkas L, Myllykangas O, Niskanen M, Saloniemi H, Sandholm M, Saranpaa T. 1998. Bovine mastitis in Finland in 1988 and 1995--changes in prevalence and antimicrobial resistance. Acta Vet Scand 39:119-26.
8. Saini V, McClure JT, Leger D, Keefe GP, Scholl DT, Morck DW, Barkema HW. 2012. Antimicrobial resistance profiles of common mastitis pathogens on Canadian dairy farms. J Dairy Sci 95:4319-32.
9. Bradley AJ, Green MJ. 2004. The importance of the nonlactating period in the epidemiology of intramammary infection and strategies for prevention. Vet Clin North Am Food Anim Pract 20:547-68.
10. Drackley JK. 1999. ADSA Foundation Scholar Award. Biology of dairy cows during the transition period: the final frontier? J Dairy Sci 82:2259-73.
11. Esposito G, Irons PC, Webb EC, Chapwanya A. 2014. Interactions between negative energy balance, metabolic diseases, uterine health and immune response in transition dairy cows. Animal Reproduction Science 144:60-71.

12. Barkema HW, Schukken YH, Lam TJ, Beiboer ML, Wilmink H, Benedictus G, Brand A. 1998. Incidence of clinical mastitis in dairy herds grouped in three categories by bulk milk somatic cell counts. J Dairy Sci 81:411-9.

13. Pinedo PJ, Fleming C, Risco CA. 2012. Events occurring during the previous lactation, the dry period, and peripartum as risk factors for early lactation mastitis in cows receiving 2 different intramammary dry cow therapies. J Dairy Sci 95:7015-26.

14. Gibson H, Sinclair LA, Brizuela CM, Worton HL, Protheroe RG. 2008. Effectiveness of selected premilking teat-cleaning regimes in reducing teat microbial load on commercial dairy farms. Lett Appl Microbiol 46:295-300.

15. Gleeson D, O'Brien B, Flynn J, O'Callaghan E, Galli F. 2009. Effect of pre-milking teat preparation procedures on the microbial count on teats prior to cluster application. Ir Vet J 62:461-7.

16. Dufour S, Frechette A, Barkema HW, Mussell A, Scholl DT. 2011. Invited review: effect of udder health management practices on herd somatic cell count. J Dairy Sci 94:563-79.

17. Timonen AAE, Katholm J, Petersen A, Orro T, Motus K, Kalmus P. 2018. Elimination of selected mastitis pathogens during the dry period. J Dairy Sci 101:9332-9338.

18. Mordak R, Stewart PA. 2015. Periparturient stress and immune suppression as a potential cause of retained placenta in highly productive dairy cows: examples of prevention. Acta Vet Scand 57:84.

19. Bach A. 2011. Associations between several aspects of heifer development and dairy cow survivability to second lactation. J Dairy Sci 94:1052-7.

20. Wang B, McKittrick O, Meyers MA. 2016. Keratin: Structure, mechanical properties,occurrence in biological organisms, and effortsat bioinspiration. Progress in Materials Science 76:229-318.

21. Bragulla HH, Homberger DG. 2009. Structure and functions of keratin proteins in simple, stratified, keratinized and cornified epithelia. J Anat 214:516-59.

22. Smolenski GA, Cursons RT, Hine BC, Wheeler TT. 2015. Keratin and S100 calcium-binding proteins are major constituents of the bovine teat canal lining. Vet Res 46:113.

23. Williamson JH, Woolford MW, Day AM. 1995. The prophylactic effect of a dry-cow antibiotic against Streptococcus uberis. N Z Vet J 43:228-34.

24. USDA APHIS U. 2008a. Antibiotic use on U.S. dairy operations, 2002 and 2007 (infosheet,5p,October,2008). 2008a. Availableat: https://www. aphis.

usda.gov/animal_health/nahms/dairy/downloads/dairy07/Dairy07_is_AntibioticUse_1.pdf Accessed 3/23/2020, (Online). Rowe SM, Godden SM, Nydam DV, Gorden PJ, Lago A, Vasquez AK, Royster E, Timmerman J, Thomas MJ. 2020. Randomized controlled trial investigating the effect of 2 selective dry-cow therapy protocols on udder health and performance in the subsequent lactation. J Dairy Sci 103:6493-6503.

25. Kabera F, Dufour S, Keefe G, Cameron M, Roy JP. 2020. Evaluation of quarter-based selective dry cow therapy using Petrifilm on-farm milk culture: A randomized controlled trial. J Dairy Sci doi:10.3168/ jds.2019-17438.
26. Redding LE, Bender J, Baker L. 2019. Quantification of antibiotic use on dairy farms in Pennsylvania. J Dairy Sci 102:1494-1507.
27. Leger DF, Newby NC, Reid-Smith R, Anderson N, Pearl DL, Lissemore KD, Kelton DF. 2017. Estimated antimicrobial dispensing frequency and preferences for lactating cow therapy by Ontario dairy veterinarians. Can Vet J 58:26-34.
28. Economou V, Gousia P. 2015. Agriculture and food animals as a source of antimicrobial-resistant bacteria. Infect Drug Resist 8:49-61.
29. Pol M, Ruegg PL. 2007. Treatment practices and quantification of antimicrobial drug usage in conventional and organic dairy farms in Wisconsin. J Dairy Sci 90:249-61.
30. Sawant AA, Sordillo LM, Jayarao BM. 2005. A survey on antibiotic usage in dairy herds in Pennsylvania. J Dairy Sci 88:2991-9.
31. Kelton DF, Lissemore KD, Martin RE. 1998. Recommendations for recording and calculating the incidence of selected clinical diseases of dairy cattle. J Dairy Sci 81:2502-9.
32. Dudek K, Bednarek D, Ayling RD, Kycko A, Reichert M. 2019. Preliminary study on the effects of enrofloxacin, flunixin meglumine and pegbovigrastim on Mycoplasma bovis pneumonia. BMC Vet Res 15:371.
33. Illambas J, Potter T, Cheng Z, Rycroft A, Fishwick J, Lees P. 2013. Pharmacodynamics of marbofloxacin for calf pneumonia pathogens. Res Vet Sci 94:675-81.
34. IllambasJ,PotterT,SidhuP,RycroftAN,ChengZ,LeesP.2013.Pharmacodynamics of florfenicol for calf pneumonia pathogens. Vet Rec 172:340.
35. Constable PD. 2009. Treatment of calf diarrhea: antimicrobial and ancillary treatments. Vet Clin North Am Food Anim Pract 25:101-20, vi
36. USDA APHIS U. 2008b. United States Department of Agriculture, Animal Plant Health Inspection Service National Animal Health Monitoring System.

Highlights of Dairy 2007 Part III: reference of dairy cattle health and management practices in the United States, 2007 (Info Sheet 4p, October, 2008). 2008b. Available at https://www. aphis.usda.gov/animal_health/nahms/dairy/downloads/dairy07/Dairy07_ir_ Food_safety.pdf Accessed 3/23/2020, (Online).

37. Baggot JD. 2006. Principles of antimicrobial drug bioavailability and disposition. Baggot JD, Brown SA. 2006. Development and formation of veterinary dosage forms, 2nd edition ed. Marcel Dekker, New York. Guardabassi L, Apley M, Olsen JE, Toutain PL, Weese S. 2018.

38. Optimization of Antimicrobial Treatment to Minimize Resistance Selection. Microbiol Spectr 6. Toutain PL, Raynaud JP. 1983. Pharmacokinetics of oxytetracycline in young cattle: comparison of conventional vs long- acting formulations. Am J Vet Res 44:1203-9.

39. Aust V, Knappstein K, Kunz HJ, Kaspar H, Wallmann J, Kaske M. 2013. Feeding untreated and pasteurized waste milk and bulk milk to calves: effects on calf performance, health status and antibiotic resistance of faecal bacteria. J Anim Physiol Anim Nutr (Berl) 97:1091-103.

40. Maynou G, Chester-Jones H, Bach A, Terre M. 2019. Feeding Pasteurized Waste Milk to Preweaned Dairy Calves Changes Fecal and Upper Respiratory Tract Microbiota. Front Vet Sci 6:159.

41. Maynou G, Migura-Garcia L, Chester-Jones H, Ziegler D, Bach A, Terre M. 2017. Effects of feeding pasteurized waste milk to dairy calves on phenotypes and genotypes of antimicrobial resistance in fecal Escherichia coli isolates before and after weaning. J Dairy Sci 100:7967-7979.

42. Barkema HW, Schukken YH, Zadoks RN. 2006. Invited Review: The role of cow, pathogen, and treatment regimen in the therapeutic success of bovine Staphylococcus aureus mastitis. J Dairy Sci 89:1877-95.

43. McDougall S, Parker KI, Heuer C, Compton CW. 2009. A review of prevention and control of heifer mastitis via non-antibiotic strategies. Vet Microbiol 134:177-85.

44. Durso LM, Cook KL. 2014. Impacts of antibiotic use in agriculture: what are the benefits and risks? Curr Opin Microbiol 19:37-44.

45. Normanno G, La Salandra G, Dambrosio A, Quaglia NC, Corrente M, Parisi A, Santagada G, Firinu A, Crisetti E, Celano GV. 2007. Occurrence, characterization and antimicrobial resistance of enterotoxigenic Staphylococcus aureus isolated from meat and dairy products. Int J Food Microbiol 115:290-6.

46. Wichmann F, Udikovic-Kolic N, Andrew S, Handelsman J. 2014. Diverse antibiotic resistance genes in dairy cow manure. MBio 5:e01017.

47. Agga GE, Schmidt JW, Arthur TM. 2016. Antimicrobial-Resistant Fecal Bacteria from Ceftiofur-Treated and Nonantimicrobial-Treated Comingled Beef Cows at a Cow-Calf Operation. Microb Drug Resist 22:598-608.

48. Wittum TE, Mollenkopf DF, Daniels JB, Parkinson AE, Mathews JL, Fry PR, Abley MJ, Gebreyes WA. 2010. CTX-M-type extended-spectrum beta- lactamases present in Escherichia coli from the feces of cattle in Ohio, United States. Foodborne Pathog Dis 7:1575-9.

49. Heider LC, Funk JA, Hoet AE, Meiring RW, Gebreyes WA, Wittum TE. 2009. Identification of Escherichia coli and Salmonella enterica organisms with reduced susceptibility to ceftriaxone from fecal samples of cows in dairy herds. Am J Vet Res 70:389-93.

50. Dunne EF, Fey PD, Kludt P, Reporter R, Mostashari F, Shillam P, WicklundJ,MillerC,HollandB,StameyK, Barrett TJ, Rasheed JK, Tenover FC, Ribot EM, Angulo FJ. 2000. Emergence of domestically acquired ceftriaxone-resistant Salmonella infections associated with AmpC beta-lactamase. JAMA 284:3151-6.

51. CDC. 2019. Antibiotic Resistance Threats Report. USDA APHIS U. Part III: Health Management and Bio¬security in US Feedlots, 1999. US Department of Agriculture; 2000. Available at https:// www.aphis.usda.gov/animal_health/ nahms/dairy/downloads/dairy07/ Dairy07_ir_Food_safety.pdf accessed December 23, 2020 (online), p. In (ed),

52. Paterson DL, Bonomo RA. 2005. Extended-spectrum beta-lactamases: a clinical update. Clin Microbiol Rev 18:657-86.

53. Malloy AM, Campos JM. 2011. Extended-spectrum beta-lactamases: a brief clinical update. Pediatr Infect Dis J 30:1092-3.

54. Wyres KL, Holt KE. 2018. Klebsiella pneumoniae as a key trafficker of drug resistance genes from environmental to clinically important bacteria. Curr Opin Microbiol 45:131-139.

55. Wyres KL, Hawkey J, Hetland MAK, Fostervold A, Wick RR, Judd LM, Hamidian M, Howden BP, Lohr IH, Holt KE. 2019. Emergence and rapid global dissemination of CTX-M- 15-associated Klebsiella pneumoniae strain ST307. J Antimicrob Chemother 74:577-581.

56. Rawat D, Nair D. 2010. Extended- spectrum beta-lactamases in Gram Negative Bacteria. J Glob Infect Dis 2:263-74.

57. Ali T, Ur Rahman S, Zhang L, Shahid M, Zhang S, Liu G, Gao J, Han B. 2016. ESBL-Producing Escherichia coli from Cows Suffering Mastitis in China Contain Clinical Class 1 Integrons with CTX-M Linked to ISCR1. Front Microbiol 7:1931.

58. Teng L, Lee S, Ginn A, Markland SM, Mir RA, DiLorenzo N, Boucher C, Prosperi M, Johnson J, Morris JG, Jr., Jeong KC. 2019. Genomic Comparison Reveals Natural Occurrence of Clinically Relevant Multidrug-Resistant Extended-Spectrum-beta-Lactamase-Producing Escherichia coli Strains. Appl Environ Microbiol 85.

59. Smet A, Martel A, Persoons D, Dewulf J, Heyndrickx M, Herman L, Haesebrouck F, Butaye P. 2010. Broad- spectrum beta-lactamases among Enterobacteriaceae of animal origin: molecular aspects, mobility and impact on public health. FEMS Microbiol Rev 34:295-316.

60. Davis MA, Sischo WM, Jones LP, Moore DA, Ahmed S, Short DM, Besser TE. 2015. Recent Emergence of Escherichia coli with Cephalosporin Resistance Conferred by blaCTX-M on Washington State Dairy Farms. Appl Environ Microbiol 81:4403-10.

61. Tragesser LA, Wittum TE, Funk JA, Winokur PL, Rajala-Schultz PJ. 2006. Association between ceftiofur use and isolation of Escherichia coli with reduced susceptibility to ceftriaxone from fecal samples of dairy cows. Am J Vet Res 67:1696-700.

62. Afema JA, Ahmed S, Besser TE, Jones LP, Sischo WM, Davis MA. 2018. Molecular Epidemiology of Dairy Cattle- Associated Escherichia coli Carrying blaCTX-M Genes in Washington State. Appl Environ Microbiol 84.

63. Thaden JT, Fowler VG, Sexton DJ, Anderson DJ. 2016. Increasing Incidence of Extended-Spectrum beta-Lactamase-Producing Escherichia coli in Community Hospitals throughout the Southeastern United States. Infect Control Hosp Epidemiol 37:49-54.

64. Turnbridge J. 2004. Antibiotic use in animals-prejudices, perceptions and realities. J Antimicrob Chemother 53:26-27.

65. Oliver SP, Boor KJ, Murphy SC, Murinda SE. 2009. Food safety hazards associated with consumption of raw milk. Foodborne Pathog Dis 6:793-806.

66. Oliver SP, Jayarao BM, Almeida RA. 2005. Foodborne pathogens in milk and the dairy farm environment: food safety and public health implications. Foodborne Pathog Dis 2:115-29.

67. Fitzgerald JR. 2012a. Human origin for livestock-associated methicillin-resistant Staphylococcus aureus. MBio 3:e00082-12.

68. Fitzgerald JR. 2012b. Livestock- associated Staphylococcus aureus: origin, evolution and public health threat. Trends Microbiol 20:192-8.

69. Holmes MA, Zadoks RN. 2011. Methicillin resistant S. aureus in human and bovine mastitis. Journal of mammary gland biology and neoplasia 16:373-382.

70. Bradley AJ, Breen J, Payne B, White V, Green MJ. 2015. An investigation of the efficacy of a polyvalent mastitis vaccine using different vaccination regimens under field conditions in the United Kingdom. Journal of dairy science 98:1706-1720.

71. Piepers S, Prenafeta A, Verbeke J, De Visscher A, March R, De Vliegher S. 2017. Immune response after an experimental intramammary challenge with killed Staphylococcus aureus in cows and heifers vaccinated and not vaccinated with Startvac, a polyvalent mastitis vaccine. J Dairy Sci 100:769-782.

72. Schukken YH, Bronzo V, Locatelli C, Pollera C, Rota N, Casula A, Testa F, Scaccabarozzi L, March R, Zalduendo D, Guix R, Moroni P. 2014. Efficacy of vaccination on Staphylococcus aureus and coagulase-negative staphylococci intramammary infection dynamics in 2 dairy herds. Journal of Dairy Science 97:5250-5264.

73. Freick M, Frank Y, Steinert K, Hamedy A, Passarge O, Sobiraj A. 2016. Mastitis vaccination using a commercial polyvalent vaccine or a herd-specific Staphylococcus aureus vaccine. Tierärztliche Praxis G: Großtiere/ Nutztiere 44:219-229.

74. Landin H, Mork MJ, Larsson M, Waller KP. 2015. Vaccination against Staphylococcus aureus mastitis in two Swedish dairy herds. Acta Vet Scand 57:81.

75. Middleton JR, Ma J, Rinehart CL, Taylor VN, Luby CD, Steevens BJ. 2006. Efficacy of different Lysigin formulations in the prevention of Staphylococcus aureus intramammary infection in dairy heifers. J Dairy Res 73:10-9.

76. Middleton JR, Luby CD, Adams DS. 2009. Efficacy of vaccination against staphylococcal mastitis: a review and new data. Vet Microbiol 134:192-8.

77. Wilson DJ, Grohn YT, Bennett GJ, González RN, Schukken YH, Spatz J. 2007. Comparison of J5 vaccinates and controls for incidence, etiologic agent, clinical severity, and survival in the herd following naturally occurring cases of clinical mastitis. J Dairy Sci 90:4282-8.

78. Wilson DJ, Mallard BA, Burton JL, Schukken YH, Grohn YT. 2009. Association of Escherichia coli J5-specific serum antibody responses with clinical mastitis outcome for J5 vaccinate and control dairy cattle. Clin Vaccine Immunol 16:209-17.

79. Collado R, Montbrau C, Sitja M, Prenafeta A. 2018. Study of the efficacy of a Streptococcus uberis mastitis vaccine against an experimental intramammary infection with a heterologous strain in dairy cows. J Dairy Sci 101:10290-10302.

80. Nickerson SC, Owens WE, Tomita GM, Widel P. 1999. Vaccinating dairy heifers with a Staphylococcus aureus bacterin reduces mastitis at calving. Large Animal Practice 20:16-28.

81. Williams JM, Mayerhofer HJ, Brown RW. 1966. Clinical evaluation of a Staphylococcus aureus bacterin (polyvalent somatic antigen). Vet Med Small Anim Clin 61:789-93.

82. Williams JM, Shipley GR, Smith GL, Gerber DL. 1975. A clinical evaluation of Staphylococcus aureus bacterin in the control of staphylococcal mastitis in cows. Vet Med Small Anim Clin 70:587-94.

83. Smith GW, Lyman RL, Anderson KL. 2006. Efficacy of vaccination and antimicrobial treatment to eliminate chronic intramammary Staphylococcus aureus infections in dairy cattle. J Am Vet Med Assoc 228:422-5.

84. Luby CD, Middleton JR. 2005. Efficacy of vaccination and antibiotic therapy against Staphylococcus aureus mastitis in dairy cattle. Vet Rec 157:89-90.

85. Luby CD, Middleton JR, Ma J, Rinehart CL, Bucklin S, Kohler C, Tyler JW. 2007. Characterization of the antibody isotype response in serum and milk of heifers vaccinated with a Staphylococcus aureus bacterin (Lysigin). J Dairy Res 74:239-46.

86. O'Brien CN, Guidry AJ, Douglass LW, Westhoff DC. 2001. Immunization with Staphylococcus aureus lysate incorporated into microspheres. J Dairy Sci 84:1791-9.

87. Leitner G, Lubashevsky E, Glickman A, Winkler M, Saran A, Trainin Z. 2003. Development of a Staphylococcus aureus vaccine against mastitis in dairy cows. I. Challenge trials. Vet Immunol Immunopathol 93:31-8.

88. Leitner G, Yadlin N, Lubashevsy E, Ezra E, Glickman A, Chaffer M, Winkler M, Saran A, Trainin Z. 2003b. Development of a Staphylococcus aureus vaccine against mastitis in dairy cows. II. Field trial. Vet Immunol Immunopathol 93:153-8.

89. Rivas AL, Tadevosyan R, Quimby FW, Lein DH. 2002. Blood and milk cellular immune responses of mastitic non-periparturient cows inoculated with Staphylococcus aureus. Can J Vet Res 66:125-31.

90. Shkreta L, Talbot BG, Diarra MS, Lacasse P. 2004. Immune responses to a DNA/protein vaccination strategy against Staphylococcus aureus induced mastitis in dairy cows. Vaccine 23:114-26.

91. Carter EW, Kerr DE. 2003. Optimization of DNA-based vaccination in cows using green fluorescent protein and protein A as a prelude to immunization against staphylococcal mastitis. J Dairy Sci 86:1177-86.

92. Shkreta L, Talbot BG, Lacasse P. 2003. Optimization of DNA vaccination immune responses in dairy cows: effect of injection site and the targeting efficacy of antigen-bCTLA-4 complex. Vaccine 21:2372-82.

93. Lee JW, O'Brien CN, Guidry AJ, Paape MJ, Shafer-Weaver KA, Zhao X. 2005. Effect of a trivalent vaccine against Staphylococcus aureus mastitis lymphocyte subpopulations, antibody production, and neutrophil phagocytosis. Can J Vet Res 69:11-8.

94. O'Brien CN, Guidry AJ, Fattom A, Shepherd S, Douglass LW, Westhoff DC. 2000. Production of antibodies to Staphylococcus aureus serotypes 5, 8, and 336 using poly(DL-lactide-co-glycolide) microspheres. J Dairy Sci 83:1758-66.

95. Merrill C, Ensermu DB, Abdi RD, Gillespie BE, Vaughn J, Headrick SI, Hash K, Walker TB, Stone E, Kerro Dego O. 2019. Immunological responses and evaluation of the protection in dairy cows vaccinated with staphylococcal surface proteins. Vet Immunol Immunopathol 214:109890.

96. Benedictus L, Ravesloot L, Poppe K, Daemen I, Boerhout E, van Strijp J, Broere F, Rutten V, Koets A, Eisenberg S. 2019. Immunization of young heifers with staphylococcal immune evasion proteins before natural exposure to Staphylococcus aureus induces a humoral immune response in serum and milk.

97. BMC Veterinary Research 15. Mellaa A, Ulloa F, Valdésd I, Olivaresa N, Ceballose A, Kruzea J. 2017. Evaluation of a new vaccine against Staphylococcus aureus mastitis in dairy herds of southern Chile. I. Challenge tria. Aust J Vet Sci 49:149-160

98. Finch JM, Hill AW, Field TR, Leigh JA. 1994. Local vaccination with killed Streptococcus uberis protects the bovine mammary gland against experimental intramammary challenge with the homologous strain. Infect Immun 62:3599-603.

99. Giraudo JA, Calzolari A, Rampone H, Rampone A, Giraudo AT, Bogni C, Larriestra A, Nagel R. 1997.

100. Field trials of a vaccine against bovine mastitis. 1. Evaluation in heifers. J Dairy Sci 80:845-53.

101. Calzolari A, Giraudo JA, Rampone H, OdiernoL,GiraudoAT,FrigerioC,BetteraS, Raspanti C, Hernandez J, Wehbe M, Mattea M, Ferrari M, Larriestra A, Nagel R. 1997. Field trials of a vaccine against bovine mastitis. 2. Evaluation in two commercial dairy herds. J Dairy Sci 80:854-8.

102. Finch JM, Winter A, Walton AW, Leigh JA. 1997. Further studies on the efficacy of a live vaccine against mastitis caused by Streptococcus uberis. Vaccine 15:1138-43.

103. Fontaine MC, Perez-Casal J, Song XM, Shelford J, Willson PJ, Potter AA. 2002. Immunisation of dairy cattle with recombinant Streptococcus uberis GapC or a chimeric CAMP antigen confers protection against heterologous bacterial challenge. Vaccine 20:2278-86.

104. Leigh JA. 1999. Streptococcus uberis: a permanent barrier to the control of bovine mastitis? Vet J 157:225-38.

105. Hogan JS, Smith KL, Todhunter DA, Schoenberger PS. 1992. Field trial to determine efficacy of an Escherichia coli J5 mastitis vaccine. J Dairy Sci 75:78-84.

106. Hogan JS, Weiss WP, Smith KL, T odhunter DA, Schoenberger PS, Sordillo LM. 1995. Effects of an Escherichia coli J5 vaccine on mild clinical coliform mastitis. J Dairy Sci 78:285-90.

107. Hogan JS, Todhunter DA, Smith KL, Schoenberger PS, Wilson RA. 1992. Susceptibility of Escherichia coli isolated from intramammary infections to phagocytosis by bovine neutrophils. J Dairy Sci 75:3324-9.

108. Gillespie BE, Lewis MJ, Boonyayatra S, Maxwell ML, Saxton A, Oliver SP, Almeida RA. 2012. Short communication: Evaluation of bulk tank milk microbiological quality of nine dairy farms in Tennessee. J Dairy Sci 95:4275-9.

109. Barbano DM, Lynch JM. 2006. Major advances in testing of dairy products: milk component and dairy product attribute testing. J Dairy Sci 89:1189-94.

110. Barbano DM, Ma Y, Santos MV. 2006. Influence of raw milk quality on fluid milk shelf life. J Dairy Sci 89 Suppl 1:E15-9.

111. Parodi P. 2004. Milk fat in human nutrition. Aust J Dairy Technol 59:3-59.

112. Jayarao BM, Pillai SR, Sawant AA, Wolfgang DR, Hegde NV. 2004. Guidelines for monitoring bulk tank milk somatic cell and bacterial counts. J Dairy Sci 87:3561-73.

113. Seegers H, Fourichon C, Beaudeau F. 2003. Production effects related to mastitis and mastitis economics in dairy cattle herds. Vet Res 34:475-91.

114. Bradley AJ, Green MJ. 2009. Factors affecting cure when treating bovine clinical mastitis with cephalosporin- based intramammary preparations. J Dairy Sci 92:1941-53.

115. Ismail ZB. 2017. Mastitis vaccines in dairy cows: Recent developments and recommendations of application. Veterinary world 10:1057.

116. Riekerink RGO, Barkema HW, Scholl DT, Poole DE, Kelton DF. 2010. Management practices associated with the bulk-milk prevalence of Staphylococcus aureus in Canadian dairy farms. Preventive veterinary medicine 97:20-28.

117. USDA APHIS U. 2009. United States Department of Agriculture, Animal Plant Health Inspection Service National Animal Health Monitoring System. Injection practices on U.S. dairy opera tions, 2007 (Veterinary Services Info Sheet 4 p, February 2009). 2009. Available at https://www.aphis.usda.gov/animal_health/nahms/ dairy/downloads/dairy07/Dairy07_is_ InjectionPrac_1.pdf accessed March 23, 2020. (Online.)

118. Dufour S, Dohoo IR, Barkema HW, Descoteaux L, Devries TJ, Reyher KK, Roy JP, Scholl DT. 2012. Epidemiology of coagulase-negative staphylococci intramammary infection in dairy cattle and the effect of bacteriological culture misclassification. J Dairy Sci 95:3110-24.

119. Piessens V, Van Coillie E, Verbist B, Supre K, Braem G, Van Nuffel A, De Vuyst L, Heyndrickx M, De Vliegher S. 2011. Distribution of coagulase-negative Staphylococcus species from milk and environment of dairy cows differs between herds. J Dairy Sci 94:2933-44.

120. Gillespie BE, Headrick SI, Boonyayatra S, Oliver SP. 2009. Prevalence and persistence of coagulase-negative Staphylococcus species in three dairy research herds. Vet Microbiol 134:65-72.

121. Pyorala S, Taponen S. 2009. Coagulase-negative staphylococci- emerging mastitis pathogens. Vet Microbiol 134:3-8.

122. Fry PR, Middleton JR, Dufour S, Perry J, Scholl D, Dohoo I. 2014. Association of coagulase-negative staphylococcal species, mammary quarter milk somatic cell count, and persistence of intramammary infection in dairy cattle. Journal of Dairy Science 97:4876-4885.

123. Taponen S, Liski E, Heikkila AM, Pyorala S. 2017. Factors associated with intramammary infection in dairy cows caused by coagulase-negative staphylococci, Staphylococcus aureus, Streptococcus uberis, Streptococcus dysgalactiae, Corynebacterium bovis, or Escherichia coli. J Dairy Sci 100:493-503.

124. Taponen S, Pyorala S. 2009. Coagulase-negative staphylococci as cause of bovine mastitis- not so different from Staphylococcus aureus? Vet Microbiol 134:29-36.

125. Levison L, Miller-Cushon E, Tucker A, Bergeron R, Leslie K, Barkema H, DeVries T. 2016. Incidence rate of pathogen-specific clinical mastitis on conventional and organic Canadian dairy farms. Journal of dairy science 99:1341-1350.

126. Taponen S, Bjorkroth J, Pyorala S. 2008. Coagulase-negative staphylococci isolated from bovine extramammary sites and intramammary infections in a single dairy herd. J Dairy Res 75:422-9.

127. Taponen S, Koort J, Bjorkroth J, Saloniemi H, Pyorala S. 2007. Bovine intramammary infections caused by coagulase-negative staphylococci may persist throughout lactation according to amplified fragment length polymorphism-based analysis. J Dairy Sci 90:3301-7.

128. Leitner G, Yadlin N, Lubashevsy E, Ezra E, Glickman A, Chaffer M, Winkler M, Saran A, Trainin Z. 2003. Development of a Staphylococcus aureus vaccine against mastitis in dairy cows. II. Field trial. Vet Immunol Immunopathol 93:153-8.

129. Leitner G, Lubashevsky E, Glickman A, Winkler M, Saran A, Trainin Z. 2003a. Development of a Staphylococcus aureus vaccine against mastitis in dairy cows. I. Challenge trials. Vet Immunol Immunopathol 93:31-8.

130. Chang BS, Moon JS, Kang HM, Kim YI, Lee HK, Kim JD, Lee BS, Koo HC, Park YH. 2008. Protective effects of recombinant staphylococcal enterotoxin type C mutant vaccine against experimental bovine infection by a strain of Staphylococcus aureus isolated from subclinical mastitis in dairy cattle. Vaccine 26:2081-91.

131. Landin H, Mörk MJ, Larsson M, Waller KP. 2015. Vaccination against Staphylococcus aureus mastitis in two Swedish dairy herds. Acta Veterinaria Scandinavica 57:81.

132. Prenafeta A, March R, Foix A, Casals I, Costa L. 2010. Study of the humoral immunological response after vaccination with a Staphylococcus aureus biofilm-embedded bacterin in dairy cows: possible role of the exopolysaccharide specific antibody production in the protection from Staphylococcus aureus induced mastitis. Vet Immunol Immunopathol 134:208-17.

133. Pellegrino M, Giraudo J, Raspanti C, Nagel R, Odierno L, Primo V, Bogni C. 2008. Experimental trial in heifers vaccinated with Staphylococcus aureus avirulent mutant against bovine mastitis. Veterinary Microbiology 127:186-190.

134. Guidry AJ, O'Brien CN, Oliver SP, Dowlen HH, Douglass LW. 1994. Effect of whole Staphylococcus aureus and mode of immunization on bovine opsonizing antibodies to capsule. J Dairy Sci77:2965-74.

135. Yancey RJ, Jr. 1999. Vaccines and diagnostic methods for bovine mastitis: fact and fiction. Adv Vet Med 41:257-73.

136. Russell MW, Brooker BE, Reiter B. 1977. Eelectron microscopic observations of the interaction of casein micelles and milk fat globules with bovine

polymorphonuclear leucocytes during the phagocytosis of staphylococci in milk. J Comp Pathol 87:43-52.

137. Zadoks RN, Tikofsky LL, Boor KJ. 2005. Ribotyping of Streptococcus uberis from a dairy's environment, bovine feces and milk. Vet Microbiol 109:257-65.
138. Oliver S, Almeida R, Calvinho L. 1998. Virulence factors of Streptococcus uberis isolated from cows with mastitis. Zoonoses and Public Health 45:461-471.
139. Zadoks RN, Gillespie BE, Barkema HW, Sampimon OC, Oliver SP, Schukken YH. 2003. Clinical, epidemiological and molecular characteristics of Streptococcus uberis infections in dairy herds. Epidemiol Infect 130:335-49.
140. Douglas VL, Fenwick SG, Pfeiffer DU, Williamson NB, Holmes CW. 2000. Genomic typing of Streptococcus uberis isolates from cases of mastitis, in New Zealand dairy cows, using pulsed- field gel electrophoresis. Vet Microbiol 75:27-41.
141. McDougall S, Parkinson TJ, Leyland M, Anniss FM, Fenwick SG. 2004. Duration of infection and strain variation in Streptococcus uberis isolated from cows' milk. J Dairy Sci 87:2062-72.
142. Wieliczko RJ, Williamson JH, CursonsRT,Lacy-HulbertSJ,WoolfordMW. 2002. Molecular typing of Streptococcus uberis strains isolated from cases of bovine mastitis. J Dairy Sci 85:2149-54.
143. Phuektes P, Mansell PD, Dyson RS, Hooper ND, Dick JS, Browning GF. 2001. Molecular epidemiology of Streptococcus uberis isolates from dairy cows with mastitis. J Clin Microbiol 39:1460-6.
144. Steeneveld W, Swinkels J, Hogeveen H. 2007. Stochastic modelling to assess economic effects of treatment of chronic subclinical mastitis caused by Streptococcus uberis. J Dairy Res 74:459-67.
145. Smith KL, Todhunter D, Schoenberger P. 1985. Environmental mastitis: Cause, prevalence, prevention1, 2. Journal of Dairy Science 68:1531-1553.
146. Smith KL, Todhunter DA, Schoenberger PS. 1985. Environmental mastitis: cause, prevalence, prevention. J Dairy Sci 68:1531-53.
147. Leigh JA. 2002. Immunisation of dairy cattle with recombinant Streptococcus uberis GapC or a chimeric CAMP antigen confers protection against heterologous bacterial challenge. M.C. Fontaine et al. [Vaccine 20 (2002) 2278-2286]. Vaccine 20:3047-8.
148. Lincoln RA, Leigh JA. 1997. Characterization of a novel plasminogen activator from Streptococcus uberis. Adv Exp Med Biol 418:643-5.
149. Leigh JA, Lincoln RA. 1997. Streptococcus uberis acquires plasmin activity following growth in the presence of bovine plasminogen through the action of its specific plasminogen activator. FEMS Microbiol Lett 154:123-9.

150. Leigh JA, Finch JM, Field TR, Real NC, Winter A, Walton AW, Hodgkinson SM. 1999. Vaccination with the plasminogen activator from Streptococcus uberis induces an inhibitory response and protects against experimental infection in the dairy cow. Vaccine 17:851-7.

151. Ward PN, Field TR, Rapier CD, Leigh JA. 2003. The activation of bovine plasminogen by PauA is not required for virulence of Streptococcus uberis. Infect Immun 71:7193-6.

152. Almeida RA, Luther DA, Park HM, Oliver SP. 2006. Identification, isolation, and partial characterization of a novel Streptococcus uberis adhesion molecule (SUAM). Vet Microbiol 115:183-91.

153. Almeida RA, Oliver SP. 2001. Role of collagen in adherence of Streptococcus uberis to bovine mammary epithelial cells. J Vet Med B Infect Dis Vet Public Health 48:759-63.

154. Almeida RA, Luther DA, Kumar SJ, Calvinho LF, Bronze MS, Oliver SP. 1996. Adherence of Streptococcus uberis to bovine mammary epithelial cells and to extracellular matrix proteins. Zentralbl Veterinarmed B 43:385-92.

155. Almeida RA, Dego OK, Headrick SI, Lewis MJ, Oliver SP. 2015. Role of Streptococcus uberis adhesion molecule in the pathogenesis of Streptococcus uberis mastitis. Vet Microbiol 179:332-5.

156. Almeida RA, Dunlap JR, Oliver SP. 2010. Binding of Host Factors Influences Internalization and Intracellular Trafficking of Streptococcus uberis in Bovine Mammary Epithelial Cells. Vet Med Int 2010:319192.

157. Almeida RA, Fang W, Oliver SP. 1999. Adherence and internalization of Streptococcus uberis to bovine mammary epithelial cells are mediated by host cell proteoglycans. FEMS microbiology letters 177:313-317.

158. Patel D, Almeida RA, Dunlap JR, Oliver SP. 2009. Bovine lactoferrin serves as a molecular bridge for internalization of Streptococcus uberis into bovine mammary epithelial cells. Veterinary microbiology 137:297-301.

159. Prado ME, Almeida RA, Ozen C, Luther DA, Lewis MJ, Headrick SJ, Oliver SP. 2011. Vaccination of dairy cows with recombinant Streptococcus uberis adhesion molecule induces antibodies that reduce adherence to and internalization of S. uberis into bovine mammary epithelial cells. Vet Immunol Immunopathol 141:201-8.

160. Almeida RA, Kerro-Dego O, Prado ME, Headrick SI, Lewis MJ, Siebert LJ, Pighetti GM, Oliver SP. 2015. Protective effect of anti-SUAM antibodies on Streptococcus uberis mastitis. Veterinary research 46:133.

161. Chen X, Dego OK, Almeida RA, Fuller TE, Luther DA, Oliver SP. 2011. Deletion of sua gene reduces the ability of Streptococcus uberis to adhere to and internalize into bovine mammary epithelial cells. Vet Microbiol 147:426-34.

162. Rambeaud M, Almeida RA, Pighetti GM, Oliver SP. 2003. Dynamics of leukocytes and cytokines during experimentally induced Streptococcus uberis mastitis. Vet Immunol Immunopathol 96:193-205.

163. Swanson KM, Stelwagen K, Dobson J, Henderson HV, Davis SR, Farr VC, Singh K. 2009. Transcriptome profiling of Streptococcus uberis-induced mastitis reveals fundamental differences between immune gene expression in the mammary gland and in a primary cell culture model. J Dairy Sci 92:117-29.

164. Moyes KM, Drackley JK, Morin DE, Bionaz M, Rodriguez-Zas SL, Everts RE, Lewin HA, Loor JJ. 2009. Gene network and pathway analysis of bovine mammary tissue challenged with Streptococcus uberis reveals induction of cell proliferation and inhibition of PPARgamma signaling as potential mechanism for the negative relationships between immune response and lipid metabolism. BMC Genomics 10:542.

165. Eberhart RJ. 1984. Coliform mastitis. Vet Clin North Am Large Anim Pract 6:287-300.

166. Weinberg ED. 1978. Iron and infection. Microbiol Rev 42:45-66.

167. Jenness R. 1974. The composition of milk, vol III. Academic Press, New York. Bullen JJ, Rogers HJ, Griffiths E. 1978. Role of iron in bacterial infection. Curr Top Microbiol Immunol 80:1-35.

168. Braun V, Hantke K, Koster W. 1998. Bacterial iron transport: mechanisms, genetics, and regulation. Met Ions Biol Syst 35:67-145.

169. Neilands JB. 1984. Siderophores of bacteria and fungi. Microbiol Sci 1:9-14.

170. Nikaido H, Rosenberg EY. 1983. Porin channels in Escherichia coli: studies with liposomes reconstituted from purified proteins. J Bacteriol 153:241-52.

171. Nikaido H, Rosenberg EY. 1981. Effect on solute size on diffusion rates through the transmembrane pores of the outer membrane of Escherichia coli. J Gen Physiol 77:121-35.

172. Guerinot ML. 1994. Microbial iron transport. Annu Rev Microbiol 48:743-72.

173. Klebba PE, Rutz JM, Liu J, Murphy CK. 1993. Mechanisms of TonB- catalyzed iron transport through the enteric bacterial cell envelope. J Bioenerg Biomembr 25:603-11.

174. Neilands JB. 1981. Microbial iron compounds. Annu Rev Biochem 50:715-31.

175. Podschun R, Fischer A, Ullmann U. 1992. Siderophore production of Klebsiella species isolated from different sources. Zentralbl Bakteriol 276:481-6.

176. Tarkkanen AM, Allen BL, Williams PH, Kauppi M, Haahtela K, Siitonen A, Orskov I, Orskov F, Clegg S, Korhonen TK. 1992. Fimbriation, capsulation, and iron-scavenging systems of Klebsiella strains associated with human urinary tract infection. Infect Immun 60:1187-92.

177. Linggoood MA, Robberts M, Ford S, Parry SH, H. WP. 1987. Incidence of the Aerobactin Iron Uptake System Among Escherichiu cdi Isolates From Infections of Farm Animals Journal of General Microbiology 133:835-842.

178. Rutz JM, Abdullah T, Singh SP, Kalve VI, Klebba PE. 1991. Evolution of the ferric enterobactin receptor in gram-negative bacteria. J Bacteriol 173:5964-74.

179. Hussein S, Hantke K, Braun V. 1981. Citrate-dependent iron transport system in Escherichia coli K-12. Eur J Biochem 117:431-7.

180. Faulkner A, Peaker M. 1982. Reviews of the progress of dairy science: secretion of citrate into milk. J Dairy Res 49:159-69.

181. Murphy CK, Kalve VI, Klebba PE. 1990. Surface topology of the Escherichia coli K-12 ferric enterobactin receptor. J Bacteriol 172:2736-46.

182. Neilands JB, Bindereif A, Montgomerie JZ. 1985. Genetic basis of iron assimilation in pathogenic Escherichia coli. Curr Top Microbiol Immunol 118:179-95.

183. Lin J, Hogan JS, Aslam M, Smith KL. 1998. Immunization of cows with ferric enterobactin receptor from coliform bacteria. J Dairy Sci 81:2151-8.

184. Lin J, Hogan JS, Smith KL. 1999. Growth responses of coliform bacteria to purified immunoglobulin G from cows immunized with ferric enterobactin receptor FepA. J Dairy Sci 82:86-92.

185. Pressler U, Staudenmaier H, Zimmermann L, Braun V. 1988. Genetics of the iron dicitrate transport system of Escherichia coli. J Bacteriol 170:2716-24.

186. Lin J, Hogan JS, Smith KL. 1999. Antigenic homology of the inducible ferric citrate receptor (FecA) of coliform bacteria isolated from herds with naturally occurring bovine intramammary infections. Clin Diagn Lab Immunol 6:966-9.

187. Lin J, Hogan JS, Smith KL. 1998. Inhibition of in vitro growth of coliform bacteria by a monoclonal antibody directed against ferric enterobactin receptor FepA. J Dairy Sci 81:1267-74.

188. Takemura K, Hogan JS, Smith KL. 2004. Growth responses of Escherichia coli to immunoglobulin G from cows immunized with ferric citrate receptor, FecA. J Dairy Sci 87:316-20.

189. Takemura K, Hogan JS, Lin J, Smith KL. 2002. Efficacy of immunization with ferric citrate receptor FecA from Escherichia coli on induced coliform mastitis. J Dairy Sci 85:774-81.

190. Petzl W, Zerbe H, Gunther J, Seyfert HM, Hussen J, Schuberth HJ. 2018. Pathogen-specific responses in the bovine udder. Models and immunoprophylactic concepts. Res Vet Sci 116:55-61.

191. Petzl W, Zerbe H, Gunther J, Yang W, Seyfert HM, Nurnberg G, Schuberth HJ. 2008. Escherichia coli, but not Staphylococcus aureus triggers an early increased expression of factors contributing to the innate immune defense in the udder of the cow. Vet Res 39:18.

192. Zhao Y, Zhou M, Gao Y, Liu H, Yang W, Yue J, Chen D. 2015. Shifted T Helper Cell Polarization in a Murine Staphylococcus aureus Mastitis Model. PLoS One 10:e0134797.

193. Porcherie A, Gilbert FB, Germon P, Cunha P, Trotereau A, Rossignol C, Winter N, Berthon P, Rainard P. 2016. IL-17A Is an Important Effector of the Immune Response of the Mammary Gland to Escherichia coli Infection. J Immunol 196:803-12.

194. Herry V, Gitton C, Tabouret G, Reperant M, Forge L, Tasca C, Gilbert FB, Guitton E, Barc C, Staub C, Smith DGE, Germon P, Foucras G, Rainard P.

195. 2017. Local immunization impacts the response of dairy cows to Escherichia coli mastitis. Sci Rep 7:3441.

196. DeGraves FJ, Fetrow J. 1991. Partial budget analysis of vaccinating dairy cattle against coliform mastitis with an Escherichia coli J5 vaccine. J Am Vet Med Assoc 199:451-5.

197. Allore HG, Erb HN. 1998. Partial budget of the discounted annual benefit of mastitis control strategies. J Dairy Sci 81:2280-92.

11 Chapter THE IMPACT OF CALF-SEX ON BOVINE MILK PRODUCTION

1. INTRODUCTION: AN OVERVIEW

Reproduction in female mammals requires significant energy expenditure, necessitating the mobilization of fat reserves throughout both gestation and lactation. [1]. In evolutionary biology, numerous hypotheses defend a sex-biased allocation of these resources by the pregnant and nursing females, to maximize the reproductive success of their male and female offspring. Some of these theories support their reasoning in the local resource competition [2, 3], local resource enhancement [4], "advantaged daughters" [5], the "safe bet"/reproductive value [6, 7] and the sex-differentiated sources of mortality [8].

The most well-known and tested theory remains the Trivers-Willard hypothesis that predicts that: 1) females in good body condition will allocate her offspring sex ratio towards males; 2) and that mothers in good body condition will also invest more per son than per daughter if males exhibit greater variation in reproductive value when males exhibit greater variation in reproductive value [9] According to this hypothesis, female mammals are able to adjust the sex of their offspring based on their own condition as a form to maximize reproductive success in the next generation. This theory also states that the mother will adapt her milk production to offspring gender, for example, by increasing milk production or changing its composition when she is nursing an offspring of the gender that has higher chances of producing future descendants. This strategy is particularly beneficial in species whose males compete for mating, like bovine, with dominant bulls leaving abundant off- spring and weaker ones having no offspring at all. On the other side, this hypothesis also describes that investment in female offspring will be more profitable when the mothers are in poor condition because the chance of producing competitive male offspring is low. Well-nourished mothers invest more in male offspring, as strong sons will more likely leave more offspring, whereas even weaker daughters will produce more progeny than weak sons [10].

In agreement with this theory it has been shown that, in humans, the milk produced for males is more energy dense in well-nourished mothers [11], while mothers with low socioeconomic status, when nursing daughters produce milk with a higher fat content than when nursing sons [12]. However, evidence for systematic sex-biased favoring males has been equivocal [13–17]. Post-natal, sex-biased nursing care has been investigated as a possible reason for sex-biased milk production in several mammalians, including humans. Several studies reported evidence of sexbiased milk synthesis in different species but drawing definitive conclusions from these studies has been difficult for several reasons [11, 12, 18–30].

This chapter aims to examine the data for and against the possibility of a sex bias in cow milk production, emphasizing the potential impacts of calf gender on subsequent lactations, particularly in dairy cows. Despite being non-consensual, its existence would provide new insights on the economic effects of utilizing sex-sorted semen to improve agricultural yield.

2. EVOLUTION OF DAIRY MILK PRODUCTION

In the last decades, industrial intensive milk production system uses the Holstein-Friesian breed, known as highest milk producing cow in the world. It is well documented that, with almost no exceptions, there has been a continuous increase in milk yield per cow. In all countries milk production and milk composition evolved over the years, due to a higher genetic merit and better management of the cows [31–32]. For example, from 2002 to 2013, in Denmark, all but two years showed a significant increase in the milk production compared to the previous year [33]. In São Miguel island, Azores, the same evolution was observed [34].

Also, in all countries, seasonal variations in milk production and composition were observed, both in intensive [35, 36] and pasture-based systems [37]. Previous studies have also proven that milk production varies with parity. It is generally observed a progressive increase in milk production in the first three to four parities and then a progressive decrease [38, 39].

3. BOVINE SEX-BIASED MILK PRODUCTION

The main source of income in a dairy farm is, by far, milk sale and any factor that can increase or decrease the production affect significantly the farmers income. Even though external factors like feeding, rearing and management are an important part of profitability, other factors, intrinsic to animals can have an important impact on profitability of a farm. The genetic merit [40] and sex of the calf are some of those factors. Beside the intrinsic difference in the commercial value of a female or a male offspring in a commercial farm, if the female milk production is indeed affected by the calf gender, then it could be a major factor for maximizing profits [41].

Calf-sex biased milk production is the capability of a cow to adapt milk production and composition to the sex of her offspring, a phenomenon well documented in diverse mammalian species [19]. The milk yield and the quality of milk produced are two important characteristics in dairy cow production and are also of great impact in beef production. Any favoring of one sex over the other in bovine offspring can lead to a great increase in the use of sex sorted semen, despite its lower conception rate [42]. In dairy cows, birth sex-ratio is biased, with more males being born, which suggests underlying mechanisms operating to favor more male offspring [43, 44].

Bull calves in dairy farms are mostly unwanted, due to their low value; in some countries, they are euthanized after birth, raising an ethical and social concern for the industry. On the other side, the used of sexed semen has higher costs and lower fertility. The fertility of sexed semen is estimated to be 8 to 17.9% lower in heifers compared to the conventional and not advisable to use in multiparous cows [42, 45, 46]. If a specific calf sex is associated with higher milk yield, this would have obvious consequences in the value and widespread use of sexed semen [46].

The growth rate of a suckling a male calf is higher than in females [47]. Therefore, it would be expected cows to have higher milk production or more energy dense milk when nursing a male. Despite differences in milk quantity or composition, cows do not show any sex biases in nursing behavior [29]. Since in most dairy farms, contrasting to most beef operations, calves are removed from the mother soon after calving, the pre and peri-natal mechanisms are the sole responsible for any observed milk-production sex-bias. Besides, cows are usually pregnant for most of the previous lactation [48], so the calf sex can potentially influence the previous lactation during its gestation or the lactation after their birth.

In Bovidae, data on the effect of calf sex in milk production are, to the least, inconsistent. Some studies reported an effect of calf sex on milk yield [1, 49–51], whereas other studies found no association [52]. One of the studies found that cows with a given genotype had higher milk yield in case of a male calf than a heifer calf [51]. In buffalos no effect between calf sex and milk production was reported [53].

In dairy cows in particular, studies addressing milk production sex-bias so far led to different results. While most studies described an advantage of female offspring, this effect was not observed for all the populations and a significant difference was not always observed [1, 33, 34, 40, 41, 54, 55]. Canadian and Iranian data for calf-sex bias in milk production found milk yield to be increased when a heifer was calved [41, 56]. However, a higher milk yield after calving a female offspring was only seen in the second lactation in New Zealand Holstein-Friesians [40], and only in the first lactation in French Holstein-Friesians [54] (Table 1).

However, Hinde et al. [1], with the largest study done so far on this topic, documented sex-biased milk production in US Holstein cattle. In his population, cows favor daughters, producing significantly more milk for daughters than for sons across lactation, suggesting that the effects of fetal sex can interact dynamically across parities. The sex of the fetus being gestated can enhance or diminish the production of milk during an established lactation. Moreover, the sex of the fetus gestated on the first parity has persistent consequences for milk synthesis on the subsequent parity. Contrastingly, Gillespie et al. [57] did not detect a significant effect of the sex of the calf being gestated on the mother milk production. Dallago et al. [55]. found only a calf-sex effect on the lactose and total solids, with an advantage to the females.

On a population of 1.49 million cows from the late 90's, primiparous cows giving birth to a female produced, on average, additional 142 kg (1.3% increase) of milk over a standardized 305-day lactation period compared with those calving a male [1]. The fetal sex on the first parity had also persistent effects on milk production during the second lactation. Calving a female on the first parity, increases milk production by 445 kg over the first two lactations, identifying a dramatic and sustained programming of mammary function by the offspring in utero. On the other side, cows calving a male son on their first parity produced less milk on their second lactation ($P < 0.001$), particularly if they also gestated a male calf on the second pregnancy (Table 2). According to the same study, the milk composition was similar whether the gestation produced a gestation of a son or daughter; the fat concentration was 3.61% after gestation of a daughter and 3.62% after gestation of a son; protein concentrations were the same (3.17%) [1].

Table 1. Studies done so far to evaluate the effect of calf sex in Holstein cows' milk production.

Country	Years analyzed	N (lactations)	Breed	Main results	Study (chronologically)
USA	1995-1999	2,390,000	Holstein	Cows favor daughters, producing significantly more milk for daughters across lactation. Effects of fetal sex interact dynamically across parities, whereby the sex of the fetus being gestated can enhance or diminish the production of milk during an established lactation. Sex of the fetus gestated on the first parity has persistent consequences for milk synthesis on the subsequent parity. Specifically, gestation of a daughter on the first parity increases milk production by, 445 kg over the first two lactations	[1]
France	2000-2008	8,901,000	Montbéliarde and Holstein	The effect of the calf sex hardly affected milk production. A small effect in favor of males was observed in parity 2 and 3 and was similar across breeds. The estimated effect of the sex of the calf in gestation on the simultaneous lactation was also very small.	[53]
Iran	1992-2008	402,716	Holstein	Cows with female calves had higher milk and fat yield, persistency of milk and fat yield and longer lactation length, while cows that gave birth to male calves had shorter calving interval and longer productive life. Also, cows with female calves had higher milk yield per day of lactation in the first two parities, but there was no difference in milk yield per day of lactation for parities ≥3.	[40]

Country	Years analyzed	N (lactations)	Breed	Main results	Study (chronologically)
Denmark	till 2013	71,088	Holstein	Cows produced higher volumes of milk if they had a bull calf, with a significantly higher milk production of 0.28% in the first lactation period for cows giving birth to a bull calf. Such difference was even higher when cows gave birth to another bull calf, so having two bull calves resulted in a difference of 0.52% in milk production compared to any other combination of sex of the offspring.	[32]
New Zealand	1995-2005	578,912	Holstein and Jersey	The lactation initiated by the birth of a female calf was associated with a 0.33–1.1% ($p < 0.05$) higher milk yield. Female calf gender present carryover effects associated with higher milk yield in second lactations for Holstein Friesians (0.24%; $p = 0.01$) and third lactations for Jerseys (1.1%; $p = 0.01$).	[39]
UK	2013-2014	211,932	Holstein	Giving birth to a heifer calf conferred a 1% milk yield advantage in first lactation heifers, whilst giving birth to a bull calf conferred a 0.5% advantage in second lactation.	[46]
Azores, Portugal	2009-2017	45,712	Holstein	Whether calving a male or a female, cows roughly produced the same amount of milk and protein content. However, the content of fat was slightly higher when they calved females ($P < 0.001$).	[33]

Gillespie et al. [57] also showed that, in the UK, calving a heifer was associated with a 1% milk yield advantage in first lactation heifers, but calving a bull calf conferred a 0.5% advantage in second lactation. Heifer calves were also associated with a 0.66 kg reduction in saturated fatty acid content of milk in first lactation, even though there was no significant difference between genders in the second lactation. Interestingly, the effects of calf gender observed on both the yield and saturated fatty acid content were considered minor compared to the nutritional and genetic influences. Aspects that affect milk production, such as mastitis [58] or lameness [59], seem to have a deeper impact on milk production than calf gender.

An Iranian study, using 402,716 Holstein milk records from 1991 to 2008, report that cows calving a female offspring present a higher milk and fat yield and longer persistency of milk and fat yield, as well as a longer lactation length [41]. Cows calving a male offspring presented shorter calving interval and an overall longer reproductive life. The observed higher daily milk yield after calving a female in the first two parities was not maintained for the next parities [60]. However, a higher occurrence of dystocia in male calving was not taken into consideration and was most likely a factor for the higher milk production observed after calving a female calf [41]. In contrast, both a French [54] and a Danish [33] studies found a small increase in milk yield in both Holstein and Montbéliarde dams calving a male offspring. On the French study, the sex-bias favoring males effect reached 40 kg milk (0.5% of the mean), 0.6 kg fat, 0.6 kg protein. A small difference was also noticed for fat and protein contents (from 0.01 to 0.02%) in parity 2 and 3. Similarly, the estimated effect of the sex of the calf in gestation on the simultaneous lactation is very small [54].

Græsbøll et al. [33] also reported significantly higher milk productions (0.28%) in first lactating cows producing a bull calf. This difference was even higher when cows calved another bull calf, with a difference of 0.52% in milk production compared to any other possible combinations of offspring sex. The same study pointed that dams would favor a bull fetus by decreasing milk production during the second pregnancy if the calf born in the first parity was a heifer, which diluted the positive effect on milk production of calving a male in the first pregnancy. Being pregnant with a bull fetus may reduce milk production to possibly increase the energy spent on the bull fetus. Also, cows seem to favor living bull offspring over unborn bull offspring, but unborn bull offspring over living heifer offspring [33].

The magnitude of sex bias milk production, when observed in other species, seems to be stronger among first parity females [11, 26, 27, 30, 59]. The fetal sex effect may be disguised in multiparous females because of the cumulative effects of sequential gestations with fetuses of different sexes on the mammary gland architecture [1]. It is also possible that maternal investment tactics may change according to the residual reproductive value of the offspring [1, 61] or transmit a targeted effort during a critical window of mammary gland preparation for a new lactation [1, 62]. Interaction effects were observed between calf gender across the first three parities, with the lowest second parity milk yield observed when a cow gave birth to male calves in all three parities. First parity calf sex did not have a significant effect on the third lactation milk yield. Disparities between the effects for calf sex sequences that differed only by the calf gender in the first parity were not significantly different from each other [40].

Table 2. Effect of the calf gender combination at the first and second lactation (305d) according to Hinde et al. [1].

Differences Kg (%)	Calf gender combination at the first and second lactation		
	Female-female vs. male-male	Female-male vs. male-male	Male-female vs. male-male
at first lactation	24 (0.3)	7 (0.1)	13 (0.2)
at second lactation	52 (0.6)	5 (0.1)	53 (0.6)
Cumulative effect	76 (0.9)	12 (0.2)	66 (0.8)

In cows' populations were a daughter-biased milk production was observed, this may involve life-history tradeoffs for both cows and their daughters. High milk production in dairy cows has been associated with reduced fertility, health, and survival depending on environmental conditions [63]. It was also observed that cows gestated during lactation have moderately reduced survival and milk production in their own adulthood [48, 64].

Some of the differences found across different studies could be partly explained by differences in the datasets used; Hess et al. [40] used total lactational yield, calculated using the test interval method; Hinde et al. [1] and Barbat et al. [54] used the test day model rather than predicting 305 day milk yields; Graesboll et al. [33] adopted a farm-based approach using Wilmink curves to calculate 305 day milk yields and Gillespie et al. [47] used the Milkbot lactation model, that can be affected by environment and genetics [65]. Also, the use of sexed semen was not known in most of the studies and it can have a significant impact in the results obtained. Sexed semen is mainly used to breed heifers with higher genetic merit [54, 66] and this creates an obvious bias towards female calves. This can be aggravated by the fact that heifers inseminated with sexed semen tend to have lower fertility and become pregnant later, consequently calving in an older age, which is associated with a higher milk production [67].

The effect of the calf gander can further interact with other factors, like parity or seasonality, making it difficult to evaluate it in a precise way. It was observed that after the third calving, the mother milk production was independent of the calf gender. This observation might be related to larger pelvic dimensions of older cows and by consequence a lower incidence of dystocia [41].

A significant difference between the dairy industry in Azores [34] or New Zealand [40] compared with other populations is that both are primarily pasturebased. The production and calving in Azores are not, however, as seasonal as the one observed in New Zealand [34, 40]. In the non-seasonal pasture-based system no calf-sex bias in milk yield was observed, even though a slight increase in fat percentage was associated with the birth of a male calf [34].

In Denmark, the difference observed in milk production due to the sex of the offspring was generally smaller than the difference between farms. Other management related aspects are more important for the milk yield registered and the differences identified might be due to size of the offspring rather than the sex, but size and sex might also have separated effects [33]. So far, no relation was observed among mean somatic cells count and the sex of the calf born [41, 68, 69], even though this parameter is often associated with the cow body condition [70].

Modeling complex biological features, such as milk production, is challenging due to the number of inherent and environmental aspects that can influence them. Also, the statistical model used for analysis may influence to a certain point the results and data interpretation. One explanation for the differences of the several studies on calf-sex biased milk production can be related to the models used. For example, in one of the studies, Holstein Friesian cows calving males in the first three parities had significantly lower first lactation milk yield than cows calving two males followed by a female in the first three parities, but this observation is biased if models do not include lactation length. Also, there are no reasonable biological reasons why to test the effect of the gender of the third calf on the first lactation yield. In fact, the observed effect of calf gender on milk yield is due to an association between calf gender and milk yield rather than calf gender triggering a difference in milk yield. The alleged effect of the third parity calf gender on the first lactation milk yield was not apparent when lactation length was included in the models [40].

In beef cows, studies with limited samples led to different sex-biased milk production, pointing to either favors a son [71], or a daughter [72], or not show any sex-biases [73]. A study in the red Chittagong cattle found no effect of the calf-sex in milk production [74].

4. PREGNANCY AND LACTATION LENGTH

In New Zealand, with a seasonal calving system, the calf gender was reported to influence milk yield possibly through the increased gestation length of male calves [40]. In that study, the milk production tests were performed on the same date for all cows, so those calving a male would have their tests performed, on average, 2 days earlier. However, when the lactation length (reported longer in male calves) was included in the model, no effects existed of the calf gender over the increased production of milk [40]. At least part of the reported difference in milk production due to calf gender, was really due to methodological issues. The interval-centering method used provide a 10.8 ± 4.0 L higher milk yield if herd tests are 2 days later in lactation. However, the observed calf sex variance is too large to be explained only by this difference in herd test dates. When lactation length shortens depending on calving date, as well as the herd tests occurring 2 days earlier, the difference in milk yield is 26.9 ± 6.2 L. This difference is similar to the observed effect of calf gender on milk yield, further supporting that this effect is, at least partially, due to the different lactation length when male calves are born 2 days later [40].

It is difficult to establish any association between the calf gender and a presumed sex-biased milk production or a sex-biased pregnancy length, because of various existing confounder factors that may permeate such interaction. Mean pregnancy in length male calves is longer than in females, the difference also being affect by breed and parity [40, 75]. Also, primiparous cows tend to present shorter pregnancies than multiparous cows, the calves born lighter [76], albeit the risk for dystocia is also higher for first calving cows.

Recently, Atashi and Asaadi [77], using 252,798 lactations on 108,077 Holstein dairy cows in Iran showed that multiparous cows with longer gestations performed better in lactation than primiparous cows. This study also showed that multiparous cows with short gestation length had a lower yield at the beginning of lactation and higher raising and declining slopes of the lactation curve compared with cows presenting longer or average length of pregnancy.

The production system may also interfere with milk production performance of dairy cows. In seasonal breeding systems, late calving cows usually have a shorter lactation since the entire herd ceases lactation on the same day [40]. The lactation length is usually longer in non-seasonal systems because the lactation can continue until the milk yield of an individual cow drops below a point when it is more economical to dry the cow. In these conditions a weaker negative correlation between gestation and lactation length is observed compared with seasonal systems where all the cows are dried of on a single day [40]. However, even in non-seasonal systems lactation length was observed to be approximately four days shorter following the birth of a male calf compared to a female calf across the first four lactations [41]. Chegini et al. [41] found that cows calving female offspring had more persistent lactations than those that calving male offspring, suggesting that the lactation curves are different.

Still, there is some controversy regarding the best methodology to apply when modeling the milk production (whether in milk yield or composition) to adequately account the effects of the gender of the calf. This is not an easy task, because it establishes a complex interaction with other parameters (e.g., pregnancy length, dystocia, and some cow related factors) that may act as confounding factors. Lactation length is one important factor affecting milk yield per lactation, leading to the need to introduce correction factors for lactation length in the models for milk production in cows. Lactation length in itself has a negative relationship with the annualized production of milk and milk solids [78]. Also, the milk yield and milk production curves change according to the lactation number, the persistency of the peak and lactational length, the cow genetics and the number or milking frequency, among other factors. Such aspects should also be considered in the lactation modeling studies. Models construct evaluate the lactation curves should be used that take all possible confounders into account simultaneously. Therefore, further investigation is necessary to confirm whether the shape of lactation curves differ based on calf gender and identify potential biological explanations for any such difference.

5. CALVING DIFFICULTY

Calving difficulty is higher with larger calves [79]. It is also known that there is a higher frequency of dystocia in male calves' birth [60, 74, 79]. Dystocia significantly reduces the whole lactation milk yield [40, 50, 54, 69, 75–77], besides increasing veterinary treatment costs [76], and reducing cow fertility. After dystocia there is a higher incidence of metritis [77], ketosis [80, 81], both associated with a decrease in milk production. Also, an easy calving presumably leads to a higher milk production because it is associated with reduced stress and pain during calving, consequently leading to a lower energy imbalance that can cause more metabolic disorders [41].

Male calves are typically larger than females, and pose a greater risk of dystocia [1, 79, 82]. However, Hinde et al. [1] reported that sex-biased milk synthesis remained when analysis was restricted to a subset of females without record of dystocia, and included information on individual cows across the first and second parity, favoring females.

A Danish study found different results. Farmer assisted calving were associated with a higher milk yield while cows with no farmer assistance or with veterinary assistance during the most recent calving produced less milk. This means that mildly to moderate calving difficulties improved milk yield, while no assistance or the need for veterinary assistance decreased subsequent milk production. In the same study the interaction between sex of offspring and difficulty of calving was found to be insignificant [33]. Still, it must be also considered that dystocia might go unnoticed, nevertheless affecting milk production, which could lead to misreading of the sex-bias towards higher production after female calving because of unidentified or unrecorded dystocia [40]. The effect of the different degrees of dystocia in milk production or for how long they persist remain unclear [83–85].

In UK Holstein-Friesian cows, moderate calving difficulties resulted in higher milk production. It is possible that some births not needing help and human supervision may experience real difficulties that go unnoticed and are wrongly registered as an easy calving, when they might have had some difficulties without the farmer's notice. Furthermore, it is likely that cows with highly valuated genetic material may be offered calving assistance from the farmer more often [67].

A reduction in milk production was observed between days in milk 10 and 90 after veterinary-assisted calving compared with non-assisted calving, leading to the conclusion that non-assisted cows presented a flatter lactation curve after peak yield [69]. One of the reasons is a reduced dry matter intake in the months postpartum [86].

In Jerseys the effects of calf gender in mothers milk production were not as pronounced as in Holstein-Friesians [40], which can point to a genetic selection of calf-sex biased milk production.

6. BIOLOGICAL PATHWAYS OF SEX-BIASED MILK PRODUCTION

Dairy calves are usually separated from their mothers right after or within hours of birth and artificially reared; therefore, the differences observed on milk production of the mother should relate to factors affecting the lactogenesis in pre- or peri-natal period [40]. The pathways through which fetal sex may influence milk production are not yet fully understood. Sex-biased milk production may reflect differential cellular capacity in the mammary gland, programmed via hormonal signals from the fetal-placental unit, or post-natal through sex-biased nursing behavior [87]. Several hypothetical mechanisms have been explored in an attempt to explain the mechanisms that may explain a sex-biased milk production in bovine, albeit with discrepant results.

One possible mechanism may relate to the translocation of fetal hormones to the cow mammary gland via the maternal circulation [1]. The concentrations of sexual hormones differ between male and female fetuses and can potentially enhance or inhibit mammary milk synthesis if they get access to the maternal circulation. In the bovine species, fetal steroid hormones are present from the first trimester [1, 88, 89]. The hormones produced by the bovine fetus can cross the placenta to the cow circulation and calf sex influences hormonal levels in the mother [76, 90–94]. Thereby, variations in the blood levels of the hormones involved in lactogenesis may influence milk, dependent on the sex of the calf born [40]. In humans, higher concentrations of circulating androgens during the second trimester were associated with a lower probability of sustaining breastfeeding to three months post-partum, but the effect of fetal sex on the milk production was not directly analyzed [1, 95].

Also, it is possible that the sex of the first parity calf affects milk production for the duration of the productive life of a cow due to the differences in the level of the hormones that influence mammary development, as it has been reported in mice [96], since dairy cows are first bred before they are fully mature, usually with only 60% of their adult weight.

Xiang and colleagues [97] showed gender variations in the placenta weight in both Bos taurus and Bos indicus pregnancies; the placenta of the male fetus present heavier total placenta weight, better placenta efficiency heavier fetus weight than female fetus. These differences might explain and favor the fact that male calves are usually heavier than the female's.

Differences in the amount of placental lactogen produced between female and male fetus could differently prime the mammary gland of the cow [1]. It is accepted that prolactin and placental lactogens have roles in mammogenesis and lactogenesis but the mechanisms of action of those hormones act are still in discussion, and the role of the calf gender is still unclear [98, 99]. Albeit the information available for bovine is scarce, in humans, differences were found in the levels of placental lactogen in the umbilical cord blood in female and male pregnancies [100]. It was also been shown that glucose-to-insulin ratios were lower in women bearing a female vs. those bearing a male fetus [101]. Both insulin and glucose are important modulators of milk production. The fetal Insulin-like peptide 3 (INSL3) are raised in maternal circulation during pregnancy in male-pregnant dairy cows and diminished in female-pregnant cows [102]. It was also demonstrated that the level of this hormone directly affects milk production [103, 104]. In cows, Insulin and IGF-I concentrations, important metabolic mediators of the energetic metabolism and body condition, are negatively associated with milk yield during the production phase of the lactation [105].

Hienddleder et al. [106] showed that total thyroxine concentrations were higher in male pregnancies, while triiodothyronine concentrations were unaffected by fetal gender. Contrastingly, free thyroxine concentrations were higher in female pregnancies of Bos indicus genetics, while in the Bos taurus, the values for that hormone tend to be higher in male pregnancies. No gender-associated differences were found regarding the Insulin-like growth factors in this study. The changes in the thyroid hormones' concentrations may contribute to a different pattern in gene expression at the mammary gland, due to their galactopoietic role that sets the mammary gland´ s metabolic priority during lactation [107].

Exploring another route, Chew et al. [108] showed that larger calves are associated with higher milk production, maybe related to higher concentrations of estrogen and placental lactogens during gestation. Indirectly, this could be one of the reasons why, in some cases, male calves are associated with higher milk production, since male calves are usually heavier at birth [109]. However, a negative correlation between birthweight and milk production during gestation was also found, leading to the hypothesis that the competition for nutrient between the fetus in gestation and the milk production for the current one would drive a diminished milk production. Yet, it cannot be ruled out that a high milk production is in itself responsible for a smaller birthweight of the calf in gestation [110].

Women giving birth to daughters show upregulation of epithelial/lactocyte genes, which may be associated with increased milk yield [111]. Also, in dairy cattle a sex-biased in nitrogen and energy metabolism during the transition period was observed [112]. Higher odds exist for a male birth in cows that lose less body condition after calving [113, 114]. The depth of the Negative Energetic Balance (NEB) experienced by these cows may affect the sex-biased production of milk to favor one sex or the other. The usually higher NEB that cows go through in more intensive systems may account for the results obtained under highly intensive conditions compared to the ones obtained under less stressful management. Roche et al. [113] showed that a higher loss of body condition score by the cow was associated with a higher rate of born females. Higher milk producer cows usually lose more body condition score and have a higher rate of female calves' gestation [114]. This might be the reason why it seems that the birth of a female is positive to milk production; however, the relationship between these factors might be the inverse, with higher producers having a higher rate of female calves [34].

Cow's milk production increases with the weight of the calf born [115], and male calves mean weight at birth is higher [82]. This difference in calf-sex birth weight can lead to the idea that the milk production is related to sex, when in fact it only reflects the birth weight [40]. Chew et al. [108] found no calf-sex bias in milk production when birth weight was included in the model.

The sex of the calf whose birth initiates lactation can influence the milk production in the subsequent lactation because of the hormonal influences on the mammary gland development or due to the calf sex effects on pregnancy length. Also, fetal sex can influence lactation production during pregnancy because cows become pregnant at peak lactation [109].

In the Cervus elaphus species, the red reindeer, dominant females give birth to a higher proportion of males than their subordinates. It is known that these dominant hinds produce higher levels of progesterone in the early days of pregnancy, and male blastocysts secrete interferon-tau earlier than females, so the hypothesis is that maternal recognition of pregnancy in dominant hinds is therefore more likely to be successful if the blastocyst is male [116]. Factors such as this at the time of maternal recognition of pregnancy in cattle could also affect calf sex, but this has not been studied yet.

Holstein heifers in the USA, even after administration of bST (bovine somatotropin) still produced significantly higher milk yield if they calve a female offspring, but sex-biased milk synthesis was not observed in parities two through five [1]. Even though hormones can cause sex-biased milk production, other factors such as birth, weight, lactation length and dystocia probably have a higher impact [40].

7. THE USE OF SEXED SEMEN

Sexed semen produces 90% of offspring of the desired sex, but the fertility is reduced in between 75 to 80% compared with conventional frozen semen [117], because the sorting process produces a higher level of damaged to the spermatozoa [118]. Usually, sexed semen is applied more frequently in heifers, to profit from their higher fertility. Also, the heifers selected to be inseminated with sexed semen are usually the ones with higher genetic merit, so they are the ones producing the replacement animals [66].

The use of sorted semen in dairy industry screws the gender ratios into the female sex, seeking the production of future genetically superior replacement animals. Under the sex-biased milk production framework, and according to some studies [1, 41, 57], it would be expected to observe an increase in milk yield in cows that calved a female in their first and eventually in the second parity. This effect would overcome any negative effects exerted by the calving of a larger male fetus (increasing the stress over nutrients partitioning between the fetus and the mother during pregnancy, and increasing the risk for dystocia) and variations in pregnancy length. On the other hand, the sorted semen being applied more often in heifers or primiparous cows, the former tending to present shorter pregnancy lengths [76], may also influence the results if the type of semen used does not enter in the model used. Attention should be paid when analyzing data from most studies, because usually the type of semen used in artificial insemination is not considered as a variable in the statistical model, which could affect the results.

After investigating the effect of sex-bias in milk production, using simulated data and considering different intensities of sexed semen in three different scenarios, two studies concluded that including sex-bias could increase profitability between €4.0 and €9.9 per cow per year [58, 119] (Table 3). On the other hand, it was also concluded that any increase in milk yield from cows calving a female calf was insufficient to warrant the use of sexed semen. The real influence of sex-biased milk production using sexed semen must be further studied before recommendations can be made into its economic impact [40]. Also, two different studies concluded that, even though there might be an effect of calf gender on a cows' milk production, the impact was not large enough to influence profit [54] or encourage the use of sexed semen [56].

Table 3. Effects of the use of sex sorted semen on milk yield per cow/year considering two different simulation scenarios [109].

Differences in milk yield per cow/year	Without sex bias	With sex bias	Simulation scenario
Milk yield (kg of ECM)	36	48	Sorted semen used in 30% of heifers and 30% of cows
Net return (€)	3.0	7.0	
Milk yield (kg of ECM)	66	99	Sorted semen used in 100% of heifers and 50% of cows
Net return (€)	3.1	13.0	

8. CONCISE SUMMARY

Sex-biased milk production in dairy cows may exist, with the bias potentially favoring one sex over the other, or occasionally neither. It appears to preferentially benefit females in intensive production systems, but this was not evident in less intense systems.

The contradictory findings from several research regarding the cow's influence on offspring sex indicate that systems where cows are typically in optimal and competitive condition yield more milk production for bull calves. They also appear to suggest that cows in poorer condition, or of a genetically divergent strain, seemingly allocate more milk to heifer calves. To date, contradictory data have been submitted to the scientific community; nevertheless, discrepancies among the employed models hinder the establishment of a definitive correlation between offspring gender and cow productivity. The observed variations in results are likely attributable to differences in methodological approaches, the diverse influencing parameters employed to compute lactation milk output, and potential confounding factors that may not be fully recognized. Additionally, other factors, including distinct housing and feeding practices, may influence the bias in calf-sex milk production through mechanisms yet to be elucidated.

Further investigation is required to examine this notion, incorporating additional cow populations and linking the investment approach with an animal wellbeing index. Should the calf sex effect on milk production exist within a population, the selection of bull mothers and progeny-tested bulls may be skewed by the sex of the offspring, hence enhancing genetic advancement towards more lucrative cows, provided that this calf-gender bias is considered in breeding value estimate.

REFERENCES

1. Hinde K, Carpenter AJ, Clay JS, Bradford BJ. Holsteins favor Heifers, not Bulls: biased milk production programmed during pregnancy as a function of fetal sex. PloS one. 2014;9(2):e86169. DOI: 10.1371/journal. pone.0086169

2. Clark AB. Sex ratio and local resource competition in a prosimian primate. Science. 1978;201(4351): 163-165. DOI: 10.1126/science.201.4351.163

3. Silk JB. Local resource competition and facultative adjustment of sex ratios in relation to competitive abilities. American Naturalist. 1983;121(1): 56-66. DOI: 10.1086/284039

4. Emlen ST, Emlen JM, Levin SA. Sex- ratio selection in species with helpers- at-the-nest. American Naturalist. 1986;127(1): 1-8

5. Simpson MJ, Simpson AE. Birth sex ratios and social rank in rhesus monkey mothers. Nature. 1982;300(5891):440- 441. DOI: 10.1038/300440a0

6. Shibata F, Kawamichi T. Female- biased sex allocation of offspring by an Apodemus mouse in an unstable environment. Behavioral Ecology and Sociobiology. 2009;63(9):1307-1317. DOI: 10.1007/s00265-009-0772-z

7. Leimar O. Life-history analysis of the Trivers and Willard sex-ratio problem. Behavioral Ecology. 1996;7(3):316-325. DOI: 10.1093/beheco/7.3.316

8. Smith JM. A new theory of sexual investment. Behavioral Ecology and Sociobiology.1980;7(3):247-251. DOI: 10.1007/BF00299371

9. Veller C, Haig D, Nowak, MA. The Trivers-Willard hypothesis: sex ratio or investment? Proceedings. Biological sciences. 1996, 283(1830), 20160126. https://doi.org/10.1098/rspb.2016.0126.

10. Trivers RL, Willard DE. Natural selection of parental ability to vary the sex ratio of offspring. Science. 1973;179(4068):90-92. DOI: 10.1126/ science.179.4068.90

11. Powe CE, Knott CD, Conklin-Brittain N. Infant sex predicts breast milk energy content. American Journal of Human Biology. 2010;22(1): 50-54. DOI: 10.1002/ajhb.20941

12. Fujita M, Roth E, Lo YJ, Hurst C, Vollner J, Kendell A. In poor families, mothers' milk is richer for daughters than sons: A test of Trivers–Willard hypothesis in agropastoral settlements in Northern Kenya. American Journal of Physical Anthropology. 2012;149(1):52- 59. DOI: 10.1002/ajpa.22092

13. Pélabon C, Gaillard JM, Loison A, Portier C: Is sex-biased maternal care limited by total maternal expenditure in polygynous ungulates? Behavioral Ecology and Sociobiology. 1995;37(5):311-319. DOI: 10.1007/ BF00174135

14. Hewison AJ, Gaillard JM. Successful sons or advantaged daughters? The Trivers-Willard model and sex-biased maternal investment in ungulates. Trends in Ecology & Evolution. 1999;14(6):229-234. DOI: 10.1016/ s0169-5347(99)01592-x
15. Cockburn A, Legge S, Double MC. Sex ratio in birds and mammals: can the hypothesis be disentangled. In: Hardy ICW, editor. Sex Ratios: Concepts and Research Methods. Cambridge: Cambridge University Press, Cambridge; 2002. p. 266-286.
16. Cameron EZ. Facultative adjustment of mammalian sex ratios in support for the Trivers-Willard hypothesis: evidence for a mechanism. Proceedings of the Royal Society B: Biological Sciences 2004;271:1723-1728. DOI: 10.1098/ rspb.2004.2773
17. Sheldon BC, West SA. Maternal dominance, maternal condition, and offspring sex ratio in ungulate mammals. American Naturalist. 2004;163(1): 40-54. DOI: 10.1086/381003
18. Clutton-Brock TH, Albon SD, Guinness FE. Parental investment in male and female offspring in polygynous mammals. Nature. 1981;289(5797):487-489. DOI: 10.1038/289487a0
19. Byers JA, Moodie JD. Sex-specific maternal investment in pronghorn, and the question of a limit on differential provisioning in ungulates. Behavioral Ecology and Sociobiology. 1990;26(3):157-164. DOI: 10.1007/ BF00172082
20. Hogg JT, Hass CC, Jenni DA. Sex-biased maternal expenditure in Rocky Mountain bighorn sheep. Behavioral Ecology and Sociobiology 1992;31(4):243-251. DOI: 10.1007/ BF00171679
21. Cameron EZ. Is suckling behaviour a useful predictor of milk intake? A review. Animal Behaviour. 1998;56(3):521-532. DOI: 10.1006/ anbe.1998.0793
22. Cameron EZ, Stafford KJ, Linklater WL, Veltman CJ. Suckling behavior does not measure milk intake in horses, Equus caballus. Animal Behaviour. 1999; 57(3):673-678. DOI: 10.1006/anbe.1998.0997
23. Brown GR. Sex-biased investment in nonhuman primates: can Trivers & Willard's theory be tested? Animal Behaviour 2001;61(4):683-694. DOI: 10.1006/ anbe.2000.1659
24. Bercovitch FB. Sex-biased parental investment in primates. International Journal of Primatology. 2002;23(4): 905-921. DOI: 10.1023/A:1015585117114
25. Landete-Castillejos T, García A, López-Serrano FR, Gallego L. Maternal quality and differences in milk production and composition for male and female Iberian red deer calves (Cervus elaphus hispanicus). Behavioral Ecology and Sociobiology. 2005: 57(3):267-274. DOI: 10.1007/ s00265-004-0848-8

26. Hinde K. First-time macaque mothers bias milk composition in favor of sons. Current Biology. 2007;17(22): R958–R959. DOI: 10.1016/j. cub.2007.09.029

27. Robert KA, Braun S. Milk composition during lactation suggests a mechanism for male biased allocation of maternal resources in the tammar wallaby (Macropus eugenii). PloS One. 2012;7(11): e51099. DOI: 10.1371/ journal. pone.0051099

28. Quinn EA. No evidence for sex biases in milk macronutrients, energy, or breastfeeding frequency in a sample of filipino mothers. American Journal of Physical Anthropology. 2013;152(2):209-216. DOI: 10.1002/ ajpa.22346

29. Stěhulová, Špinka M, Šárová R, Máchová L, Kněz R, Firla P. Maternal behaviour in beef cows is individually consistent and sensitive to cow body condition, calf sex and weight. Applied Animal Behaviour Science Sci 2013;144(3-4):89-97. DOI: 10.1016/j. applanim.2013.01.003

30. Thakkar SK, Giuffrida F, Cristina CH, De Castro CA, Mukherjee R, Tran LA, Steenhout P, Lee le Y, Destaillats F. Dynamics of human milk nutrient composition of women from Singapore with a special focus on lipids. American Journal of Human Biology. 2013;25(6):770-779. DOI: 10.1002/ajhb.22446

31. Roche JR, Berry DP, Bryant AM, Burke CR, Butler ST, Dillon PG, Donaghy DJ, Horan B, Macdonald KA, Macmillan KL. A 100-Year review: a century of change in temperate grazing dairy systems. Journal of Dairy Science. 2017;100:10189-10233. DOI: 10.3168/ jds.2017-13182

32. Salfer IJ, Dechow CD, Harvatine KJ. Annual rhythms of milk and milk fat and protein production in dairy cattle in the United States. Journal of Dairy Science. 2019;102:742-753. DOI: 10.3168/jds.2018-15040.

33. Græsbøll K, Kirkeby C, Nielsen SS, Christiansen LE. Danish Holsteins Favor Bull Offspring: Biased Milk Production as a Function of Fetal Sex, and Calving Difficulty. PLoS ONE. 2015;10(4):e0124051. DOI: 10.1371/ journal.pone.0124051

34. Quaresma M, Rodrigues M, Medeiros-Sousa P, Martins A. Calf-sex bias in Holstein dairy milk production under extensive management. Livestock Science. 2020;235:104016. DOI: 10.1016/j.livsci.2020.104016

35. Bouraoui R, Lahmarb M, Majdoubc A, Djemalic M, Belyead R. The relationship of temperature-humidity index with milk production of dairy cows in a Mediterranean climate. Animal Research. 2002;51(6):479-491. DOI: 10.1051/ animres:2002036

36. Bertocchi L, Vitali A, Lacetera N, Nardone A, Varisco G, Bernabucci U. Seasonal variations in the composition of Holstein cow's milk and temperature- humidity index relationship. Animal. 2014;8:667-674. DOI: 10.1017/ S1751731114000032

37. Nantapo CWY, Muchenje V. Winter and spring variation in daily milk yield and mineral composition of Jersey, Friesian cows and their crosses under a pasture-based dairy system. South African Journal Of Animal Science. 2013;43(5). DOI: 10.4314/sajas. v43i5.3

38. Ray DE, Halbach TJ, Armstrong DV. Season and lactation number effects on milk production and reproduction of dairy cattle in Arizona. Journal of Dairy Science. 1992;75:2976-2983. DOI: 10.3168/jds.S0022-0302(92)78061-8

39. Yang L, Yang Q, Yi M, Pang ZH, Xiong BH. Effects of seasonal change and parity on raw milk composition and related indices in Chinese Holstein cows in northern China. Journal of Dairy Science. 2013;96(11):6863-6869. DOI: 10.3168/jds.2013-6846

40. Hess MK, Hess AS, Garrick DJ. The Effect of Calf Gender on Milk Production in Seasonal Calving Cows and Its Impact on Genetic Evaluations. Plos One. 2016;11(3). DOI: 10.1371/ journal.pone.0169503

41. Chegini A, Hossein-Zadeh NG, Hosseini-Moghadam H. Effect of calf sex on some productive, reproductive and health traits in Holstein cows. Spanish Journal of Agricultural Research. 2015;13(2). DOI: 10.5424/ sjar/2015132-6320

42. Norman HD, Hutchison JL, Miller RH. Use of sexed semen and its effect on conception rate, calf sex, dystocia, and stillbirth of Holsteins in the United States. Journal of Dairy Science. 2010;93(8):3880-3890. DOI: 10.3168/jds.2009-2781

43. Foote RH. Sex ratios in dairy cattle under various conditions. Theriogenology. 1977;8(6):349-356. DOI: 10.1016/0093-691X(77)90186-8

44. Silva del Rio N, Stewart S, Rapnicki P, Chang YM, Fricke PM. Mont: An observational analysis of twin births, calf sex ratio, and calf mortality in Holstein dairy cattle. Journal of Dairy Science. 2007;90(3): 1255-1264. DOI: 10.3168/jds.s0022-0302(07)71614-4

45. DeJarnette JM, Nebel RL, Marshall CE. Evaluating the success of sex-sorted semen in US dairy herds from on farm records. Theriogenology. 2009;71(1):49-58. DOI: 10.1016/j. theriogenology.2008.09.042

46. Healy AA, House JK, Thomson PC. Artificial insemination field data on the use of sexed and conventional semen in nulliparous Holstein heifers. Journal of Dairy Science. 2013;96(3):1905±1914. DOI: 10.3168/jds.2012-5465

47. Fortin A, Simpfendorfer S, Reid J, Ayala H, Anrique R, Kertz A. Effect of level of energy intake and influence of breed and sex on the chemical composition of cattle. Journal of Animal Science. 1980;51(3):604-614. DOI: 10.2527/jas1980.513604x

48. González-Recio O, Ugarte E, Bach A. Trans-generational effect of maternal lactation during pregnancy: a Holstein cow model. PloS One. 2012;7(12):e51816. DOI: 10.1371/journal. pone.0051816

49. Quesnel FN, Wilcox CJ, Simerl NA, Sharma AK, Thatcher WW. Effects of fetal sex and sire and other factors on periparturient and postpartum performance of dairy cattle. Brazilian Journal of Genetic. 1995;18(4):541-545.

50. Gaafar HMA, Shamiah ShM, Abu El-Hamd MA, Shitta AA, Tag El-Din MA. Dystocia in Friesian cows and its effects on postpartum reproductive performance and milk production. Tropical Animal Health and Production. 2011;43(1):229-234. DOI: 10.1007/s11250-010-9682-3

51. Yudin NS, Aitnazarov RB, VoevodaMI,GerlinskayaLA,MoshkinMP. Association of polymorphism harbored by tumor necrosis factor alpha gene and sex of calf with lactation performance in cattle. Asian-Australasian Journal of Animal Science. 2013;26:1379-1387. DOI: 10.5713/ajas.2013.13114

52. Atashi H, Zamiri MJ, Sayyadnejad MB. Effect of twinning and stillbirth on the shape of lactation curve in Holstein dairy cows of Iran. Archives fur Tierzucht. 2012;55(3):226- 233. DOI: 10.5194/aab-55-226-2012

53. Afzal M, Anwar M, Mirza MA. Some factors affecting milk yield and lactation length in Nili Ravi buffaloes. Pakistan Veterinary Journal. 2007;27(3):113-117.

54. Barbat A, Lefebvre R, Boichard D. Replication study in French Holstein and Montbeliarde cattle data. Post comment regarding the paper from Hinde et al., 2014. [Internet] Available from: http://www.plosone.org/annotation/listThread.action?root=78955. [Accessed: 2020-05-02]

55. Dallago GM, Barroso L, Alves G, Vieira J, Guimarães L, Santos C, Maciel L, Santos R, Figueiredo D, Santos D. The Influence of Calf 's Sex on Total Milk Yield and Its Constituents of Dairy Cows. Proceedings of the 14th Internacional Conference on Precision Agriculture. 2018; Quebéc, Canada.

56. Beavers L, Van Doormaal B. Is Sex- Biased Milk Production a Real Thing? [Internet] 2014. Available from: https:// dairyresearchblog.ca/2014/03/29/sex- biased-milk-production-real-thing/ [Accessed: 2020-05-02]

57. Gillespie AV, Ehrlich JL, Grove-White DH. Effect of Calf Gender on Milk Yield and Fatty Acid Content in Holstein Dairy Cows. PLoS ONE. 2017;12 (1):e0169503. DOI: 10.1371/journal.pone.0169503

58. Seegers H, Fourichon C, Beaudeau F. Production effects related to mastitis and mastitis economics in dairy cattle herds. Veterinary Research. 2003;34(5):475-491. DOI: 10.1051/ vetres:2003027

59. Green LE, Hedges VJ, Schukken YH, Blowey RW, Packington AJ. The impact of clinical lameness on the milk yield of dairy cows. Journal of Dairy Science. 2002;85(9):2250-2256. DOI: 10.3168/jds. S0022-0302(02)74304-X

60. Sawa A, Jankowska M, Glowska M. Effect of some factors on sex of the calf born, and of sex of the calf on performance of dairy cows. Acta Scientiarum Polonorum Zootechnica. 2014;13:75-84.

61. Williams GC. Adaptation and natural selection. New Jersey: Princeton University Press, Princeton; 1966.307 p. Cameron EZ, Linklater WL, Stafford KJ, Minot EO. Aging and improving reproductive success in horses: declining residual reproductive value or just older and wiser? Behavioral Ecology and Sociobiology. 2000;47(4):243-249. DOI:10.1007/ s002650050661

62. Winding JJ, Calus MPL, Beerda B, Veerkamp RF. Genetic correlations between milk production and health and fertility depending on herd environment. Journal of Dairy Science. 2006: 89(5):1765-1775. DOI: 10.3168/jds. S0022-0302(06)72245-7

63. Berry DP, Lonergan P, Butler ST, Cromie AR, Fair T, Mossa F, Evans AC. Negative influence of high maternal milk production before and after conception on offspring survival and milk production in dairy cattle. Journal of Dairy Science. 2008;91(1):329-337. DOI: 10.3168/jds.2007-0438

64. Cole JB, Ehrlich JL, Null DJ. Short communication: Projecting milk yield using best prediction and the MilkBot lactation model. Journal of Dairy Science. 2012;95(7):4041-4044. DOI: 10.3168/jds.2011-4905

65. Weigel KA. Exploring the role of sexed semen in dairy production systems. Journal of Dairy Science.2004;87(Suppl. 13):120-130. DOI: 10.3168/jds. S0022-0302(04)70067-3

66. Brickell JS, Bourne N, McGowan MM, Wathes DC. Effect of growth and development during the rearing period on the subsequent fertility of nulliparous Holstein- Friesian heifers. Theriogenology. 2009;72 (3):408-416. DOI: 10.1016/j. theriogenology.2009.03.015

67. Berry DP, Lee JM, Macdonald KA, Roche JR. Body condition score and body weight effects on dystocia and stillbirths and consequent effects on postcalving performance. Journal of Dairy Science. 2007;90:4201-4211. DOI: 10.3168/ jds.2007-0023

68. Eaglen S, Coffey M, Woolliams J, Mrode R, Wall E. Phenotypic effects of calving ease on the subsequent fertility and milk production of dam and calf in UK Holstein-Friesian heifers. Journal of Dairy Science. 2011;94(11):5413-5423. DOI: 10.3168/jds.2010-4040.

69. Van Straten M, Friger, M, Shpigel N Y. Events of elevated somatic cell counts in high-producing dairy cows are associated with daily body weight loss in early lactation. Journal of Dairy Science. 2009, 92(9):4386-4394. DOI:10.3168/jds.2009-2204

70. Minick JA, Buchanan DS, & Rupert SD. Milk production of crossbred daughters of high-and low-milk EPD Angus and Hereford bulls. Journal of Animal Science. 2001;79(6):1386-1393. DOI: 10.2527/2001.7961386x

71. Rutledge JJ, Robison OW, Ahlschwede WT, Legates JE. Milk yield and its influence on 205-day weight of beef calves. Journal of Animal Science. 1971;33(3):563-567. DOI: 10.2527/ jas1971.333563x

72. Christian LL, Hauser ER, Chapman AB. Association of preweaning and postweaning traits with weaning weight in cattle. Journal of Animal Science. 1965;24(3):652-656. DOI: 10.2527/jas1965.243652x

73. Habib MA, Afroz MA, Bhuiyan AK. Lactation performance of red Chittagong cattle and effects of environmental factors. Bangladesh Veterinarian. 2010;27:18-25. DOI: 10. 3329/bvet.v27i1.5911

74. Fitch J, McGilliard P, Drumm G. A study of the birth weight and gestation of dairy animals. Journal of Dairy Science. 1924;7(3):222-233. DOI: https://doi.org/10.3168/jds. S0022-0302(24)94016-1

75. Vieira-Neto A, Galvão KN, Thatcher WW, Santos JEP. Association among gestation length and health, production, and reproduction in Holstein cows and implications for their offspring. Journal of Dairy Science. 2017;100(4):3166-3181. DOI: 10.3168/ jds.2016-11867

76. Atashi H, Asaadi A. Association between gestation length and lactation performance, lactation curve, calf birth weight and dystocia in Holstein dairy cows. Iran. Animal Reproduction. 2019;16(4):846-852. DOI: 10.21451/1984-3143-AR2019-0005

77. Auldist MJ, O'Brien G, Cole D, Macmillan KL, Grainger C. (2007). Effects of Varying Lactation Length on Milk Production Capacity of Cows in Pasture-Based Dairying Systems. Journal of Dairy Science. 2007; 90(7):3234-3241. DOI: 10.3168/ jds.2006-683

78. Johanson JM, Berger PJ. Birth weight as a predictor of calving ease and perinatal mortality in Holstein cattle. Journal of Dairy Science. 2003;86(11):3745±3755. DOI: 10.3168/ jds.S0022-0302(03)73981-2

79. Drackley JK. Biology of Dairy Cows During the Transition Period: The Final Frontier? Journal of Dairy Science. 1999;82(11):2259-2273. DOI: 10.3168/ jds. S0022-0302(99)75474-3

80. Bobe G, Young JW, Beitz DC. Invited review: pathology, etiology, prevention, and treatment of fatty liver in dairy cows. Journal of Dairy Science. 2004;87(10):3105-3124. DOI: 10.3168/ jds.S0022-0302(04)73446-3

81. Gianola D, Tyler WJ. Influences on birth weight and gestation period of Holstein-Friesian cattle. Journal of Dairy Science. 1974;57(2):235-240. DOI: 10.3168/jds.S0022-0302(74)84864-2

82. Fourichon C, Seegers H, Bareille N, Beaudeau F. Effects of disease on milk production in the dairy cow: a review. Preventive Veterinary Medicine. 1999;41(1):1-35. DOI: 10.1016/ s0167-5877(99)00035-5

83. Deluyker HA, Gay JM, Weaver LD, Azari AS. Change of milk-yield with clinical-diseases for a high producing dairy-herd. Journal of Dairy Science. 1991;74(2):436-445. DOI: 10.3168/jds. S0022-0302(91)78189-7

84. Thompson JR, Pollak EJ, Pelissier CL. Interrelationships of parturition problems, production of subsequent lactation, reproduction,and age at 1st calving. Journal of Dairy Science. 1983;66(5):1119-1127. DOI: 10.3168/jds. S0022-0302(83)81909-2

85. Bareille N, Beaudeau F, Billon S, Robert A, Faverdin P. Effects of health disorders on feed intake and milk production in dairy cows. Livestock Production Science. 2003;83(1):53-62. DOI: 10.1016/S0301-6226(03)00040-X

86. Hinde K. Richer milk for sons but more milk for daughters: Sex-biased investment during lactation varies with maternal life history in rhesus macaques. American Journal of Human Biology. 2009;21(4):512-519. DOI: 10.1002/ajhb.20917

87. Yang MY, Fortune JE. The capacity of primordial follicles in fetal bovine ovaries to initiate growth in vitro develops during mid-gestation and is associated with meiotic arrest of oocytes. Biology of Reproduction. 2008;78(6): 1153-1161. DOI: 10.1095/ biolreprod.107.066688

88. Nilsson EE, Skinner MK. Progesterone regulation of primordial follicle assembly in bovine fetal ovaries. Molecular and Cellular Endocrinology. 2009;313(1):9-16. DOI: 10.1016/j. mce.2009.09.004

89. Dematawena CMB, Berger PJ. Effect of dystocia on yield, fertility, and cow losses and an economic evaluation of dystocia scores for Holsteins. Journal of Dairy Science. 1997;80(4):754-761. DOI: 10.3168/jds.s0022-0302(97)75995-2

90. Correa MT, Erb H, Scarlett J. Path- analysis for 7 postpartum disorders of Holstein cows. Journal of Dairy Science. 1993;76(5):1305-1312. DOI: 10.3168/ jds. S0022-0302(93)77461-5

91. Barrier A, Haskell M. Calving difficulty in dairy cows has a longer effect on saleable milk yield than on estimated milk production. Journal of Dairy Science. 2011;94(4):1804-1812. DOI: 10.3168/jds.2010-3641

92. Coleman DA, Thayne WV, Dailey RA. Factors affecting reproductive performance of dairy cows. Journal of Dairy Science. 1985;68:1793-1803. DOI: 10.3168/jds. S0022-0302(87)80296-5

93. Ivell R, Bathgate RAD. Reproductive biology of the relaxin-like factor (RLF/ INSL3). Biology of Reproduction. 2002;67(3):699-705. DOI: 10.1095/ biolreprod.102.005199

94. Carlsen SM, Jacobsen G, Vanky E. Mid-pregnancy androgen levels are negatively associated with breastfeeding. Acta Obstetricia et Gynecologica Scandinavica. 2010;89(1):87-94. DOI: 10.3109/00016340903318006

95. Hadsell DL. Genetic manipulation of mammary gland development and lactation. In: Pickering LK, Morrow AL, Ruiz-Palacios GM, Schanler RJ, editors. Protecting Infants through Human Milk. Advances in Experimental Medicine and Biology, vol 554. Boston, MA: Springer; 2004. P. 229-251. DOI: 10.1007/978-1-4757-4242-8_20

96. Xiang R, Estrella C, Fitzsimmons C, Kruk Z, Burns B, Roberts CT, Hiendleder S. Sex-specific placental and fetal phenotypes in bovine at Midgestation. Proceedings of the SRB Orals - Epigenetics & gene networks in reproduction. http://esa-srb-2013.m.asnevents.com.au/schedule/ session/1522/ abstract/7586

97. Akers RM. Lactogenic hormones binding-sites, mammary growth, secretory-cell differentiation, and milk biosynthesis in ruminants. Journal of Dairy Science. 1985;68(2):501-519. DOI: 10.3168/jds.s0022-0302(85)80849-3

98. Knight CH. Overview of prolactin's role in farm animal lactation. Livestock Production Science. 2001;70(1-2):87-93. DOI: 10.1016/S0301-6226(01)00200-7

99. Houghton DJ, P. Shackleton, B.C. Obiekwe, T. Chard. Relationship of maternal and fetal levels of human placental lactogen to the weight and sex of the fetus. Placenta. 1984;5(5):455-458. DOI: 10.1016/ s0143-4004(84)80026-0

100. Xiao L, Zhao JP, Nuyt AM, Fraser WD, Luo ZC. Female fetus is associated with greater maternal insulin resistance in pregnancy Diabetes Medicine. 2014;31(12):1696-1701. DOI: 10.1111/dme.12562.

101. Anand-Ivell R, Hiendleder S, Viñoles C, Martin GB, Fitzsimmons C, Eurich A, Hafen B, Ivell R. INSL3 in the ruminant: a powerful indicator of gender and genetic-specific feto-maternal dialogue. PloS one. 2011;6(5):e19821. DOI: 10.1371/journal.pone.0019821

102. Hammon HM, Bellmann O, Voigt J, Schneider F, Kühn C. Glucose- dependent insulin response and milk production in heifers within a segregating resource family population. Journal of Dairy Science. 2007;90:3247- 3254. DOI: 10.3168/jds.2006-748

103. Zinicola M, Bicalho RC. Association of peripartum plasma insulin concentration with milk production, colostrum insulin levels, and plasma metabolites of Holstein cows. Journal of Dairy Science. 2019;78:1153-1161. DOI: 10.3168/jds.2017-14029

104. Kamal MM, Van Eetvelde M, Depreester E, Hostens M, Vandaele L, Opsomer G. Age at calving in heifers and level of milk production during gestation in cows are associated with the birth size of Holstein calves. Journal of Dairy Science. 2014;97(9):5448-5458. DOI: 10.3168/jds.2014-7898

105. Hiendleder S, Shuaib E, Owens JA, Kennaway DJ, Gatford KL, Kind KL. Effects of conceptus sex and genetics on circulating thyroid hormones and IGFs in heifers at mid gestation depend on maternal genetic background. In: Proceedings of the World Congress on Genetics Applied to Livestock Production. Volume Biology - Reproduction 1. 2018; 979.

106. Capuco AV, Connor EE, Wood DL. Regulation of mammary gland sensitivity to thyroid hormones during the transition from pregnancy to lactation. Experimental biology and medicine (Maywood, N.J.). 2008;233(10):1309-1314. DOI:10.3181/0803-RM-85

107. Chew BP, Maier LC, Hillers JK, Hodgson AS. Relationship between calf birth-weight and dams subsequent 200-day and 305-day yields of milk, fat, and total solids in Holsteins. Journal of Dairy Science. 1981;64(12):2401-2408. DOI:10.3168/ jds.S0022-0302(81)82863-9

108. Kertz AF, Reutzel LF, Barton BA, Ely RL. Body weight, body condition score, and wither height of prepartum Holstein cows and birth weight and sex of calves by parity: A database and summary. Journal of Dairy Science. 1997;80(3):525-529. DOI: 10.3168/jds. S0022-0302(97)75966-6

109. Swali A, Wathes DC. Influence of the dam and sire on size at birth and subsequent growth, milk production and fertility in dairy heifers. Theriogenology. 2006;66(5):1173-1184. DOI: 10.1016/j. theriogenology.2006.03.028

110. Twigger AJ, Hepworth AR, Lai CT, Chetwynd E, Stuebe AM, Blancafort P, Hartmann PE, Geddes DT, Kakulasa F. Gene expression in breastmilk cells is associated with maternal and infant characteristics. Scientific Reports. 2015;5:12933. DOI: 10.1038/srep12933

111. Alberghina D, Piccione G, Giannetto C, Morgante M, Gianesella M. Sex of offspring influences metabolism during early transition period in dairy cows. Archiv Fur Tierzucht-Archives of Animal Breeding. 2015;58:73-77. DOI:10.5194/aab-58-73-2015

112. Roche JR, Lee JM, Berry DP. Pre-conception energy balance and secondary sex ratio–partial support for the Trivers-Willard hypothesis in dairy cows. Journal of Dairy Science. 2006;89:2119-2125. DOI: 10.3168/jds. S0022-0302(06)72282-2

113. Meier S, Williams YJ, Burke CR, Kay JK, Roche JR. Short communication: feed restriction around insemination did not alter birth sex ratio in lactating dairy cows. Journal of Dairy Science. 2010;93:5408-5412. DOI: 10.3168/ jds.2009-2935

114. Erb RE, Chew BP, Malven PV, Damico MF, Zamet CN, Colenbrander VF. Variables associated with peripartum traits in dairy- cows. VII. Hormones, calf traits and subsequent milk-yield. Journal of Animal Science. 1980;51(1):143-152. DOI: 10.2527/jas1980.511143x

115. Flint APF, Albon SD, Jafar SI. Blastocyst development and conceptus sex selection in red deer (Cervus elaphus): Studies of a free-living population on the Isle of Rum. General and Comparative Endocrinology. 1997;106(3):374-383. DOI: 10.1006/ gcen.1997.6879

116. DeJarnette JM, Nebel RL, Meek B, Wells J, Marshall CE. Commercial application of sex-sorted semen in Holstein heifers. Journal of Animal Science. 2007;90(Suppl.1):228

117. Garner DL, Seidel GE. History of commercializing sexed semen for cattle. Theriogenology. 2008; 69 (7):886-95. DOI: 10.3168/jds.2014-8774

118. Ettema JF, Ostergaard S. Short communication: Economics of sex- biased milk production. Journal of Dairy Science. 2015;98(2):1078-1081. DOI: 10.3168/ jds.2014-8774

12 Chapter REPRODUCTIVE TOXICITY OF INSECTICIDES

1. INTRODUCTION: AN OVERVIEW

Over decades, consumption of pesticides has slightly increased year by year; over 4 million tons of pesticides were used worldwide in 2017. Asia (52.8%) followed by USA (30.2%) and Europe (13.8%) were the highest amount of pesticide used obtain the most excessive amount of pesticide used continents. Insecticides, a subgroup of pesticides, constitute nearly 100ooo tons per year [1]; and, carbamates, chlorinated hydrocarbons, organophosphates and pyrethroids are most commonly used insecticides. Although these chemicals increase crop yields and provide economic benefits by reducing pest-borne diseases, their harmful effects on human health and environment still have the attention; and, considering these effects less toxic alternatives continue to be developed. Pesticide exposure alone or in mixture via environmental contamination could have important acute and chronic adverse effects on living organisms. Pesticide usage in agriculture is increasing every passing day and becoming a confusing issue due to the use of new chemical compounds that come into the market.

Chronic or delayed insecticide exposure exerts its toxicity on several systems such as nervous, immune, respiratory and reproductive. Reproductive toxicity of insecticides may affect either men or women; reduced fertility, spontaneous abortion, birth defects and developmental retardation have been linked to insecticide toxicity [2, 3]. For livestock industry, decreasing reproductive functions is rising problem; and, common problems can be listed as infertility, sub-fecundity, ovarian cycle failures, decreased pregnancy rates, altered germ cell quality, reduced sperm motility as well as structural damage of testes or ovaries [4]. Furthermore, insecticides have important impacts on HPG axis and that qualifies them as endocrine disrupters. Endocrine-disrupting insecticides alter hormone synthesis or impair hormonal metabolic pathway by acting as hormonal receptor agonist or antagonists [5].

This chapter describes the reproductive system toxicity of commonly used insecticides based on each male and female; furthermore, it focuses on endocrine disruption.

2. THE FUNDAMENTALS OF INSECTICIDES

Insecticides are described as "chemicals used to control insects by killing them or preventing them from engaging in undesirable or destructive behaviors" by United States Environmental Protection Agency (EPA) [6]. Insecticides provide substantial benefits during agriculture by controlling or preventing pests that could harm to crops and food causing nutritional and economic losses.

Additionally, pests could damage wooden constructions and reduce the beauty and attractiveness of landscapes. Furthermore, insects could carry various diseases such as malaria [7, 8]. Insecticides play a crucial role in producing safe and quality food at affordable prices, home and gardening as well as controlling pest-borne diseases for public health.

Insecticides can be classified in varying ways such as their chemical structure, natural or synthetic origin, application requirement or mode of action. The chemical structure is particularly important for toxicology, since insecticides could exert similar toxicological effects due to their common chemical properties. Considering the chemical structure, insecticides could be divided into five groups: (i) organo- chlorines, (ii) organophosphates, (iii) carbamates, (iv) pyrethrins/pyrethroids and (v) nicotine/neonicotinoids.

Organochlorines have chlorinated hydrocarbon structures with high lipophilicity and persistence in the environment. Most exert their effects by disrupting sodium/potassium imbalance and others affect γ-aminobutyric acid (GABA) receptors; eventually, they cause hyperexcitation in the nervous system. Organophosphates, as another major class of insecticides, are phosphoric acid esters that cause acetylcholine accumulation at neuromuscular junctions by irreversible acetylcholinesterase (AChE) inhibition [6, 9, 10]. The other AChE inhibitor insecticide group carbamates are carbamic acid derivatives and show their effects reversibly, unlike organophosphates [11]. Pyrethrins are isolated from the flowers of Chrysanthemum cinerariaefolium; and, pyrethroids are synthetic analogs of pyrethrins. Both keep open the sodium channels, cause hyperexcitation in peripheral and central nervous systems and ultimately lead to paralysis. Pyrethrins and pyrethroids have lower environmental bioaccumulation and mammalian toxicity [12, 13]. Nicotine and neonicotinoids, as a newer class of insecticides widely used all over the world, have selectively neurotoxic effects on nicotinic acetylcholine receptor (nAChRs) [14].

High levels of exposure to several insecticides due to lack of legislations, regulations and education with ignorant behaviors may cause serious consequences on the human health and environment. Many studies showed that the misuse or overuse of insecticides lead to harmful effects in various systems such as nervous, respiratory and reproductive. The rest of this chapter gives details of the effects of selected insecticides on the female and male reproductive systems.

3. TOXICITY OF INSECTICIDES ON REPRODUCTIVE SYSTEM

Toxic effects of insecticides on male and female reproductive system and HPG axis are shown in Figure 1.

3.1 Hormonal system disruption

Insecticides could be characterized as "endocrine disrupters" due to their adverse effects on reproductive hormone pathway [15]. The half-life of endocrine disrupting insecticides changes from hours to months in the environment.

Insecticides may have toxic effects on synthesis, secretion, transport, binding to target receptors, intracellular transmission and elimination processes of reproductive hormones. In addition, insecticides alter hormone-receptor binding via chancing receptor affinity or agonist/antagonist effects, since, they mimic hormones.

Thus, many of insecticides have estrogenic, androgenic or anti-estrogenic and anti- androgenic effects. Furthermore, insecticides could bind several types of receptors such as membrane, nuclear, orphan and neurotransmitter receptors. Endocrine disrupting insecticides also exert toxic effects via inducing cell death in reproductive system cells playing a role from hormone synthesis to germ cell axis. Different studies confirmed that insecticides irreversibly affect hypothalamic-pituitary axis due to their mimicking properties of hormones or undesired inhibition or activation of metabolic pathways [15–17].

Pyrethroids, synthetic esters of pyrethrins, widely used worldwide are important endocrine-disrupting chemicals. In animal studies, contradictory results were obtained about the effects of pyrethroids on HPG axis. It has been shown that permethrin, fenvalerate and cypermethrin exposure decreased serum testosterone levels and increased follicle stimulating hormone (FSH) and luteinizing hormone (LH) levels. Lower levels of testosterone constitute negative feedback in HPG axis resulting in increased levels of FSH and LH. However, in another study, delthamethrin exposure caused increased levels of testosterone, FSH and LH [18].

Elbetieha et al. [19] demonstrated that cypermethrin exposure decreased the serum testosterone, FSH and LH levels in male rats. On the other hand, different studies reported that pyrethroids have no effects on hypothalamus functions and gonadotropin releasing hormone (GnRH) levels. There are few studies demonstrating that gonadotropic cells' function and expression of LH and FSH coding genes have changed with pyrethroids exposure [20]. Dohlman et al. [21] reported that permethrin caused reduction in progesterone levels in beef heifers. Overall, it has been concluded that changes of hormone production due to exposure of pyrethroids depend on dose and duration of the exposure.

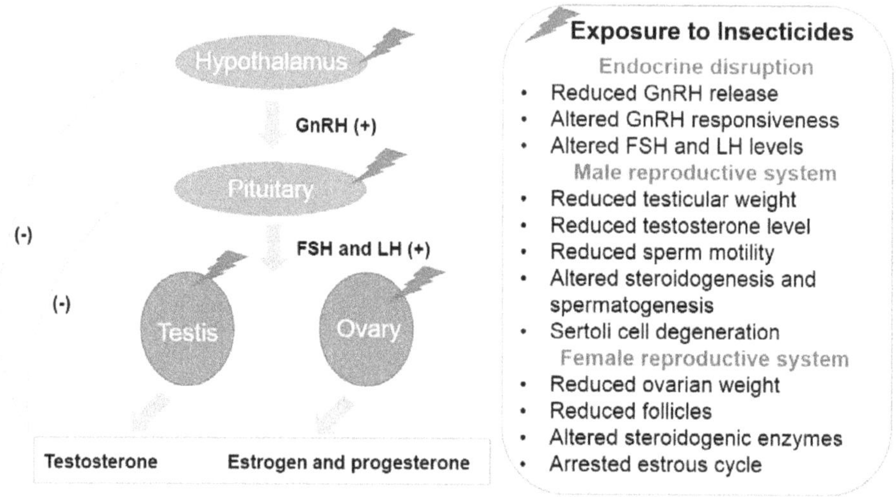

Figure 1. Schematic representation of insecticides on male and female reproductive system via HPG axis (32).

Soljjou et al. [22] demonstrated that thiacloprid, a neonicotinoid, and delthamethrin, a pyrethroid, exposure decreased GnRH, LH, FSH and testosterone serum levels in the hypothalamus in a dose-dependent manner; and, interfered with steroidogenesis in testicular tissues. Annabi and Dhouib [23] showed that imidacloprid, a neonicotinoid, affected the biochemical pathways of hypothalamic pituitary-adrenal (HPA) axis via induction of oxidative stress.

Heptachlor, an organochlorine, may induce testosterone synthesis via 16-α and 16-β hydroxylases. Thiram, sodium N-methyldithiocarbamate and other dithiocarbamate insecticides inhibit the dopamine-β-hydroxylase activity and result in higher LH production, which prolonged proestrus stage. It has been reported that chlordimeform and amitraz interfere with the norepinephrine by binding to α2-andrenoreceptors and disrupt the GnRH release. Some other insecticides such as methoxychlor, DDT endosulfan, toxaphene, dieldrin, triadimefon, aldrin, methiocarb, chlordecone, malathion and sumithrin affect the HPA axis via binding receptors, mimicking the hormones and have shown estrogenic effects [24, 25]. In Table 1 [3], selected insecticides and their endocrine-disrupting effects are listed.

3.2 Toxicity on male reproductive system

Dysfunction of male reproductive system represents a fundamental issue for livestock industry. Impairment of spermatogenesis, anti-androgenic effects, alterations in reproductive enzyme pathways, decreased sperm quality and motility are key elements in insecticide-induced male infertility [5]. Insecticides exert their toxic outcomes on male reproductive system by directly affecting reproductive organs (testes, sertoli cells, leydig cells) and germ cells or impairing hormonal balance in secondary endocrine system [26].

Table 1. Selected insecticides and their effects on endocrine system.

Pesticide	Hormone disruption effects
Aldicarb	17 beta-estradiol and progesterone inhibition
Aldrin	Androgen receptor binding
Bioallethrin	Estrogen-sensitive cells proliferation inhibition
Carbofuran	Estradiol and progesterone increase; testosterone decrease
Chlordane	Androgen receptor binding, estrogenic pathway inhibition
Chlorpyrifos-methyl	Androgen activity antagonism
Cypermethrin	Estrogenic effect increase
Deltamethrin	Estrogenic activity
Dieldrin	Androgen receptor binding, inducing estrogen receptor production in the cell
Endosulfan	Androgen receptor binding, inducing estrogen receptor production in the cell
Fenoxycarb	Testosterone metabolism disruption
Lindane	Luteal progesterone decrease, androgen, estrogen and progesterone receptor binding
Methoxychlor	Estrogenic effect, pregnane X cellular receptor binding
Parathion	Gonadotrophic hormone synthesis inhibition
Tetramethrin	Estrogen antagonism in females

It has been demonstrated in laboratory animals that carbamates have toxic effects on male reproductive system. Alterations of testicular weight and male accessory gland morphology, degeneration of seminiferous tubules and epididymis, spermatogenesis arrest, abnormalities of sperm motility and number, impairment of serum hormone and total proteins levels and estrogen receptor expressions were observed in several studies. However, detailed underlying molecular mechanisms of carbamate toxicity on male reproductive organs are still unclear [26–29].

Organophosphates could alter the spermatozoon chromatin structure, DNA, acrosome, motility and, have toxic effects on HPG axis. Reduced levels of testosterone were measured with organophosphate exposure due to inhibition of testosterone synthesis, which possibly occurs via reduction of steroidogenic enzymes' expression levels [5]. Organophosphates have dose-dependent detrimental effects on the morphology of testis and seminiferous tubules by causing atrophy and inducing germ cell death [26]. Additionally, organophosphate exposure is associated with decreased levels of sialic acid, glycogen alkaline phosphatase activity and increased levels of total protein, cholesterol and acid phosphatase. These imbalances could lead to induction of oxidative stress in male reproductive system by triggering inflammation, mitochondrial deficiency, DNA fragmentation and apoptosis [30, 31]. In wild birds such as parakeets and munias, organophosphate administration resulted in testicular dysfunctions [32]. Organophosphate insecticides induce DNA damage in sperm chromatin and that alters spermatogenesis pathway and causes infertility in male animals. Germ cell genetic material is protected by structure of male reproductive organs; however, it has been demonstrated that organophosphate insecticide disrupted the germ cell DNA integrity [32].

DDT, methoxychlor, chlordane, heptachlor, aldrin, dieldrin, endrin, toxaphene, mirex and lindane are commonly used organochlorines. Organochlorines have shown their toxic effects via inducing oxidative stress in the epididymis and decreasing antioxidant defense. It has been demonstrated that endosulfan caused abnormal sperm maturation in the epididymis. In addition, organochlorines disrupt male reproductive maturation in adolescence. TCDD (2,3,7,8-tetrachlorodibenzo-p-dioxin), the most dangerous compound in world history, causes reduced fertility, delayed puberty and reproductive organ weights alterations, and also induces oxidative stress resulting in abnormal sperm morphology, motility and sperm number decrease [26].

Pyrethroids are generally accepted as safe; however, their weak toxic effects on reproductive system were demonstrated in limited studies. Pyrethroids have adverse effects such as reducing sperm count and motility, aneuploidy in germ cells, reducing sex hormone levels and reducing semen quality and sperm morphological abnormalities in human [33].

3.3 Toxicity on female reproductive system

Toxic effects of insecticides on female reproductive system were shown in different studies; and, it is concluded that insecticides disrupt female endocrine system and cause alterations in reproductive organs and germ cells [24]. Insecticides disrupt ovarian physiology. This is a two-way street as altering organ functions causes hormone secretion changes and this endocrine changes mostly affect the female reproductive system and result with dysfunctions via HPG axis.

Disrupted hormone synthesis, altered follicular maturation, disrupted ovarian cycle, pregnancy time prolong, stillbirth and infertility are linked to oxidative imbalance in the cells, and eventually lead to DNA damage, inflammation and apoptosis induction [34].

It has been speculated that pesticides have important role in slaughtering buffaloes reproductive defects. This could be associated with follicle membrane permeability features that permit xenobiotics entrance to the system. Higher concentrations of insecticides including DDT, eldrine, endosulphan and butachlor were detected in ovary than serum. This could make a way for follicular wall alterations and more insecticide entrance to the cellular system. In addition, insecticides could affect germ cells at primordial phases resulting in infertility in adult stage [5].

In wild birds such as female bobwhite quail (Colinus virginianus), parathion exposure caused reduction of egg production, impairment of follicular cycle, and reduction of LH and progesterone levels. Organophosphate (methyl parathion/ phosphamidon/quinalphos) administration of white-throated munia (Lonchura malabarica) caused inhibition of two important enzymes: Δ5-3β- hydroxysteroid dehydrogenase (3βHSD) and 17β-hydroxysteroid dehydrogenase (17βHSD), playing key role in estrogen and progesterone production inhibition [32].

Endosulfan, an organochlorine, triggered apoptosis via oxidative stress induction in the follicle cells. Moreover, it induced the expressions of steroidogenic acute regulatory protein (StAR), CYP19A1a and aromatase, causing improper ovarian maturation. DDT exposure caused ovulation time alterations via inhibiting CYP450-side chain cleavage enzyme, progesterone receptor, estrogen sulfotransfer- ase, cyclooxygenase-2 (COX-2) and epidermal growth factor (epiregulin) [34].

In female reproductive system, chlorpyrofos cause alterations in uterine weight and morphology via inducing surface epithelium and myometrium thickness

[35]. In addition, chlorpyrofos could qualify as an ovotoxic and embryotoxic agent while mimicking estrogen and altering embryonic hatching, cell proliferation and apoptosis in zebrafish. Furthermore, chlorpyrifos reduces the levels of serum sex hormones such as LH, estrogen and progesterone [36, 37].

Toxic effects mechanisms of insecticides in female reproductive system are schematized in Figure 2.

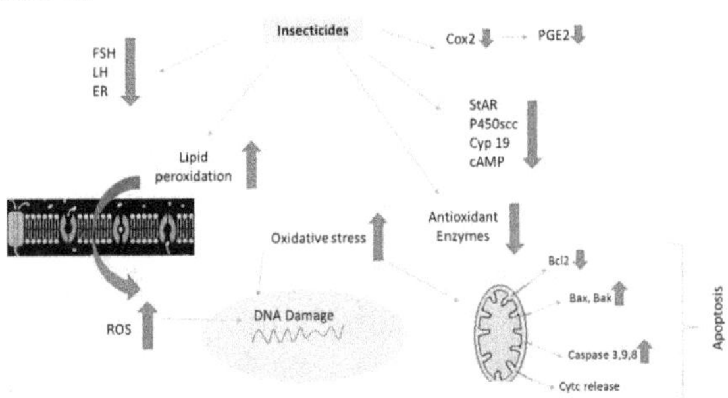

Figure 2. Toxic effects mechanisms of insecticides in female reproductive system (FSH; follicle-stimulating hormone, LH; luteinizing hormone, ER; estrogen, ROS; reactive oxygen species, Cox2; Cyclooxygenase-2, StAr; Steroidogenic acute regulatory protein) [34].

4. CONCISE SUMMARY

The potential impact of insecticides on the reproductive systems of both males and females, along with their ability to disrupt endocrine balance, underscores the ongoing worry regarding the reduction or elimination of insecticide usage. Literature indicates that numerous insecticides induce infertility or developmental defects through various mechanisms, necessitating the urgent need for knowledge. Given that a substantial portion of the data was derived from rodent studies, additional research is required to elucidate the harmful effects of pesticides on livestock. Moreover, elucidating the potential molecular processes of pesticides could facilitate the development of more efficient and cost-effective livestock breeding practices.

REFERENCES

1. FAOSTAT. The pesticides use database, Food and Agriculture Organization of the United Nations [Internet]. 2020. Available from: http:// www.fao.org/ faostat/en/#data/RP [Accessed: 08 April 2020]
2. Frazier LM. Reproductive disorders associated with pesticide exposure. Journal of Agromedicine. 2007;12:27-37. DOI: 10.1300/J096v12n01_04
3. Manif W, Hassine AIH, Bouaziz A, Bartegi A, Thomas O, Roig B. Effect of endocrine disruptor pesticides:
4. A review. International Journal of Environmental Research and Public Health. 2011;8:2265-2303. DOI: 10.3390/ ijerph8062265
5. Campagna C, Guillemette C, Paradis R, Sirard MA, Ayotte P, Bailey JL. An environmentally relevant organochlorine mixture impairs sperm function and embryo development in the porcine model. Biology of Reproduction. 2002;67:80-87. DOI: 10.1095/biolreprod67.1.80
6. Ghuman SPS, Ratnakaran U, Bedi JS, Gill JPS. Impact of pesticide residues on fertility of dairy animals: A review. The Indian Journal of Animal Sciences. 2013;83:1243-1255
7. EPA. Insecticides, CADDIS Volume 2 by United States Environmental Protection Agency [Internet]. 2020. Available from: https://www.epa.gov/ caddis-vol2/ insecticides#main-content [Accessed: 08 April 2020]
8. Aktar W, Sengupta D, Chowdhury A. Impact of pesticides use in agriculture: Their benefits and hazards. Interdisciplinary Toxicology. 2009;2:1-12. DOI: 10.2478/ v10102-009-0001-7
9. Marrs TC. Mammalian toxicology of insecticides (No. 12). In: Issues in Toxicology. Royal Society of Chemistry. UK. 2012. pp. 1-13. ISBN: 978-1-84973-191-1

10. Coats JR. Mechanisms of toxic action and structure-activity relationships for organochlorine and synthetic pyrethroid insecticides. Environmental Health Perspectives. 1990;87:255-262. DOI: 10.1289/ehp.9087255

11. Jayaraj R, Megha P, Sreedev P. Organochlorine pesticides, their toxic effects on living organisms and their fate in the environment. Interdisciplinary Toxicology. 2016;9: 90-100. DOI: 10.1515/intox-2016-0012

12. Fukuto TR. Mechanism of action of organophosphorus and carbamate insecticides. Environmental Health Perspectives. 1990;87:245-254. DOI: 10.1289/ehp.9087245

13. Ensley SM. Pyrethrins and pyrethroids. In: Gupta RC, editor. Veterinary Toxicology. 3rd Edn. USA: Academic Press; 2018. pp. 515-520. ISBN: 978-0-12-811410-0

14. Oztas E, Ulus B, Özhan G. In vitro investigation on the toxic potentials of commonly used synthetic pyrethroids, especially esbiothrin. Applied In Vitro Toxicology. 2015;1:302 307. DOI: 10.1089/aivt.2015.0022

15. Matsuda K, Buckingham SD, Kleier D, Rauh JJ, Grauso M, Sattelle DB. Neonicotinoids: Insecticides acting on insect nicotinic acetylcholine receptors. Trends in Pharmacological Sciences. 2001;22:573-580. DOI: 10.1016/S0165-6147(00)01820-4

16. Sweeney T, Nicol L, Roche JF, Brooks AN. Maternal exposure to octylphenol suppresses ovine fetal follicle stimulating hormone secretion, testis size, and Sertoli cell number. Endocrinology. 2000;141:2667-2673. DOI: 10.1210/endo.141.7.7552

17. Zama AM, Uzumcu M. Epigenetic effects of endocrinedisrupting chemicals on female reproduction: An ovarian perspective. Frontiers in Neuroendocrinology. 2010;31:420-439. DOI: 10.1016/j.yfrne.2010.06.003

18. Rivas A, Fisher JS, McKinnell C, Atanassova N, Sharpe RM. Induction of reproductive tract developmental abnormalities in the male rat by lowering androgen production or action in combination with a low dose of diethylstilbestrol: Evidence for importance of the androgenestrogen balance. Endocrinology. 2002;143: 4797-4808. DOI: 10.1210/ en.2002-220531

19. Ye X, Li F, Zhang J, Ma H, Ji D, Huang X, et al. Pyrethroid insecticide cypermethrin accelerates pubertal onset in male mice via disrupting hypothalamic–pituitary–gonadal axis. Environmental Science & Technology. 2017;51:10212-10221. DOI: 10.1021/acs. est.7b02739

20. Elbetieha A, Da'as SI, Khamas W, Darmani H. Evaluation of the toxic potentials of cypermethrin pesticide on some reproductive and fertility parameters in

the male rats. Archives of Environmental Contamination and Toxicology. 2001;41:522-528. DOI: 10.1007/s002440010280

21. Ye X, Liu J. Effects of pyrethroid insecticides on hypothalamic-pituitarygonadal axis: A reproductive health perspective. Environmental Pollution. 2019;245:590-599. DOI: 10.1016/j. envpol.2018.11.031
22. Dohlman TM, Phillips PE, Madson DM, Clark CA, Gunn PJ. Effects of label-dose permethrin administration in yearling beef cattle: I. Bull reproductive function and testicular histopathology. Theriogenology. 2016;85:1534-1539. DOI: 10.1016/j. theriogenology.2016.02.014
23. Solhjou KA, Hosseini SE, Vahdati A, Edalatmanesh MA. Changes in the hypothalamic-pituitary-gonadal axis in adult male rats poisoned with Proteus and Biscaya insecticides. Iranian Journal of Medical Sciences. 2019;44:155-162
24. Annabi A, Dhouib IEB. Mechanisms of imidacloprid-induced alteration of hypothalamic-pituitary-adrenal (HPA) axis after subchronic exposure in male rats. Recent Advances in Biology and Medicine. 2015;1:51-59. DOI: 10.18639/RABM.2015.01.195931
25. Bretveld RW, Thomas CM, Scheepers PT, Zielhuis GA, Roeleveld N. Pesticide exposure: The hormonal function of the female reproductive system disrupted? Reproductive Biology and Endocrinology. 2006;4:30. DOI: 10.1186/1477-7827-4-30
26. Rezg R, Mornagui B, Benahmed M, Chouchane SG, Belhajhmida N, Abdeladhim M, et al. Malathion exposure modulates hypothalamic gene expression and induces dyslipedemia in Wistar rats. Food and Chemical Toxicology. 2010;48:1473-1477. DOI: 10.1016/j. fct.2010.03.013
27. Ngoula F, Ngouateu OB, Kana JR, Defang HF, Watcho P, Kamtchouing P, et al. Reproductive and developmental toxicity of insecticides. In: Perveen F, editor. Insecticides, Advances in Integrated Pest Management. UK: IntechOpen; 2012. pp. 429-457. ISBN: 978-953-307-780-2
28. Archana R, Sahai A, Srivastava AK, Rani A. Carbaryl induced histopathological changes in the testis of albino rats. Journal of the Anatomical Society of India. 2007;56:4-6
29. Shalaby MA, El Zorba HY, Ziada RM. Reproductive toxicity of methomyl insecticide in male rats and protective effect of folic acid. Food and Chemical Toxicology. 2010;48: 3221-3226. DOI: 10.1016/j. fct.2010.08.027
30. Han J, Park M, Kim JH, Kim A, Won M, Lee DR, et al. Increased expression of the testicular estrogen receptor alpha in adult mice exposed to low doses of methiocarb. Journal of Applied Toxicology. 2009;29:446-451. DOI: 10.1002/jat.1417

31. Choudhary N, Goyal R, Joshi SC. Reproductive toxicity of endosulfan in male albino rats. Bulletin of Environmental Contamination and Toxicology. 2003;70:285-289. DOI: 10.1007/s00128-002-0189-0

32. Harchegani AB, Rahmani A, Tahmasbpour E, Kabootaraki HB, Rostami H, Shahriary A. Mechanisms of diazinon effects on impaired spermatogenesis and male infertility. Toxicology and Industrial Health. 2018;34:653-664. DOI: 10.1177/0748233718778665

33. Mitra A, Maitra SK. Reproductive toxicity of organophosphate pesticides. Annals of Clinical Toxicology. 2018;1:1004-1012

34. Meeker JD, Barr DB, Hauser R. Human semen quality and sperm DNA damage in relation to urinary metabolites of pyrethroid insecticides. Human Reproduction. 2008;23:1932- 1940. DOI: 10.1093/humrep/den242

35. Sharma RK, Singh P, Setia A, Sharma AK. Insecticides and ovarian functions. Environmental and Molecular Mutagenesis. 2020;61:369- 392. DOI: 10.1002/em.22355

36. Nishi K, Hundal SS. Chlorpyrifos induced toxicity in reproductive organs of female Wistar rats. Food and Chemical Toxicology. 2013;62:732-738. DOI: 10.1016/j.fct.2013.10.006

37. Ventura C, Nieto MRR, Bourguignon N, Lux-Lantos V, Rodriguez H, Cao G, et al. Pesticide chlorpyrifos acts as an endocrine disruptor in adult rats causing changes in mammary gland and hormonal balance. The Journal of Steroid Biochemistry and Molecular Biology. 2016;156:1-9. DOI: 10.1016/j.jsbmb.2015.10.010

38. Nandi S, Gupta PSP, Roy SC, Selvaraju S, Ravindra JP. Chlorpyrifos and endosulfan affect buffalo oocyte maturation, fertilization, and embryo development in vitro directly and through cumulus cells. Environmental Toxicology. 2011;26:57-67. DOI: 10.1002/tox.2052

Index

www.ingramcontent.com/pod-product-compliance
Lightning Source LLC
LaVergne TN
LVHW062119200926
848484LV00007B/1715
9781787155992